One Century of Karl Jaspers' *General Psychopathology*

International Perspectives in Philosophy and Psychiatry

Series editors: Bill (K.W.M.) Fulford, Katherine Morris, John Z. Sadler, and Giovanni Stanghellini

Volumes in the series:

Portrait of the Psychiatrist as a Young Man: The Early Writing and Work of R.D. Laing, 1927–1960
Beveridge

Mind, Meaning, and Mental Disorder 2e
Bolton and Hill

What is Mental Disorder?
Bolton

Delusions and Other Irrational Beliefs
Bortolotti

Postpsychiatry
Bracken and Thomas

Philosophy, Psychoanalysis, and the A-Rational Mind
Brakel

Unconscious Knowing and Other Essays in Psycho-Philosophical Analysis
Brakel

Psychiatry as Cognitive Neuroscience
Broome and Bortolotti (eds.)

Free Will and Responsibility: A Guide for Practitioners
Callender

Reconceiving Schizophrenia
Chung, Fulford, and Graham (eds.)

Darwin and Psychiatry
De Block and Adriaens (eds.)

Nature and Narrative: An Introduction to the New Philosophy of Psychiatry
Fulford, Morris, Sadler, and Stanghellini (eds.)

Oxford Textbook of Philosophy and Psychiatry
Fulford, Thornton, and Graham

The Mind and its Discontents
Gillett

Thinking Through Dementia
Hughes

Dementia: Mind, Meaning, and the Person
Hughes, Louw, and Sabat (eds.)

Talking Cures and Placebo Effects
Jopling

Philosophical Issues in Psychiatry II: Nosology
Kendler and Parnas

Discursive Perspectives in Therapeutic Practice
Lock and Strong (ed.)

Schizophrenia and the Fate of the Self
Lysaker and Lysaker

Responsibility and Psychopathy
Malatesti and McMillan

Body-Subjects and Disordered Minds
Matthews

Rationality and Compulsion: Applying action theory to psychiatry
Nordenfelt

Philosophical Perspectives on Technology and Psychiatry
Phillips (ed.)

The Metaphor of Mental Illness
Pickering

Mapping the Edges and the In-between
Potter

Trauma, Truth, and Reconciliation: Healing Damaged Relationships
Potter (ed.)

The Philosophy of Psychiatry: A Companion
Radden

The Virtuous Psychiatrist
Radden and Sadler

Autonomy and Mental Disorder
Radoilska (ed.)

Feelings of Being
Ratcliffe

Recovery of People with Mental Illness: Philosophical and Related Perspectives
Rudnick (ed.)

Values and Psychiatric Diagnosis
Sadler

Disembodied Spirits and Deanimated Bodies: The Psychopathology of Common Sense
Stanghellini

One Century of Karl Jaspers' General Psychopathology
Stanghellini and Fuchs

Emotions and Personhood
Stanghellini and Rosfort

Essential Philosophy of Psychiatry
Thornton

Empirical Ethics in Psychiatry
Widdershoven, McMillan, Hope, and Van der Scheer (eds.)

The Sublime Object of Psychiatry: Schizophrenia in Clinical and Cultural Theory
Woods

One Century of Karl Jaspers' *General Psychopathology*

Edited by

Giovanni Stanghellini

and

Thomas Fuchs

OXFORD
UNIVERSITY PRESS

OXFORD
UNIVERSITY PRESS

Great Clarendon Street, Oxford, OX2 6DP,
United Kingdom

Oxford University Press is a department of the University of Oxford.
It furthers the University's objective of excellence in research, scholarship,
and education by publishing worldwide. Oxford is a registered trade mark of
Oxford University Press in the UK and in certain other countries

First Edition published in 2013

Impression: 1

Published in the United States of America by Oxford University Press
198 Madison Avenue, New York, NY 10016, United States of America

British Library Cataloguing in Publication Data
Data available

Library of Congress Control Number: 2013937979

ISBN 978–0–19–960925–3

Printed and bound in Great Britain
by CPI Group (UK) Ltd, Croydon, CR0 4YY

Acknowledgements

The list of people we would like to mention for their help in preparing this book is very long. We will confine to our closest assistants: Alexander Englert, Rixta Fambach, Alessandro Longo, Milena Mancini, Simona Presenza, and Laerte Vetrugno. Their assistance had several forms including contacts with authors, secretarial support, text editing, organization of references, as well as personal encouragement. We are very grateful for their generosity. A special thank you must go to Charlotte Green and the entire staff of Oxford University Press for their precious work of editorial assistance. We also would like to express our gratitude to Bill Fulford with whom in the last two decades we had the privilege to share the project of the renaissance of the philosophy of psychiatry.

Contents

Contributors

Matthias Bormuth
Institute for Philosophy
University of Oldenburg
Oldenburg, Germany

Matthew R. Broome
Department of Psychiatry,
University of Oxford, Oxford, UK;
Highfield Adolescent Unit,
Warneford Hospital, Oxford Health NHS
Foundation Trust, Oxford, UK

Otto Doerr-Zegers
Director of the Center of
Studies on Phenomenology and Psychiatry,
University Diego Portales,
Santiago de Chile

Thomas Fuchs
Psychiatric Clinic
Center for Psychosocial Medicine
University of Heidelberg
Heidelberg, Germany

Bill (K.W.M) Fulford
Fellow of St Catherine's College and
Member of the Philosophy Faculty
University of Oxford and
Emeritus Professor of Philosophy and
Mental Health
University of Warwick, UK

S. Nassir Ghaemi
Tufts Medical Center
Boston, MA, USA

Christoph Hoerl
Department of Philosophy
University of Warwick
Coventry, UK

Alfred Kraus
Psychiatric Clinic
Center for Psychosocial Medicine
University of Heidelberg
Heidelberg, Germany

Mario Maj
Department of Psychiatry, University of
Naples SUN, Naples, Italy

Christoph Mundt
Psychiatric Clinic
Center for Psychosocial Medicine
University of Heidelberg
Heidelberg, Germany

Josef Parnas
Center For Subjectivity Research
University of Copenhagen
and Psychiatric Center Hvidovre
University of Copenhagen
Copenhagen, Denmark

Héctor Pelegrina-Cetrán
Universidad Autónoma de Madrid
Madrid, Spain

Matthew Ratcliffe
Department of Philosophy
Durham University
Durham, UK

Mario Rossi Monti
University of Urbino
Urbino, Italy

Henning Sass
Department of Psychiatry
University of Technology RWTH
Aachen, Germany

Louis A. Sass
Rutgers University
New Brunswick, NJ, USA

Jann E. Schlimme
Psychiatric University Hospital Charité
Berlin, Germany

Michael Alan Schwartz
Texas AMHSC
School of Medicine
Austin, TX, USA

Giovanni Stanghellini
'G.d'Annunzio' University
Chieti, Italy
and 'Diego Portales' University
Santiago, Chile

Umberto Volpe
Department of Psychiatry
University of Naples SUN
Naples, Italy

Chris Walker
Consultant Psychiatrist, retired

Osborne P. Wiggins
Department of Philosophy
University of Louisville
Louisville, KY, USA

Abbreviations

DSM	*Diagnostic and Statistical Manual of Mental Disorders*
ICD	International Classification of Diseases
MDD	major depressive disorder
WHO	World Health Organization

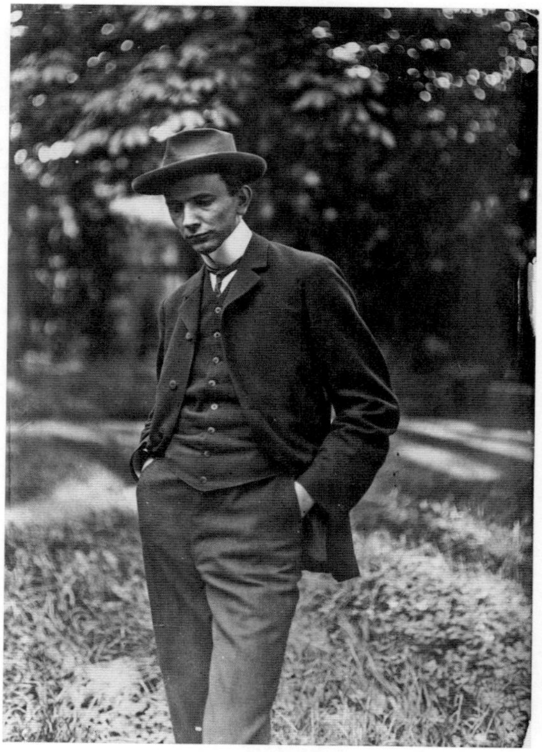

Karl Jaspers
(photographer unknown;
by courtesy of Hans Saner, Basel)

Editors' introduction

Giovanni Stanghellini and Thomas Fuchs

> But the healthy person who keeps his psyche marginally exposed and who investigates the psychopathological will find there what he potentially is.
>
> *(Jaspers 1997: 786)*

The year 2013 is the centenary of Karl Jaspers' foundation of psychopathology as a science in its own right.

In 1913, Jaspers published his psychiatric *opus magnum—Allgemeine Psychopathologie* (*General Psychopathology*). The idea inspiring his book was very simple: to bring order into the chaos of abnormal psychic phenomena by rigorous description, definition, and classification, and to empower psychiatry with a valid and reliable method to assess and make sense of abnormal human subjectivity. To this purpose, Jaspers blended Diltheyian hermeneutic approaches with Husserlian concepts of intuition, description, and presuppositionless methodology in order to create an approach that enables psychiatrists to determine the pathological mental states in their patients. The resulting descriptive phenomenology has served as the basis for psychopathology until today.

Jaspers from today's perspective

Jaspers was working at a time like our own of rapid expansion in the neurosciences and responding to the philosophical challenges that this raised. His foundation of psychopathology rested not least on the rejection of scientific reductionism which attempted to attribute the phenomena of mental illness to putative substrates in the brain. This reductionism, Jaspers argued, placed the question 'Why?' before the question 'What?', thus omitting the careful description and understanding of the pathological alterations of mental life. Psychopathology as a science, however, should be based on the assumption that mental life even in its pathologies always displays a meaningful, holistic, and gestalt-like character.

Therefore psychopathology, according to Jaspers, is not exhausted by listing symptoms that could be regarded as a direct reflection of underlying brain disturbances. In contrast to neurology which correlates single clinical defects with circumscribed organic lesions, psychopathology starts where the unified experience of self and world itself suffers an alteration. This disturbance of the very constitution of experience may not be described in the way of single symptoms but requires an in-depth investigation of the structure of conscious experience. Only when this is achieved through careful and comprehensive phenomenological description, the search for organic, biographical, or other causes may proceed on a methodically well-funded basis.

In the introduction to *General Psychopathology*, Jaspers emphasized that his book 'is not enslaved to neurology and medicine on the dogmatic grounds that "psychic disorder is cerebral disorder"' (Jaspers 1997: 4). This dogma, established by the German psychiatrist Wilhelm Griesinger (1861), had led many psychiatrists to the conviction that 'if only we had an exact knowledge of the brain, we would then know the psychic life and its disturbances. This has induced psychiatrists to abandon psychopathological studies as unscientific, so that they have lost whatever psychopathological knowledge had been gained up to then' (Jaspers 1997: 459). Jaspers characterized this attitude as 'somatic prejudice' which tacitly presupposes 'that the actual reality of human existence is a somatic event. Man is only comprehensible when he is understood in somatic terms' (Jaspers 1997: 18). All talking of the psychic were only preliminary and meant nothing but a stopgap without any epistemic value. This attitude leads, according to Jaspers, to an overhasty identification of morphological or physiological data with subjective experience and, thus, to hazardous constructions which he termed 'brain mythologies'.

Jaspers' criticism of biological reductionism is closely connected to his well-known confrontation of understanding and explanation. On the one hand, he assigned a crucial role to causal explanation; on the other hand he strongly opposed any tendency to make it into an absolute, thus believing to have 'recognized the "essence" of psychic illness in the physical illness' (Jaspers 1997: 461). For the psychopathologist this would mean a betrayal of his task of representing and understanding mental life 'in an orderly and penetrating way' (Jaspers 1997: 461). 'The tendency to make causal speculation the main thing has a disastrous effect on our empirical knowledge of the varied forms of psychic abnormality' (Jaspers 1997: 461).

But Jaspers even carries the opposition forwards into the therapeutic domain. The desire for causal explanation, he argues, is essentially grounded in the striving for 'the greatest therapeutic power' (Jaspers 1997: 461). Where the material causes of mental disturbances become graspable, their immediate medical manipulation comes within reach. But 'causal knowledge, which grasps the non-understandable as it arises from its causes, can influence therapy decisively by measures in which the psyche which is wanting help need take no active part' (Jaspers 1997: 461). In stark contrast to such a therapy which, though efficient, remains external and indifferent to the individual person, Jaspers postulates an existential therapy through personal influence on the patient and his development. This approach via understanding is based on empathy, re-enactment, and on the affinity with the patient which the therapist feels as a fellow human being. 'Causal thinking impinges on what is alien, non-understandable and on what can be manipulated; understanding of meaning impinges on myself in the other and what is closest to me in the other'. In this encounter lies 'the most intense presentation of what is entirely individual' (Jaspers 1997: 461).

In times of a dominance of the neurobiological paradigm, criteriological diagnostic menus and a corresponding decline of psychopathological expertise, such considerations seem more relevant than ever. On the other hand, it must not be overlooked that Jaspers' approach also had its limitations. First, his concept of phenomenology, derived from the early Husserl and his 'Logical Investigations' (1900), remained restricted to a description of experience as verbally presented by the patient. In Jaspers' view, phenomenology was only a subdiscipline within psychopathology. Its primary task consisted in providing a basic taxonomy of psychopathological phenomena, thus performing a preparatory work for other subdisciplines of psychopathology and psychiatry. Jaspers was all the more anxious to keep his approach free from all explanatory claims which he thought would contaminate the purity of description by premature inferences, theories, and speculations. He never took notice of the further development of phenomenology toward eidetic, constitutional, or genetic approaches, not to mention the phenomenology of the bodily subject in Sartre's or Merleau-Ponty's accounts. Similarly, Jaspers took a rather deprecating position against all attempts of later anthropological and existential psychiatry to understand the patients' condition on the background of their overall being-in-the-world, their existential orientation or their projection of *Dasein*.

Moreover, there are limits to understanding *sensu* Jaspers, namely vis-à-vis the delusional experiences of schizophrenic patients which resist any attempt to understand them by empathic, intuitive, or psychological methods. For Jaspers, even the gradual changes of self-awareness apparent in the early stages of schizophrenia were due to an incomprehensible 'process'—as opposed to the understandable 'development' of the normal or neurotic personality. This (perhaps reductive) understanding of Jaspers' doctrine of incomprehensibility not only had an authoritative influence on German and international psychopathology, it also paved the way for treating schizophrenia merely as an epiphenomenon of some underlying brain dysfunction.

Further problems arise from Jaspers' tendency to draw too firm or even dualistic distinctions between domains such as explanation and understanding, or mind and body. Thus, he restricted the notion of explanation to causal reduction of mental phenomena to their biological underpinnings, which in turn meant that phenomenological analyses could not have an explanatory value for the psychiatrist. Moreover, by strictly limiting his descriptive psychopathology to conscious mental experience—'We should picture only what is really present in the patient's consciousness' (Jaspers 1968: 1316)—he apparently discarded any approach to unconscious dimensions of subjectivity. Jaspers remained very critical to the search for the understandable in unconscious processes or symptom patterns as psychoanalysis did. Nor did his dualistic approach encourage any possibility to look for the repercussion of subjective experience on neurophysiological events or brain structures.

Thus, on one side, the sphere of subjectivity remained an unconquerable citadel in whose investigation the psychopathologist could delve ad libitum. However, with the increase of causal knowledge relevant for medical interventions, this careful investigation was in danger of losing its relevance for the progress of psychiatry. In the second half of the last century, a growing crisis of psychopathology was clearly recognizable. In 1960, Kurt Schneider assumed that with the completion of the description and ordering of symptoms the 'mine of psychopathology was depleted' (Schneider 1960), and there was no use in engaging in psychopathological research any more. Gradually cut down to an ancillary role for nosological and syndromatic diagnosis, psychopathological research and expertise in clinical psychiatry suffered an alarming decline (Andreasen 1998; Hojaij 2000).

At least on the level of research, however, this has changed over the last decade. Present phenomenological psychopathology has gained new ground by investigating the basic structures and constitutive moments of conscious experience in mental health and illness. After almost one century, many of the concepts challenged by Jaspers are again at issue, and his investigations provide the ground for new analyses and discussions. Methodological issues like understanding and incomprehensibility, and clinical topics like defining delusions or self-awareness and its disorders are the core matter of twenty-first-century psychopathology. The velvet revolution kindled at the turn of the last century by the renaissance of the philosophy of psychiatry has given new strength to Jaspers' project of the foundation of psychiatry on *psychopathology*—the basic knowledge for the many schools, and the common language for the many dialects spoken by clinicians in the field of mental health.

However, after one century since its birth, there is a quite a confusion about the meaning of psychopathology. The aim of the following sections is to shed light on these issues: 'What psychopathology is not', 'What psychopathology really is', and 'What psychopathology is for'.

What psychopathology is not

Psychopathology is not mental pathology

In current literature, the word 'psychopathology' is used to refer to the subject matter of psychiatry, that is, pathologies of the psyche. A SCOPUS search reveals that over 30,000 studies have been published in the last 100 years which include the word 'psychopathology' in the title, abstract, or keywords. In the majority of studies, 'psychopathology' is used to talk about the subject matter of psychiatry, that is, pathologies of the psyche. This use of the term 'psychopathology' is trivial for the following main reasons: it ignores the origin and history of the discipline named 'psychopathology', it is ill-defined and confusingly overlaps with other concepts (e.g. symptom, syndrome, etc.), it overlooks basic epistemological distinctions (e.g. it conflates different concepts like 'illness' and 'disease', to be kept rigorously distinct), and evades the problem of defining the nature of the entities that are being diagnosed and classified. Psychopathology is not the *opus operatum* of psychiatry and clinical psychology. Rather, it is a discipline—a science—that provides clinicians with basic knowledge about the phenomena that affect the human mind and with a valid and reliable modus operandi.

Psychopathology is not symptomatology

Symptomatology is the study of isolated symptoms in view of their clinical, i.e. diagnostic and aetiological, significance. The use of the term 'symptom' in psychiatry is the consequence of a model of psychic illness derived from the natural sciences being used to relate objective data to specific aetiologies. In biological medicine, a symptom is the epiphenomenon of an underlying pathology. Within the biomedical paradigm, a symptom is first of all an index for diagnosis, i.e. it is used by clinicians to establish that the person who shows that symptom is sick (rather than healthy), and that he or she is affected by a particular illness or disease. The principal utility of any system of medical taxonomy relies on its capacity to identify specific entities to allow prediction of natural history and response to therapeutic intervention (Stanghellini, in press). Psychopathology is also about that, but *not just* about that. Whereas symptomatology is strictly *morbus* oriented since it deals with symptoms in a strict biomedical sense, psychopathology is also *person* oriented since it attempts to describe the special modes of experience and behaviour of a patient and his relationship to himself and to the world (Kraus 1994: 156). Psychopathology is not merely about assessing symptoms, it is about understanding a given type of experience and a given way of being in the world.

Psychopathology is not nosography

The aim of nosography is the description of single illnesses to allow their diagnosis. Nosography outlines provisional and conventional characteristics of a syndrome and thereby serves the goal of an empirical diagnosis. Psychopathology is not merely about diagnosis. Diagnosis, as Jaspers wrote, is the last point to be considered in the comprehension of a psychiatric case, since what matters most is that the 'chaos of phenomena' should not be buried under a diagnostic label, but rather should stand out in an evident way and in multiple connections. Blankenburg pointed out that the too tight association between psychopathology and nosology characterizing psychiatric tradition from Kahlbaum to Kraepelin did not constantly operate in favour of these two directions of research (Blankenburg 1971).

At present, the existing classifications of mental illnesses are merely provisional diagnostic conventions. Since no extra-clinical (e.g. aetiological or biological) indexes of putative nosological discontinuities are available, our nosography is necessarily based on exclusively psychopathologically defined syndromes. Thus, it is true that there is a strong link between psychopathology and nosography, since due to this lack of extra-clinical markers psychopathology aimed at becoming a doctrine linking symptoms and diagnosis. However, psychopathologists had to admit to the serious difficulties that we must occasionally overcome to 'build, from a psychopathological finding, a psychiatric diagnosis' and recommend the use of psychopathological concepts as 'floating buoys' useful as marks of reference for clinical navigation (Schneider 1959). Psychopathology is necessary, but not sufficient to establish diagnosis. Notwithstanding Schneider's warning, psychopathology is at risk of being too much diagnosis oriented and too much under the influence of the dominant nosographical grid. The result is that if psychopathology is conflated with nosography, only those symptoms that are supposed to have diagnostic value are investigated, in a sort of nosography-focused twilight state (Rossi Monti and Stanghellini 1996). The dominant focus on diagnosis disregards the attention to real people's experiences. As a consequence, clinical utility is confined to ad hoc bits of information useful for clinical decision-making. This excludes the scrutiny of the manifold manifestations of what is really there in the patients' experience, the essential prerequisite to understanding the worlds they live in.

Psychopathology is not a specialty in the field of mental health

Psychopathology is not one of numerous approaches to the classification and treatment of mental symptoms and syndromes; it is not one among the many theories aiming at illuminating the aetio-pathogenesis of mental disorders—as it is the case with psychoanalysis or the cognitive sciences.

Psychoanalytic psychopathology, as well as cognitive psychopathology, are disciplines in their own right, and cannot be conflated with psychopathology itself. These approaches use specific concepts and theories, meta-psychological or about the functioning of the mind, in order to explain the genesis and the development of mental disorders. Their main focus is on the aetio-pathogenesis of symptoms and syndromes. For instance, psychoanalytic psychopathology in describing a given neurotic symptom assumes that this symptom is produced by a given unconscious mechanism of defence. Its main focus is on the process producing a symptom. It seems that psychoanalytically oriented psychopathologists cannot refrain from asking 'Why?' before having answered to the (more basic) question 'How?'. Thus, psychopathology must be clearly demarcated from explanatory psychopathologies. The latter aims to explain how a symptom occurred and why it should be that particular symptom, mainly on the evidence of that person's experience in early life. This is stigmatized as 'prescient understanding' (Oyebode 2008: 21), indicating presumed foreknowledge of how events of mental life must unfold because they will necessarily conform with theoretical postulates. All interpretative constructs represent a paradigm different from that of psychopathology and tend to impede true knowledge of the phenomena of experience.

Psychopathology is not uninterested in the pathogenesis of symptoms and syndromes. But first and foremost it focuses on the precise description, definition, and classification of these—which psychoanalytic and cognitive psychopathologies instead take for granted.

Psychopathology assumes that, in order to dig into the hidden abyss of the sick mind, one needs first to have a precise map of its surface. This is the reason why we assume that psychopathology is not a specialty in the field of mental health, but the basic science in psychiatry and clinical psychology. As poet William Yeates writes, 'Though leaves are many/The root is one'. Psychopathology is—or better: should be—the common root, the basic, indispensable educational pre-requisite in the curriculum for psychiatrists and clinical psychologists.

What psychopathology really is

Now, as in Jaspers' times, the relevance of the discipline of psychopathology for psychiatry is threefold: it is the common language (*koiné*) that allows specialists, belonging to different schools each one speaking its own dialect or jargon, to understand each other; it is the ground for diagnosis and classification in a field where all major conditions are not aetiologically defined disease entities, but exclusively clinically defined syndromes; it makes an indispensable contribution to understanding, a special kind of intelligibility based on the meanings of personal experiences. We can distinguish three types of psychopathologies: descriptive, clinical and structural psychopathology (Stanghellini 2009).

Descriptive psychopathology can be defined as the precise description and categorization of abnormal experiences as recounted by the patient and observed in his behaviour. It is a detailed unfolding of the patient's field of consciousness whose aim is bringing into view his subjectivity. Jaspers was very clear in stating that 'we expect to account for *every* psychic phenomenon. In no circumstances should we rest satisfied with a general impression or a set of details collected ad hoc' (Jaspers 1997: 56, emphasis added). Jaspers' *General Psychopathology* is the breeding ground of descriptive psychopathology. Jaspers delimited its field, which he called 'phenomenology'. The main purpose of descriptive psychopathology is the systematic study of conscious experiences, ordering and classifying them, and creating valid and reliable terminology. To obtain this, it focuses on the patients' states of mind as they are experienced and narrated by them; expressions and behaviours are considered important, but less specific than personal experiences. The form in which a content is given to consciousness is considered more important than the content itself.

Descriptive psychopathology relies on two main methodological assumptions. The first, quintessential methodological prerequisite is avoiding theoretical explanations, as well as presuppositions and prejudices. 'We confine ourselves solely to the things that are present to the patients' consciousness. Conventional theories, psychological constructions, interpretations and evaluations must be left aside' (Jaspers 1997: 56). The second methodological assumption is about the use of empathy, and its limitations. Descriptive psychopathology attempts to use empathy as a clinical instrument to recreate in the psychopathologist the subjective experience of a patient to obtain a valid and reliable description of his experience. 'Since we never can perceive the psychic experience of the other in any direct fashion, there has to be an act of empathy' (Jaspers 1997: 55). It is empathy that makes it possible for us to know what it is like for another person to be in a particular mental state. Empathy is a special kind of intentional experience in which my perception of the other leads me to grasp (or to feel that I grasp) his personal experience. It implies a special kind of (feel of) immediate resonance between myself and the other person.

Clinical psychopathology is essentially aimed at the identification of symptoms that are significant in view of nosographical distinctions. K. Schneider, in the preface to the fourth edition of his *Clinical Psychopathology*, affirms that clinical psychopathology aims at becoming the 'psychopathological doctrine of symptoms and diagnosis'. Clinical psychopathology aims at becoming the link between descriptive psychopathology and nosography. The assessment made following the principles of clinical psychopathology is chiefly of pragmatic diagnostic use. Lanteri-Laura pointedly stated that, in the Schneiderian view, 'psychopathology tends, contrarily to symptomatology, to select pathognomonic signs' (Lanteri-Laura 1998: 606). It restricts the task of the psychopathological inquiry to the search for diagnostically relevant symptoms. This means that clinical psychopathology is interested in eliciting, during the psychopathological interview, first and foremost those abnormal psychic phenomena that help the clinician to establish a reliable diagnosis.

Although clinical psychopathology is at risk of flattening the practice of psychopathology to that of nosographical diagnosis, it also serves an epistemologically important function. Clinical psychopathology is concerned with generalizing the individual case and subsuming it into a general category. It complements the view of descriptive psychopathology (which keeps the individual and its complexity in focus) in that the patient here is also an 'instantiation of a general category', rather than merely 'a primordially real individual' (Broome 2008: 114). Psychopathology is not only about the description of phenomena idiosyncratically taking place in a single individual—although its first aim is to do justice to the *individuum*. In addition to that, it also envisions the individual as an exemplar of a given general type. Although its form of intelligibility is different from that of the natural sciences, psychopathology is a kind of scientific knowledge since it allows generalizations. It keeps in tension the knowledge about the real, single individual (e.g. this person with schizophrenia) with the horizonal knowledge of an abstract kind (e.g. what psychopathology knows about the condition called 'schizophrenia'). Knowledge emerges as the mutual, dialectic enlightenment between the individual and the genre he is attributed to.

Structural psychopathology subscribes to the view that the manifold of phenomena of a given form of existence is a meaningful whole, that is, a structure. Psychopathology in general is chiefly about experiences and their meanings. Structural psychopathology assumes that the symptoms of a syndrome have a meaningful coherence.

Meaningfulness emerges from a structure via a dialogue-oriented process of unfolding. With 'unfolding' we mean the explication of a single form of existence which does not transform it into something else, but lets it manifest itself. To unfold or explicate means to grasp the fleeting entanglement of interlaced parts of a given structure, for example, inter-related actions in a narrative or interconnected symptoms in a syndrome. To explicate or unfold the field of experience or the pattern of actions of a given person is to bring out or lay bare its structure, that is, the internal relations of dependence which constitute its immanent pattern.

In a structure, meaningfulness is not the outcome of the action of an external subject who artificially cuts-and-pastes separate elements. Rather, meaningfulness ideally comes into sight and emerges via a spiral of approximations leading to a kind of epiphany or manifestation. The role of the knowing subject is that of letting this manifestation happen. Rather than being the product of an active construction, meaningfulness preferably emerges from an act of receptiveness or voluntary inaction—a 'wise passiveness' in the words of the poet Wordsworth that lets the links between the parts of the structure become manifest.

Meaningfulness is the product of this holistic view. This attitude aspires to collecting a range of phenomena that point to multiple facets of a potentially significant concept, letting tacit, implicit, and opaque phenomena and their meanings emerge to the surface of awareness (Uehlein 1992). The final aim of this meaning-oriented and contextually sensitive approach is sometimes referred to as 'thick description' (Geertz 1979).

Structural psychopathology aims to grasp the motivational relationships that lend coherence and continuity to that person's consciousness' (Parnas and Sass 2008: 264), focusing on formal (rather than content) aspects of experience—like lived space and time, and qualities of the object-world and self-experience. The connections between the manifold phenomena are neither logical, nor law-like causal connections, but *phenomenological*, since each phenomenon 'carr[ies] the traces of the underlying formal alterations of subjectivity' (Parnas and Sass 2008: 267). Looking for structural relationships consists in the unfolding of the basic structure(s) of subjectivity, that is, the way consciousness appropriates phenomena.

Thus, starting with first-person accounts, structural psychopathology is certainly no longer descriptive, but proceeds to investigate the *constitutive processes* that build up subjective experience, such as the formation of perceptual meaning, temporal continuity, or implicit bodily action. It analyses the basic structures of consciousness such as self-awareness, embodiment, spatiality, temporality, intentionality, and intersubjectivity. This allows detection of the critical points where the constitution of self and world is vulnerable and open to deviations or derailments. Particularly in psychotic disorders, the patient may lose his ground in the lived body as the ensemble of dispositions and habitualities, his anchoring in temporal continuity and in intersubjective common sense. On the other hand, despite the erosion of the constitutional processes, the patients still strive for a coherent world view, though this may sometimes only be possible in the form of delusion or autistic withdrawal. Accordingly, structural phenomenology also explores the modes by which the patients try to make sense of their basic disturbances and to re-establish some form of meaningful coherence (Fuchs 2010; Stanghellini 2010).

What psychopathology is for

With all that in place, we are sure that it has become fully comprehensible why psychiatry and clinical psychology are in strong need for psychopathology (Stanghellini and Rosfort, in press):

- Psychiatry is a heterogeneous discipline since its adepts approach its 'object' from many different angles, as for instance neuroscience, depth psychology, sociology, and philosophy, each of which has its own language, methodology, and practice. Thus psychiatrists need a common ground and a common language. To Jaspers, disturbing mental phenomena are the main relevant facts for psychiatry, and psychopathology is the shared language that allows clinicians with different theoretical backgrounds to understand each other when debating about mental disorders.
- Psychiatry addresses abnormal human subjectivity. Psychopathology attempts to define what is abnormal (rather than taking for granted common-sense views) as well as grasp what is human in apparently non-human (e.g. irrational) phenomena.

- Psychiatry aims at establishing rigorous diagnosis. Psychopathology is still highly useful in a field where all major disorders are not neuroscientifically defined disease entities, but exclusively syndromes that can be defined according to characterizing symptoms and among them especially abnormal subjective experiences.
- Psychiatry is about understanding disturbed human experience, rather than simply diagnosing and classifying it. Psychopathology functions as a bridge between human and clinical sciences, providing the basic tools to make sense of mental suffering.
- Psychiatry is about caring for troubled human existence, rather than judging, marginalizing, punishing, and stigmatizing it. Psychopathology connects understanding with caring and endeavours to establish an epistemological as well as ethical framework for this.
- Psychiatry looks for a way to connect, or at least think together, first-person subjective experience with impersonal brain functioning. As Jaspers saw with admirable clarity, psychopathology is about bridging understanding (*Verstehen*) and explaining (*Erklären*) both in research and clinical settings.

Outline of the volume

This volume, celebrating the centennial of Karl Jaspers' *General Psychopathology*, develops these issues. Three sections are included:

Section 1: the first section sets Jaspers' work in its historical, cultural, institutional, psychiatric, psychotherapeutic, and philosophical background, especially illuminating its controversial relationship with Freud's psychoanalysis and with the philosophy of Edmund Husserl. This section also shows how Jaspers' *General Psychopathology* was received in more recent times. It includes the following chapters:

- Federico Leoni: 'Jaspers in his time'.
- Osborne P. Wiggins and Michael Alan Schwartz: 'Phenomenology and psychopathology: in search of a method'.
- Mario Rossi Monti: 'Karl Jaspers' "Critique of Psychoanalysis": between past and future'.
- Christoph Mundt: 'Impact of Karl Jaspers' *General Psychopathology*: the range of appraisal'.

Section 2: the second section deals with basic methodological issues and concepts: Jaspers' conception of phenomenology, the use of Jaspersian phenomenology for clinical practice, the emphasis of Jaspers' phenomenology on subjectivity and on the formal aspects of subjective experiences, meaningful connections, the dichotomy of explaining versus understanding and the related issues of incomprehensibility and brain mythology, and finally Jaspers' ideas on characterology and his caveat against the ambition to understand human existence as a whole. Also, two special topics are addressed: pathography and psychotherapy. This section includes:

- Otto Doerr-Zegers and Héctor Pelegrina-Cetrán: 'Karl Jaspers' *General Psychopathology* in the framework of clinical practice'.
- Chris Walker: 'Form and content in Jaspers' psychopathology'.
- Louis A. Sass: 'Jaspers, phenomenology, and the "ontological difference"'.

- Christoph Hoerl: 'Jaspers on explaining and understanding in psychiatry'
- Matthew R. Broome: 'Jaspers and neuroscience'.
- Matthias Bormuth: 'Karl Jaspers the pathographer'.
- Jann E. Schlimme: 'Karl Jaspers' existential concept of psychotherapy'.
- Giovanni Stanghellini: 'The ethics of incomprehensibility'.

Section 3: the last section is about those clinical concepts that Jaspers for the first time analysed in a rigorous, systematic, and philosophically grounded way, and that are still at the core of our understanding of mental disorders. These concepts include delusions, delusional mood, ego-disorders, mood and its disorders, principles of classification, and the relationship between personality and psychosis. The chapters in this section do not merely provide an outline and a commentary to Jaspers' ideas, but set these topics within the landscape of contemporary debate and controversies in psychopathology:

- Henning Sass and Umberto Volpe: 'Karl Jaspers' hierarchical principle and current psychiatric classification'.
- Josef Parnas: 'On psychosis: Karl Jaspers and beyond'.
- Matthew Ratcliffe: 'Delusional atmosphere and the sense of unreality'.
- Thomas Fuchs: 'The self in schizophrenia: Jaspers, Schneider, and beyond'.
- S. Nassir Ghaemi: 'Understanding mood disorders: Karl Jaspers' biological existentialism'.
- Alfred Kraus: 'Reaction and development in manic and melancholic-depressive patients'.

References

Andreasen, N. (1998). 'Understanding Schizophrenia: A Silent Spring?', *American Journal of Psychiatry*, **155**(12): 1657–1659.

Blankenburg, W. (1971). *Der Verlust der natuerlichen Selbstverstaendlichkeit. Ein Beitrag zur Psychopathologie symptomarmer Schizophrenien*. Stuttgart, Germany: Enke.

Broome, M. (2008). 'Philosophy as the Science of Value: Neo-Kantianism as a Guide to Psychiatric Interviewing', *Philosophy, Psychiatry, & Psychology*, **15**: 107–116.

Fuchs, T. (2010). 'Phenomenology and Psychopathology', In S. Gallagher, D. Schmicking (eds), *Handbook of Phenomenology and the Cognitive Sciences*. Dordrecht: Springer, 547–573.

Geertz, C. (1979). *The Interpretation of Cultures*. New York, NY: Basic Books.

Griesinger, W. (1861). *Die Pathologie und Therapie der psychischen Krankheiten für Ärzte und Studirende* (2nd edn). Stuttgart: Krabbe.

Hojaij, C.R. (2000). 'Reappraisal of dementia praecox: focus on clinical psychopathology', *World Journal of Biological Psychiatry*, **1**:43–54.

Jaspers, K. (1968). 'The phenomenological approach in psychopathology', *British Journal of Psychiatry*, **114**: 1313–1323.

Jaspers, K. (1997). *General Psychopathology* (7th edn) (J. Hoenig, M.W. Hamilton, trans.). Baltimore, MD: Johns Hopkins University Press.

Kraus, A. (1994). 'Phenomenological and Criteriological Diagnosis: Different or Complementary?', in J.Z. Sadler, O.P. Wiggins, M.A. Schwartz (eds), *Philosophical Perspectives on Psychiatric Classification*. Baltimore, MD: John Hopkins University Press, 148–162.

Lanteri-Laura, G. (1998). *Essay on the Paradigms of Modern Psychiatry*. Paris: Editions du Temps.

Oyebode, F. (2008). *Symptoms in the Mind. An Introduction to Descriptive Psychopathology* (4th edn). Edinburgh: Elsevier

Parnas, J., Sass, L.A. (2008). 'Varieties of "Phenomenology." On Description, Understanding, and Explanation in Psychiatry', in K.S. Kendler, J. Parnas (eds), *Philosophical Issues in Psychiatry; Explanation, Phenomenology, and Nosology*. Baltimore, MD: Johns Hopkins University Press, 239–278.

Rossi Monti, M., Stanghellini, G. (1996). 'Psychopathology: An Edgeless Razor?'. *Comprehensive Psychiatry*, 37(3): 196–204.

Schneider, K. (1959). *Clinical Psychopathology* (5th edn). New York, NY: Grune & Stratton.

Schneider, K. (1960). *Psychiatrie Heute*. Stuttgart: Thieme.

Stanghellini, G. (2009). 'The Meanings of Psychopathology', *Current Opinion in Psychiatry*, **22**: 559–564.

Stanghellini, G. (2010). 'A Hermeneutic Framework for Psychopathology', *Psychopathology*, **43**: 319–326.

Stanghellini, G. (in press). 'Philosophical Resources for the Psychiatric Interview', In K.W.M Fulford, M. Davies, R. Gipps, G. Graham, J.Z. Sadler, G. Stanghellini, T. Thornton (eds), *Oxford Handbook of Philosophy and Psychiatry*. Oxford: Oxford University Press.

Stanghellini, G., Rosfort, R. (in press). 'Toward a Person-Centered Psychopathology of Emotions. Jaspers in Between Moods and Affects', in T. Fuchs, C. Mundt, T. Breyer (eds), *Karl Jaspers' Philosophy and Psychopathology*. New York, NY: Springer.

Uehlein, F.A. (1992). 'Eidos and Eidetic variations in Husserl's phenomenology', in M. Spitzer, F.A. Uehlein, M.A. Schwartz, C. Mundt (eds), *Phenomenology, Language, and Schizophrenia*. New York, NY: Springer, 88–102.

Introduction: The relevance of Karl Jaspers' *General Psychopathology* to current psychiatric debate

Mario Maj

One hundred years after the appearance of its first edition, Karl Jaspers' *General Psychopathology* (1913) remains highly relevant to at least three areas of psychiatric inquiry: the epistemology of psychiatry, the classification of mental disorders, and the exploration of subjective experiences in people with schizophrenia. All of them are highlighted in the present volume.

In the realm of epistemology, a first basic assertion made in the text is that psychiatry does need a philosophy. 'If anyone thinks he can exclude philosophy and leave it aside as useless he will eventually be defeated by it in some obscure form or other' (Jaspers 1997: 770). 'If we are not clearly conscious of our philosophy we shall mix it up with our scientific thinking quite unawares' (Jaspers 1997: 769). These statements forerun the ongoing debate about the alleged 'atheoretical' attitude of the *Diagnostic and Statistical Manual of Mental Disorders* (DSM), the lack of a guiding philosophy in contemporary psychiatry, and the need to be aware of our conceptual assumptions in order to prevent their distorting effects (Fulford et al. 2004; Ghaemi 2007).

Related to this is the acknowledgement that an essential, invariable feature of the psychiatric discipline is the coexistence of a variety of research methods, whose 'presuppositions' and limitations need to be recognized, but none of which can be ignored. 'No theory or viewpoint is ignored. I try to grasp each different view of the whole and give it place according to its significance and limitations' (Jaspers 1997: 41). 'There is no system of elements and functions to be applied generally in psychopathological analysis […] we must simply be satisfied with a number of different methods of approach' (Jaspers, 1997: 42). These statements resonate with the contemporary critique of 'antitheoretical eclecticism' (Ghaemi 2007; Havens 1973/2004) as well as with the argument that the existence of different theoretical orientations in psychiatry should not be regarded as a weakness, but as an evidence of the peculiar integrative nature of the discipline and a consequence of the complexity of the mind and its disorders. Other disciplines may have a clearer identity and appear less divided than psychiatry, but one of the reasons for this is that their vision and approach are more unilateral, thus being not sufficient to address the complexity of mental disorders (Maj 2010).

Also highlighted in the present volume is Jaspers' view of the relationship between psychopathology and neuroscience (Broome, Chapter 9). Jaspers recognizes that 'in every individual event soma and psyche form an inseparable unity' (Jaspers 1997: 3). 'There are somatic phenomena, universally accepted as such, which are in part dependent on psychic events [...] On the other hand, the most complex psychic events originate in part from somatic sources' (Jaspers 1997: 4). However, 'neither line of enquiry encounters the other so directly that we can speak of some specific psychic event as directly associated with some specific somatic event or of an actual parallelism' (Jaspers 1997: 4). Indeed, 'the further neurology advances, the further the psyche recedes' (Jaspers 1997: 4). These statements resonate with the currently growing evidence of the multiple interrelationships between mental and physical diseases, with the ongoing debate about whether it is possible to fully 'explain' complex mental disorders at a biological level (Maj 2001) and with the recent revival of the discussion (which has obvious political as well as scientific implications) on whether mental disorders do represent 'brain diseases' (Bolton, 2013; Maj, 2013; White et al. 2012). Actually, there are clear analogies between the present ideological climate and that of the beginning of the twentieth century (Broome 2013; Fulford et al. 2004), when the enthusiasm brought about by the progress in neuroscience—and some reductionistic excesses generated by that enthusiasm, indeed epitomized by Griesinger's statement that 'mental illnesses are brain diseases'—was being followed by some disillusionment, due to the limited relevance of that progress to the elucidation of the aetiopathogenesis of mental disorders.

In the area of classification of mental disorders, Jaspers' *General Psychopathology* contains first of all an acknowledgement of the 'provisional' nature of classification in psychiatry, 'a fiction which will discharge its function if it proves to be the most apt for the time' (Jaspers 1997: 605). This statement is remarkably endorsed in the preface to the International Classification of Diseases (tenth revision, ICD-10) chapter on mental disorders (World Health Organization 1992: vii). Furthermore, Jaspers' text introduces the subdivision of mental disorders into three groups ('real disease entities', i.e. known somatic illnesses with psychic disturbances, in which 'there are no transitions between disease and health'; 'circles', such as schizophrenia and manic-depressive illness, in which 'we can still draw a sharp line between what is health and what is not', but which are not 'clearly delineated from each other'; and 'types', including neuroses and abnormal personalities, among which 'there is no sharp line to be drawn' and there is no 'decisive borderline in every case between what is healthy and what is not') (Jaspers 1997: 605–611). This subgrouping, and in particular the conceptualization of 'ideal types' as opposed to 'disease entities', resonates with the current argument that the DSM-III and its successors, in spite of their declared 'atheoretical' stance, implicitly treat all mental disorders as equivalent to biologically-based natural disease entities (Ghaemi 2009; Wiggins and Schwartz 1994).

Less widely known, but also highlighted in the present volume (Sass and Volpe, Chapter 13), is Jaspers' critique of the assumption that mental disorders represent 'mosaic-like structures composed from a variety of individual and identical pieces', so that 'we only need to name those generally identical pieces to see in which illness each fragment appeared most frequently'. 'This method of living mosaic [...] turns psychopathological investigation and diagnosis into something mechanical and petrifies discovery' (Jaspers 1997: 563). This criticism is clearly relevant to the current trend to regard psychopathological symptoms as 'building blocks', which recur exactly with the same characteristics (and presumably with the same biological correlates) in all the various mental disorders. This assumption lies at the heart of some ongoing research projects (e.g. Sanislow et al. 2010), but is currently being criticized exactly along Jaspers' lines (e.g. Ghaemi 2009).

Also striking is Jaspers' acknowledgement of both a 'factual' and a 'value' component in the conceptualization of mental illness (Jaspers 1997: 784), and of the essential role of social functioning ('social usefulness') in that conceptualization (Jaspers 1997: 789), forerunning the current debate on 'what is mental disorder' (e.g. Wakefield 2007).

The most widely acknowledged contribution of Jaspers' *General Psychopathology* to the psychiatric discipline is the delineation of phenomenology as an 'empirical method of enquiry', providing 'a concrete description of the psychic states which patients actually experience' (Jaspers 1997: 55). Indeed, Jaspers' characterization of 'subjective phenomena of morbid psychic life', and especially of the 'activity of the self' and its disorders, has given rise to a line of inquiry, concerning in particular schizophrenia, that has developed throughout the past century up to our days.

According to Jaspers, 'every psychic manifestation […] carries this particular aspect of "being mine," of having an "I"-quality, of "personally belonging"' (Jaspers 1997: 121). In people with schizophrenia, this 'awareness of performing one's own actions' is basically altered, so that 'any mode of activity may acquire the sense of being "artificially made"' (Jaspers 1997: 123). This concept, supported in the text by a variety of examples and passages from patients' self-descriptions, has been extensively developed during the past century by the phenomenological school, leading to the current view that impairment of pre-reflexive self-awareness is the core feature of schizophrenia, already evident in the prodromal phase of the disease (e.g. Parnas 2012). The 'basic tone of selfhood' is supposed to be 'granted in the brain by a continuous source of internally generated input' (e.g. Kircher and David 2003), and the search for the neural correlates of its 'trait alteration' in schizophrenia is currently an active area of neuroscientific inquiry.

A reflection of this view can be found in the ICD-10 definition of schizophrenia ('The disturbance involves the most basic functions that give the normal person a feeling of individuality, uniqueness and self-direction' (World Health Organization 1992: 78)), as well as in the texts of the DSM-III and DSM-III-R ('The sense of self that gives the normal person a feeling of individuality, uniqueness, and self-direction is frequently disturbed in schizophrenia' (American Psychiatric Association 1980, 1987: 189)), while there is no trace of it in either the DSM-IV or the current DSM-5 draft.

Although very influential, the notion that disorders of self-awareness represent the core feature of schizophrenia raises some practical concerns, which will have to be addressed by future research (Maj 2012). These regard the feasibility and reliability of the ascertainment of these disorders under ordinary clinical conditions (as opposed to their assessment by experts or super-experts), their diagnostic specificity for schizophrenia, and whether they are amenable to currently available treatments (or should be viewed as an essentially unmodifiable constitutional deficit). The concern about reliability becomes even deeper if the approach is going to be adopted in the very sensitive area of early diagnosis of psychosis. It is important, in this respect, to emphasize that Jaspers himself was acutely aware of the possible misapplication of his proposed phenomenological method, and of the need for a high level of expertise and supervision to use it ('Experience shows us that this is by no means easy to do'; 'It is not something which one just has, but it has to be acquired painfully through much critical effort and frequent failure' (Jaspers 1997: 56)).

When I was a young psychiatrist, Jaspers' *General Psychopathology* was a prescribed reading for every resident. My familiarity with that book (and some other classic texts) helped me to see the DSM-III and its successors in the appropriate light (i.e. as synopses of available knowledge to be used for clinical purposes). I could use, for instance, the twenty-two words composing the DSM-IV diagnostic criteria for schizophrenia as a useful algorithm, easy to memorize and to recall. This may not be the case for current residents in psychiatry, who are unlikely to have read *General Psychopathology* as well as some other key classic texts. For these young colleagues, those twenty-two words are likely to remain what they are, with a high risk of misunderstanding and oversimplification.

But Jaspers' *General Psychopathology* is not an easy text to read. Especially nowadays, in the Internet era, it may appear in several parts obscure, convoluted, or repetitive. This is why the present volume has the potential to be not only attractive to scholars, but also extremely useful for young psychiatrists and busy clinicians. It may represent for them a 'guide' to the reading of that ponderous text, helping them to extract the key messages that are likely to resonate with, and at the same time enrich, their clinical practice and theoretical reflection.

References

American Psychiatric Association. (1980). *Diagnostic and Statistical Manual of Mental Disorders, 3rd Edition*. Washington, DC: American Psychiatric Association.

American Psychiatric Association. (1987). *Diagnostic and Statistical Manual of Mental Disorders, 3rd Edition, Revised*. Washington, DC: American Psychiatric Association.

Bolton, D. (2013). 'Should Mental Disorders be Regarded as Brain Disorders? 21st Century Mental Health Sciences and Implications for Research and Training', *World Psychiatry*, 12: 24–25.

Fulford, K.W.M, Morris, K.J, Sadler, J.Z, Stanghellini, G. (2003) 'Past Improbable, Future Possible: the Renaissance in Philosophy and Psychiatry', in K.W.M Fulford, K.J. Morris, J.Z. Sadler, G. Stanghellini (eds), *Nature and Narrative: An Introduction to the New Philosophy of Psychiatry*. Oxford: Oxford University Press, 1–41.

Fulford, K.W.M., Stanghellini, G., Broome, M. (2004). 'What Can Philosophy Do For Psychiatry?', *World Psychiatry*, **3**: 130–135.

Ghaemi, S.N. (2007). 'Existence and Pluralism: The Rediscovery of Karl Jaspers', *Psychopathology*, **40**: 75–82.

Ghaemi, S.N. (2009). 'Nosologomania: DSM & Karl Jaspers' Critique of Kraepelin', *Philosophy, Ethics, and Humanities in Medicine*, **4**: 10–17.

Havens, L.L. (1973/2004). *Psychiatric Movements: Approaches to the Mind*. Cambridge, MA: Harvard University Press. (Original work published in 1973.)

Jaspers, K. (1913). *Allgemeine Psychopathologie* (1st edn). Berlin: Springer.

Jaspers, K. (1997). *General Psychopathology* (7th edn) (J. Hoenig, M.W. Hamilton, trans.). Baltimore, MD: Johns Hopkins University Press.

Kircher, T., David, A.S. (2003). 'Self-Consciousness: An Integrative Approach from Philosophy, Psychopathology and the Neurosciences', in T. Kircher, A.S. David (eds), *The Self in Neuroscience and Psychiatry*. Cambridge: Cambridge University Press, 217–241.

Maj, M. (2001). 'Is it Possible to Explain Complex Mental Disorders at the Biological Level?', *World Psychiatry*, **10**: 1.

Maj, M. (2010). 'Are Psychiatrists an Endangered Species?', *World Psychiatry*, **9**: 1–2.

Maj, M. (2012). 'The Self and schizophrenia: Some Open Issues', *World Psychiatry*, **11**: 65–66.

Maj M. (2013). 'Mental Disorders as "Brain Diseases" and Jaspers' Legacy', *World Psychiatry*, 12: 1–3.

Parnas, J. (2012). 'The Core Gestalt of Schizophrenia', *World Psychiatry*, **11**: 67–69.

Sanislow, C.A., Pine, D.S., Quinn, K.J., Kozak, M.J., Garvey, M.A., Heinssen, R.K., *et al.* (2010). 'Developing Constructs for Psychopathology Research: Research Domain Criteria', *Journal of Abnormal Psychology*, **119**: 631–639.

Wakefield, J.C. (2007). 'The Concept of Mental Disorder: Diagnostic Implications of the Harmful Dysfunction Analysis', *World Psychiatry*, **6**: 149–156.

White, P.D., Rickards, H., Zeman, A.Z.J. (2012). 'Time to End the Distinction Between Mental and Neurological Illnesses', *British Medical Journal*, **344**: e3454.

Wiggins, O., Schwartz, M. (1994). 'The Limits of Psychiatric Knowledge and the Problem of Classification', in J. Sadler, O Wiggins, M. Schwartz (eds), *Philosophical Perspectives on Psychiatric Diagnostic Classification*. Baltimore, MD: Johns Hopkins University Press, 89–103.

World Health Organization. (1992). *The ICD-10 Classification of Mental and Behavioural Disorders: Clinical Descriptions and Diagnostic Guidelines*. Geneva: World Health Organization.

Introduction: Particular psychopathologies—lessons from Karl Jaspers' *General Psychopathology* for the new philosophy of psychiatry

K.W.M. (Bill) Fulford

The publication of this book in 2013 celebrates no less than two significant life events for psychiatry. As the title of the book indicates, 2013 is the centenary of *General Psychopathology*. But 2013 is also the year in which with Stanghellini and Fuchs' timely collection, the IPPP (International Perspectives in Philosophy and Psychiatry) book series reaches its 40th volume.

Celebrating the positives

The conjunction of these two events is historically significant. Just as Jaspers' work in the philosophy of psychiatry grew out of and was (in part) inspired by the remarkable developments in the neurosciences at the turn of the nineteenth century (psychiatry's 'first biological phase'), so the modern movement in philosophy of psychiatry has grown out of and has been (in part) inspired by the no less remarkable developments in the neurosciences at the turn of the twentieth century. Small wonder therefore that as Mario Maj so elegantly describes in his introduction, Jaspers' work remains vitally relevant today.

Maj highlights three broad areas of contemporary relevance: psychiatric epistemology, the classification of mental disorders, and phenomenological understanding of schizophrenia. In each of these areas, as Maj describes, there is still much to learn from what Jaspers said in *General Psychopathology*. Other chapters in this marvellous collection explore topics ranging from psychoanalysis and neuroscience to clinical practice, from depression and mania to delusion. It seems there is hardly a matter of importance in psychiatry today on which Jaspers' work in *General Psychopathology* has nothing to say.

On first inspection the continuing relevance of Jaspers' work might seem unsurprising. Advances in the neurosciences, as no less a neuroscientist than Nancy Andreasen pointed out in her book *Brave New Brain* (2001), raise in a peculiarly acute form many of the deepest problems of philosophy: this is one very immediate reason then why philosophy of psychiatry (in 2013 as in 1913) flourishes at times of neuroscientific progress: yet the problems of philosophy have exercised the brightest and best minds without resolution for well over two thousand years: and it is to this extent therefore no surprise to find that the problems of philosophy as they presented to a neuroscientifically-informed psychiatry at the start of the twentieth century, should be with us still unresolved a mere century later in a neuroscientifically-informed psychiatry at the start of the twenty-first century.

Learning from the negatives

Yet if there is no surprise here there is also a challenge. If the problems of philosophy are in practice if not in principle irresolvable, whither the philosophy of psychiatry? It is one thing for philosophers to adopt a two-thousand-year research time line. From this perspective the persistence of the philosophical challenges of the neurosciences from Jaspers' time a (mere) century ago to our own is indeed no surprise. But psychiatry is disciplined by the pressures of clinical necessity. At the start of the twenty-first century then, the challenge for philosophy of psychiatry is to define a research agenda which is at one and the same time both philosophically realistic and clinically relevant.

Here I believe we have as much to learn from Jaspers' failures as from his successes. The year 1913 was something of an *annus mirabilis* for the young Jaspers (he was just 30 at the time). Closely anticipated by his paper on the phenomenology method, 1913 was the year not only of *General Psychopathology* (1913a) but also of a still widely cited publication spelling out Jaspers' central message about the need for meaningful understanding as well as causal explanations in psychopathology (1913b). Yet after this extraordinary creative outburst we get, well, almost nothing. Jaspers did indeed produce a series of follow-up editions of *General Psychopathology* (the last being however edited by the clinician Kurt Schneider); and as Stanghellini (Chapter 12, this volume) has pointed out, Jaspers' later work as a philosopher was informed by his earlier studies in philosophy of psychiatry. But otherwise, aside from his pathographical studies of great historical figures published in the 1920s (Bormuth, Chapter 10, this volume), and a long running battle with psychoanalysis (Stanghellini, Chapter 12; also Rossi Monti, Chapter 3, this volume), Jaspers neither worked further on nor inspired others to work further on the philosophy of psychiatry for the remainder of his long life. He was well celebrated of course. He became a respected Professor of Philosophy in Heidelberg.[1] As such he worked on areas (like phenomenology) relevant to the philosophy of psychiatry. But on the philosophy of psychiatry as such he (and with him the field) fell essentially silent until the birth of the modern movement some 50 years later.

Cave foundations

So, what are the lessons from Jaspers' 50 years of silence for the research agenda of philosophy and psychiatry today? One very immediate lesson could be summed up aphoristically as '*cave* (beware) foundations'. Jaspers sought to put psychiatry on secure philosophical foundations: the very title of his book, *General Psychopathology*, signals his foundationalist aims. In this Jaspers was consistent with the philosophy of his day. At the time of publication of *General Psychopathology*, the English philosopher Bertrand Russell had just published with his Cambridge colleague A.N. Whitehead their *magnum opus* in which they

[1] As is well known, despite fears for his Jewish wife, Gertrud, Jaspers stood out against the Nazi regime and eventually lost his professorship to the pro-Nazi Martin Heidegger. Less well known is that the then White's Professor of Moral Philosophy in Oxford, H.J. Paten, worked hard though in the end unsuccessfully to persuade his colleagues to offer Jaspers a Visiting Professorship. Suzanne Kirkbright's (2004) intellectual biography of Jaspers told mainly through his diaries and letters provides a gripping first-hand account of these events.

sought to put mathematics on (what they believed were) secure foundations in logic: they called their book *Principia Mathematatica*. A few years earlier another British philosopher, G.E. Moore, had published a *Principia Ethica*. And in Germany and Austria a group of philosophers including Mauritz Schlick and Rudolf Carnap, influenced by the German philosopher and physicist Ernst Mach, were close to establishing their Vienna Circle the explicit aim of which was to put empirical science on secure philosophical foundations with a version of positivism they called 'logical positivism'.

It is easy to sympathize with the urge to find secure foundations—a rock, an anchor, a starting point. No less a figure after all than the seventeenth-century French philosopher and mathematician René Descartes was motivated by his ambitions for a 'first philosophy' to develop the method of doubt from which his *cogito* ('I think therefore I am') and in turn the modern discipline of philosophy of mind are derived.[2] Yet there are two reasons, one practical the other theoretical, why foundationalism is not on the research agenda of contemporary philosophy of psychiatry.

The practical reason is that as a basis for policy, clinical work, and indeed science in psychiatry, secure foundations are not all they are cracked up to be. Again, the urge to find foundations is easy to understand. To extend the earlier metaphors, in the shifting sands of psychiatric policy, practice, and research, the desire for a 'rock, an anchor, a starting point' is entirely natural. In the absence of such foundations it seems we are exposed to the idiosyncratic vagaries of epistemological and ethical relativism.

And yet, and yet … the repeated lesson of history is that many of the worst abuses of psychiatry have arisen not from relativism but from absolutism, not, that is to say, from a *laissez faire* 'anything goes' approach either in science or in ethics, but from the convictions of this or that individual or school that 'they', and only they, had 'got it right'. In our work in Oxford, for example, with the Russian psychiatrist Alex Smirnoff, Elena Snow and I (Fulford et al. 1993) showed how the notorious political abuses of psychiatry in the former Soviet Union, although amplified by systemic (legislative

[2] 'Cogito', 'I think', from which Descartes concluded 'ergo sum', 'therefore I am'. The cogito comes in Descartes' 'Discourse on Method', a methodological preface to a mainly scientific work; and the argument of the cogito is repeated (though not in quite the same words) in his later more explicitly foundational philosophical treatise, 'Meditations on First Philosophy'. Descartes took the cogito to be clearly indubitable and, hence, genuinely foundational: and 'cogito' at least, does seem to be self-verifying, i.e. to doubt that 'I think' is to have the thought 'I doubt that I think' which is itself an instance of 'I think'. But as is the way with any good philosophical (or indeed scientific) idea, far from being accepted as indubitable, the cogito generated right from the start a whole series of critiques from which many of the key questions of philosophy relevant to psychiatry and neuroscience today are ultimately derived. Such questions include, the nature of personal identity, the relationship between first and second hand knowledge of mental states, and, not least, the mind-body problem in its many aspects (including ongoing work on meanings and causes, see Hoerl, Chapter 8, this volume). Importantly, these are all areas where as well as psychiatry having much to learn from philosophy, so too does philosophy have much to learn from psychiatry: 'thought insertion' alone for example, arguably a prima facie challenge to the cogito, has generated a huge philosophical literature in recent decades. The impact of Descartes' cogito is thus with us still in the dynamic two-way 'trade' that has emerged as such a key feature of contemporary philosophy of psychiatry. (For more on this, see part V, 'Philosophy of Mind and Mental Health', in Fulford et al.'s (2006) *Oxford Textbook of Philosophy and Psychiatry*.)

and administrative) failings, were made possible in the first place by the dominance of a schizophrenia-as-just-brain-pathology disease model masking the social value judgements governing local criteria of rationality. The German historian and psychiatrist Paul Hoff (2005), has shown, similarly, how the history of psychiatric science is a history of serial collapses into 'single message mythologies'. Nor are the 'abuses of absolutism' confined to psychiatry. The Oxford philosopher, Jonathan Glover, has charted a similar history in his compendious overview of the moral history of the twentieth century: titled *Humanity* (1999), Glover's book shows how man's repeated inhumanity to man over this period was driven by this or that group's (initially at least) well-intentioned determination to impose their convictions of 'the good' on others, literally at any cost.

A natural response to the failure of foundationalism is to blame the foundations in question, to say 'sure, those chaps got it wrong, they had the wrong foundations; but in seeking foundations in the first place they had the right idea—so give us one more go then, and this time we'll get it right!'. This response however runs slap up against the second reason, the theoretical reason, why foundations are not all they are cracked up to be, namely that foundations in mathematics and science at least, are simply not to be had.

Gödel's hurdle

It will be worth looking at this second reason in a little more detail since it takes us to the heart of what modern philosophy and with it modern philosophy of psychiatry is all about. A key strand of the story runs through Bertrand Russell, one of Jaspers' philosophical foundationalist contemporaries noted earlier. Russell you will recall was seeking secure foundations for mathematics in logic. As a young philosopher working in Cambridge he had done ground-breaking research which overturned nineteenth-century work on the foundations of mathematics notably by the German logician and mathematician Gottlob Frege's reduction of numbers to set theory. Believing that in overturning Frege he had finally secured mathematics in logic, Russell went on as previously described to publish his *Principia Mathematica*. Yet within a mere two decades of this supposed mathematical 'principia', Russell's work had in turn been overturned by the next new kid on the block, the Austrian logician, Kurt Gödel. Gödel, however, who was in his mid-twenties at the time, took the game to a whole new level. For what Gödel proved was not merely that Russell had failed to secure the foundations of mathematics but that no such foundations were possible *even in principle*.

Gödel's demonstration of what might be called radical uncertainty is arguably our most valuable philosophical legacy from the twentieth century. Other perhaps better known philosophers argued to similar anti-foundationalist conclusions: perhaps most famous is the Cambridge-based Austrian philosopher, Ludwig Wittgenstein's work in linguistic philosophy (notably in his 1953 *Philosophical Investigations*); not far behind in fame but a little later in the twentieth century is the American philosopher, Willard Van Orman Quine, whose undermining of the traditional analytic-synthetic distinction (in among other publications his *Two Dogmas of Empiricism* (1951)) contributed to the final demise of the foundationalist project of logical positivism; least celebrated but directly underpinning recent practical products from the philosophy of psychiatry (see later) were continuing mid-century debates within the Oxford School of linguistic analytic philosophy about the naturalist foundations for ethics (of which Moore in his *Principia* believed he had finally disposed).[3]

What Gödel showed, however, was both simpler and more decisive. Gödel showed that any mathematical system sufficiently complex to allow just the basic procedures of addition, subtraction, multiplication, and division, must contain within itself statements the truth or falsehood of which can be determined only by drawing on the resources of a more complex mathematical system—such statements are thus said to be 'undecidable': but the problem with drawing on the resources of a more complex system is of course that that more complex system will contain undecidable statements of its own; and so on ad infinitum. So mathematics is incompletable: in this formal sense it cannot be put on secure foundations because there are no foundations to be had; and if mathematics then science as in the physical (maths-based) sciences; and if science then (likely as not) knowledge as a whole.

Against foundations

One important role of philosophy in psychiatry therefore, given the failure of foundationalism, is to help us resist premature closure on the complex problems at the heart of our so difficult field. J.L. Austin, one of those mid-century Oxford philosophers from whom as I have suggested elsewhere (1990) psychiatry has much to learn, talked of philosophy as working at the edge of understanding. So too then, as Tim Thornton, George Graham, and I argued in the first chapter of the *Oxford Textbook of Philosophy and Psychiatry* (2006), does psychiatry. This is one reason why in psychiatry perhaps more so even than in other scientific and medical disciplines, there is such a strong perceived need for 'foundations'. Our field is just *so* complex, ethically and scientifically, that the offer of 'a rock, an anchor, a starting point' is all too seductive. Remember though, *cave* foundations. As the American humorist, H.L. Mencken, so neatly put it, 'For every complex problem, there is a solution that is simple, neat, and wrong'.[4]

Avoiding premature closure is important clinically if the historical evidence of the sources of abuses in psychiatry noted earlier is to be believed. Here, as I describe further later, modern philosophy of psychiatry has already gone beyond *General Psychopathology* to particular psychopathologies as represented by developments in values-based practice. There are indications too that avoiding premature closure could be important scientifically. The editors of the American Psychiatric Association's *Research Agenda for DSM-V*, disappointed by the apparent lack of progress towards neuroscientific understanding of mental disorders in the (mere) two decades since DSM-IV, came close to calling for psychiatry to be ready to

---

3 For a clear and still helpful introduction to these issues, see the Oxford philosopher Geoffrey Warnock's (1967) *Contemporary Moral Philosophy*: illustrative of more recent work exploring the logical relationships between description and evaluation is the American philosopher Hilary Putnam's collection of essays, *The Collapse of the Fact-Value Dichotomy and Other Essays* (2002).

4 Although usually thus quoted, Wikipedia gives the original wording as: 'There is always an easy solution to every human problem—neat, plausible, and wrong'. It attributes this version of Mencken's apt witticism to his essay 'The Divine Afflatus', published in 1917.

trade reliability (the nearest we have to a basis in observation) for validity.[5] But we owe our current descriptive (i.e. observation-based) classifications to logical positivism (through the philosopher Carl Hempel[6]); small wonder therefore that since logical positivism itself failed as a way of characterizing observational science, our classifications also should turn out not to be the last word in psychiatric science. *Cave* then, indeed, foundations: for the right response to the failure of logical positivism in psychiatric classification is not to give up, to fall as it were on our observational-scientific swords. The right response is rather to turn to the successors of logical positivism for a more nuanced understanding of the nature of observational science in general and hence of psychiatric science in particular.

For progress

Giving up on foundations then, does not mean giving up on progress in philosophy. Far from it: Gödel's hurdle is best understood not as a barrier but rather as a gateway to progress. Just how philosophy as a whole has progressed in the second half of the twentieth century is beyond my scope here. But in one area at least, in the philosophy of psychiatry, progress there has been: this book you will recall is no less than the fortieth volume in the IPPP series; and the series itself is only one among a growing range of book series and journals across an increasingly diverse range of language groups.

Where we go from here only time will tell. But in the introduction to what will be the forty-first volume in the IPPP series, the *Oxford Handbook of Philosophy and Psychiatry* (in press), my editorial colleagues and I suggested five 'conditions for flourishing', 4 Ps and a Q, i.e. five conditions that we believe modern philosophy of psychiatry must satisfy if it is to continue to flourish rather than with Jaspers falling back into another 50 years of silence. Briefly, our 4 Ps and a Q were:

1. *P for particular problems*—that philosophy and psychiatry should proceed by way of disciplined attention to particular well-defined problems rather than general theory building (including foundational theory building).
2. *P for product orientation*—that we should work with practical products (for policy, training, clinical work, or empirical research) firmly in mind but, and this is an important but, always responsibly so: being 'responsibly product oriented' means practitioners and philosophers being prepared to put in the work necessary to go sufficiently deep in each others' disciplines that neither scientific nor philosophical standards of rigour become compromised by the pressures of practical necessity (however urgent these may seem at the time).
3. *P for partnership*—that as an aspect of being responsibly product oriented we should work always in partnership of one kind or another: partnerships thus might include

5 In their Introduction the editors of the Research Agenda rightly remind us that the 'major advantage of adopting a descriptive classification [is] improved reliability'; but they go on to claim that 'the primary strength of a descriptive approach [is] its ability to improve communication among clinicians and researchers, *not its established validity*' (both quotes, Kupfer et al. 2002: xviii, emphasis added).

6 Importantly, Hempel's insight was refracted through the clinical 'lens' provided at the time by Aubrey Lewis and Norman Sartorius (Fulford and Sartorius, 2009): this is an early example of the importance of partnership in the philosophy of psychiatry—see later discussion.

doubly qualified individuals (like Jaspers), different combinations of clinician/researcher-philosopher pairings, team-working of various kinds, incorporating patients and carers as experts by experience as well as clinicians and researchers as experts by training.

4. *P for process*—that we remain attentive to and reflect always on the difficult issues of process raised by cross-disciplinary research which, while being based firmly on independent peer review, should leave scope always for the occasional exceptional individual or group to cut against the grain of the crowd.
5. *Q for college*—that the field should continue to develop as a distributed collegial enterprise showing the right balance of Q: recent sociological work has shown that creative individuals tend to emerge only within groups showing the right (Q) balance of internal checks-and-balances (as through peer review) and external openness to the continued fertilization of new ideas.

We can see something of the operation of these conditions for flourishing in the contrast between the creatively high-output young Jaspers, culminating in his *annus mirabilis* of 1913, and his subsequent 50 years of silence. The young Jaspers had a particular problem in mind in writing *General Psychopathology*, the growing scientism of the neuroscientifically-informed psychiatry of his day—'quite fantastic', he called some of his contemporaries' scientistic aspirations to an aetiological psychiatric 'theory of everything'[7]; the later Jaspers however never got beyond philosophical foundationalism as a response to this problem. The young Jaspers in tackling the problem of scientism in psychiatry was responsibly product oriented—although trained as a clinician (who had also done empirical research in the neurosciences) he had 'gone deep' also in philosophy; the later Jaspers by contrast became 'just' a philosopher. For similar reasons, where the doubly-qualified young Jaspers embodied the principle of partnership between philosophy and psychiatry, the later Jaspers became a sole trader philosopher. As to process, where the young Jaspers cut to an extent at least against the grain of his (biologically-minded) psychiatric peers, the later Jaspers, by now a distinguished professor of philosophy in his own right, cut largely with the grain of his new philosophical peers.

Importantly, at neither stage in his life did Jaspers have the support of a collegiate Q group. As the fifth of our conditions for flourishing, therefore, Jaspers' lack of a creative community is perhaps the key to why he fell silent. And how differently by contrast are we placed today. Avoiding as it has the factionalism to which so many of the new intellectual movements of the twentieth century fell prey, modern philosophy of psychiatry has developed throughout as a strongly collegial discipline, always jealous of academic standards yet at the same time open and inclusive of the many different traditions of thought and practice by which philosophy and psychiatry are alike made up. The result, as this book so richly illustrates, has been a vigorously expanding international discipline distributed across a range of stakeholders including not only philosophers, clinicians, and researchers, but also and importantly, patients, carers, managers, and policymakers.

---

[7] See page 18 in the 1997 Johns Hopkins University Press edition of Hoenig and Hamilton's original 1963 translation of *General Psychopathology*.

Progress indeed then there has been at least in psychiatric theory. But there has been progress too in psychiatric practice. The development of values-based practice is a case in point. As its name implies, values-based practice is like evidence-based practice in supporting clinical decision-making in the increasingly complex environment of contemporary healthcare: evidence-based practice offers tools for working with complex and (in part) conflicting evidence; values-based practice correspondingly offers tools for working with complex and (in part) conflicting values.[8]

To see it now you might be forgiven for failing to recognize that values-based practice has philosophical origins. Based as it is primarily on learnable clinical skills, values-based practice provides a process for coming to balanced clinical decisions on individual cases within frameworks of shared values. Just another tool for the clinical tool kit then, you might think. And to this point you would be right. Values-based practice is indeed just another tool in the clinical tool kit: and the practice of values-based practice no more requires a knowledge of philosophy than the practice of prescribing requires a knowledge of pharmacology.[9] But values-based practice, nonetheless, is a direct product of progress by way of modest increments in understanding in philosophy: mid-twentieth-century Oxford analytic philosophy produced a number of modest increments in understanding of the language we use to talk about values (see, e.g. R.M. Hare's *The Language of Morals* (1952)); these modest increments in understanding the language of values in turn generated modest increments in understanding the language of medicine (as in my *Moral Theory and Medical Practice* (1989)); and it is these modest increments in understanding the language of medicine which have latterly been cashed out in the policy, service development, and training initiatives of values-based practice (Fulford and van Staden, in press, 2013).

And there is more. For values-based practice although developed first in mental health is now being extended to other areas of healthcare.[10] This is essentially because as a partner to evidence-based practice in clinical decision-making, values-based practice links generalized scientific knowledge (the evidence) with the unique values (the needs, wishes, etc.) of individual people. The need for linking science with people by way of values was evident to the pioneers of evidence-based practice.[11] This need is increasingly apparent across medicine as a whole as advances in science and technology open up an ever wider range of individual choices (and hence diversity of individual values) in medicine. And it is psychiatry, with the development of the philosophy-into-practice tool kit of values-based practice that is supplying that need. There is thus a neat reversal here of the psychiatry-second stereotype of

---

8 For more information on values-based practice see the VBP website jointly hosted by Warwick University Medical School and Cambridge University Press at: <http://www.Go.warwick.ac.uk/values-basedpractice> or via<http://www2.warwick.ac.uk/fac/med/study/research/vbp>.

9 No more but also of course no less—practice in all areas is informed and strengthened by a knowledge of underlying theory.

10 See, for example, a series of clinical case studies covering a wide range of situations in different areas of clinical medicine in Fulford et al. (2012). This book is the first in a new book series from Cambridge University Press on Values-based Practice in medicine. Again, the VBP website (see footnote 8) gives additional information.

11 Thus David Sackett, in his training manual for evidence-based practice, actually defines evidence-based medicine as combining best research evidence with clinical experience and patients' values (Sackett et al. 2000: 1).

twentieth-century medicine. In being first in the field with values-based practice, psychiatry has taken poll position in the development of a medicine for the twenty-first century that is equally science-based and person-centred. Progress indeed, then, and progress that in this instance at least, is philosophy driven.

No country for old men

In falling into 50 years of silence, Jaspers was in part a child of his times as no doubt are we all. In 1913 he could not have foreseen the abuses, locally within psychiatry and on the wider moral and political front, to which foundationalism would lead in the twentieth century; nor of course could he have anticipated the radical uncertainties to be discovered by Gödel and others in science and mathematics. The year 1913 moreover, the year of *General Psychopathology*, was also the year in which as the Australian poet and psychiatrist Russell Meares (2003) has graphically illustrated through art works of the period, the zeitgeist of European culture as a whole shifted from meaning to mechanism. Small wonder then that Jaspers, caught between an increasingly reductionist medical psychiatry and the mechanistic models of Freudian psychoanalysis, found himself Q-less and with nowhere to hide but in philosophy.

This is easy to see now with the benefit of twenty-twenty hindsight from the perspective of 2013. Our own successors, no doubt, will look back critically from the perspective of 2113 on contemporary philosophy of psychiatry. We should, nonetheless, I believe, read Jaspers today, 100 years on, as much for what we can learn from his limitations as from his strengths. This is what this book helps us to do. Yes, there is much to learn from Jaspers' attempt to put the neuroscientifically-informed psychiatry of his day on firmer intellectual foundations: his insistence in particular on the need for meanings as well as causes in psychopathology is as relevant now as it was then, arguably more so with the contemporary rise in importance of the patient's voice.[12] But where Jaspers became subordinate to the academic norms of his philosophical peers this book pushes at the boundaries of psychiatric thought and practice; where Jaspers lost touch with his scientific and clinical roots this book seeks throughout responsibly to get the science right; where Jaspers gave up on partnership and became (just) a philosopher this book illustrates the diversity of partnerships by which modern philosophy of psychiatry is characterized; and where Jaspers' ambitions for a foundationalist *general* psychopathology failed, this book's focus on particular psychopathologies promises the modest increments in understanding from which, with progress of the kind illustrated by values-based practice, psychiatry may yet emerge as a lead discipline in rising to the challenges of twenty-first-century medicine as a whole.

In the library on the top floor of the University Department of Psychiatry in Heidelberg there is a small but full-length photograph of Jaspers in his late twenties.[13] The alert young man who looks out at us from this picture, framed by the library book shelves, lean, sharp, heads-up, is a long way from the venerable benign of later more familiar images. But this is the Jaspers who wrote *General Psychopathology*. This is the Jaspers by whom the modern movement in philosophy of psychiatry is inspired. This is the Jaspers who is rightly celebrated by this wonderful book.

---

[12] Anticipated by a relatively neglected passage in *General Psychopathology*—see Stanghellini et al. (2013).

[13] Reproduced with grateful acknowledgement to Professor Christoph Mundt and Dr Peter Schoenknecht in the opening chapter of the launch volume of the IPPP series (Fulford et al. 2003: 3)

References

Andreasen, N.C. (2001). *Brave New Brain: Conquering Mental Illness in the Era of the Genome.* Oxford: Oxford University Press.

Fulford, K.W.M. (1989). *Moral Theory and Medical Practice.* Cambridge: Cambridge University Press. (Reprinted 1995 and 1999.)

Fulford, K.W.M. (1990). 'Philosophy and Medicine: The Oxford Connection', *British Journal of Psychiatry*, **157**: 111–115.

Fulford, K.W.M., Davies, M., Gipps, R., Graham, G., Sadler, J., Stanghellini, G., Thornton, T. (in press). 'The Next Hundred Years: Watching our Ps and Q,' in Fulford, K.W.M., Davies, M., Gipps, R., Graham, G., Sadler, J., Stanghellini, G., Thornton, T. (eds), *The Oxford Handbook of Philosophy and Psychiatry*. Oxford: Oxford University Press.

Fulford, K.W.M., Morris, K.J., Sadler, J.Z., Stanghellini, G. (2003). 'Past Improbable, Future Possible: The Renaissance in Philosophy and Psychiatry', in K.W.M. Fulford, K.J. Morris, J.Z. Sadler, G.Stanghellini (eds), *Nature and Narrative: An Introduction to the New Philosophy of Psychiatry.* Oxford: Oxford University Press, 1–41.

Fulford, K.W.M., Peile, E.P., Carroll, H. (2012). *Essential Values-based Practice: Clinical Stories Linking Science with People.* Cambridge: Cambridge University Press.

Fulford, K.W.M., Sartorius, N. (2009). 'A Secret History of ICD and the Hidden Future of DSM', in M. Broome, L. Bortolotti (eds), *Psychiatry as Cognitive Neuroscience: Philosophical Perspectives.* Oxford: Oxford University Press, 29–48.

Fulford, K.W.M., Smirnov, A.Y.U., Snow, E. (1993). 'Concepts of Disease and the Abuse of Psychiatry in the USSR', *British Journal of Psychiatry*, 162: 801–810.

Fulford, K.W.M., Thornton, T., Graham, G. (2006). 'Progress in Five Parts', in K.W.M. Fulford, T. Thornton, G. Graham (eds), *The Oxford Textbook of Philosophy and Psychiatry*. Oxford: Oxford University Press, pp. xxxv–xxxvii.

Fulford, K.W.M., van Staden, W., (in press, 2013) chapter 26, pp 385–412 in Fulford, K.W.M., Davies, M., Gipps, R., Graham, G., Sadler, J., Stanghellini, G., and Thornton, T. (eds). The Oxford Handbook of Philosophy and Psychiatry. Oxford: Oxford University Press.

Glover, J. (1999). *Humanity: A Moral History of the Twentieth Century*. London: Jonathan Cape. (Reprinted in 2001, London: Pimlico.)

Hare, R.M. (1952). *The Language of Morals*. Oxford: Oxford University Press.

Hoff, P. (2005). 'Die psychopathologische Perspektive', in M. Bormuth, U. Wiesing (eds), *Ethische Aspekte der Forschung in Psychiatrie und Psychotherapie*. Cologne: Deutscher Aerzte-Verlag, 71–79.

Jaspers, K. (1912). The Phenomenological Approach in Psychopathology. *Zeitschrift fur die Gesamte Neurologie und Psychiatrie*, **9**, 391–408. Published in translation, (1968) (on the initiative of J. N. Curran), *British Journal of Psychiatry*, 114, 1313–1323.

Jaspers, K. (1913a). *Allgemeine Psychopathologie* (1st edn). Berlin, Springer-Verlag.

Jaspers, K. (1913b). 'Causal and Meaningful Connexions Between Life History and Psychosis', reprinted in S.R. Hirsch, M. Shepherd (eds) (1974). *Themes and Variations in European Psychiatry*. Bristol: John Wright and Sons Ltd, 80–93.

Jaspers, K. (1963). *General Psychopathology* (7th edn) (J. Hoenig, M.W. Hamilton, trans.). Chicago, IL: University of Chicago Press.

Jaspers, K. (1997). *General Psychopathology* (7th edn) (J. Hoenig, M.W. Hamilton, trans.). Baltimore, MD: Johns Hopkins University Press.

Kirkbright, S. (2004). *Karl Jaspers, a Biography: Navigations in Truth*. New Haven, CT: Yale University Press

Kupfer, D.J., First, M.B., Regier, D.E. (2002). 'Introduction,' in D.J. Kupfer, M.B., First, D.E. Regier (eds), *A Research Agenda for DSM-V*. Washington, DC: American Psychiatric Association, xv–xxiii.

Meares, R. (2003). 'Towards a Psyche for Psychiatry', in K.W.M. Fulford, K.J. Morris, J.Z. Sadler, G. Stanghellini (eds.) *Nature and Narrative: An Introduction to the New Philosophy of Psychiatry*. Oxford: Oxford University Press, 43–56.

Moore, G.E. (1980). *Principia Ethica*. Cambridge: Cambridge University Press.

Putnam, H. (2002). *The Collapse of the Fact/Value Dichotomy and other Essays*. Cambridge, MA: Harvard University Press.

Quine, W.V.O. (1951). 'Two Dogmas of Empiricism', *Philosophical Review*, **60**(1): 20–43.

Sackett, D.L. Straus, S.E., Scott Richardson, W., Rosenberg, W., Haynes, R.B. (2000). *Evidence-Based Medicine: How to Practice and Teach EBM* (2nd edn). Edinburgh: Churchill Livingstone.

Stanghellini, G., Bolton, D., Fulford, K.W.M. (2013). 'Resources for a Person centred Psychopathology of Schizophrenia: Building on Karl Jaspers' Understanding of the Patient's Attitude Towards His Illness', *Schizophrenia Bulletin,* **39**(2): 287–294.

Warnock, G.J. (1967). *Contemporary Moral Philosophy*. London: The Macmillan Press Ltd.

Whitehead, A.N., Russell, B. (1910/1912/1913). *Principia Mathematica*, 3 vols, Cambridge: Cambridge University Press. (2nd edn, 1925 (Vol. 1) 1927 (Vols 2, 3).)

Wittgenstein, L. (1953). *Philosophical Investigations*. Oxford: Blackwell.

Section 1

Historical and cultural background

Chapter 1

Jaspers in his time

Federico Leoni

Jaspers and Goethe

The origins of things are rudimentary, as Giambattista Vico one of the founding fathers of modern historicism used to write. Only over time do things get refined and acquire their own distinctive traits. What initially prevails is cross-breedness, mixture, heterogeneity. To talk about Karl Jaspers in his time, then, amounts primarily to discussing the breeding ground in which the young psychiatrist progressively moulds himself, the manifold cultural influences that reciprocally overlap in his first writings.

At the time, Jaspers has not yet become the author of either the *Allgemneine Psychopathologie*, or the *Psychologie der Weltanschauungen*, or the monumental *Philosophie*. He is the ideal pupil of Wilhelm Dilthey, the passionate reader of Max Weber, the *connoisseur* of Georg Simmel's essays. The philosophical climate in which Jaspers shapes himself is that of German historicism, and the spiritual atmosphere he encounters is that of the *Lebensphilosophie*. 'Life' is the concept in which we find, in a nutshell, the key themes of a debate which is not only methodological and not even philosophical. Life is a unity, a form of becoming, a variation around a theme or a set of themes. It is a search which proves always imperfect inasmuch it is never warranted a priori, a path exposed to the risk of misdirection because of its being disentwined from a programme, because of its being devoted to the unceasing creation of its own forms.

To some extent, all this means that the age in which Jaspers forms himself is that of the great, fecund Goethian decline. Simmel is a great Goethian thinker, and the whole philosophy of life, the one championed by Dilthey as well as the one indirectly developed by Weber, cannot be understood if not within this symbolic and conceptual context, dominated by the themes of unity and the transformation of the living being. When the young Jaspers drops his juridical studies so as to devote himself to medical science, it is the idea of getting committed to an understanding of 'nature' in its concreteness that guides him. And the 'nature' Jaspers refers to, at the time, is not certainly Newton's or Descartes' nature. It is rather the nature expressed in the *Metamorphosen der Pflanzen* or in the *Farbenlehre*.

Only very slowly, over time, will such vitalistic suggestions turn into existential themes, so bringing to light a vein which is probably more personal, more audacious in expressing that frailty and melancholy which the young Jaspers had partially concealed in the majestic, systematic, almost triumphal construction of the *Allgemeine Psychopathologie*. Then, his Kierkegaardian soul will erupt, with all his sensitivity for the failure that lies in ambush in any faltering path, for the amorphous, baleful speckledness lurking into the magnificent becoming of forms and of sense. The leading theme of life will be displaced by the 'existence' theme, the adventure of 'living' will be displaced by the hazard of an 'existing' which is always and structurally situated 'outside itself', necessarily fashioned by the encounter with its own limits and by its being placed 'at the margins of itself'. Jaspers will get even with his juvenile Diltheyan formational background, and will develop himself, alongside Heidegger, as one of the great figures of the twentieth-century existentialism. The wide effects of the war will reverberate on Jaspers' scheme, the *Allgemeine Psychopathologie* will be far behind, and even the project, still Diltheyan, of the *Psychologie der Weltanschauungen.*

Jaspers and Kraepelin

The exordium of the young psychiatrist is tied, as it is well known, to a series of cases encountered in the Heidelberg clinic, alongside those found in the psychiatric literature of the time. Jaspers (1990b: 1-84), writes about young women, forced away from their countryside life and compelled to work in towns, at the service of rich and complicated bourgeois families; women worn out by the encounter with that hectic and undecipherable world that Simmel set out to describe in momentous texts like *Metropolis und Geistesleben*, in the outstanding *Philosophie des Geldes*, in the sharp pages on fashion. A world which Simmel describes as the source of any modern neurosis, or, better stated, as the condition which makes every modern life properly 'modern'—that is, unstable, contradictory, spasmodic, and, in a word, essentially neurotic.

Psychosis, however, is what overthrows the existence of those female patients whom Jaspers meets and describes. Women who, at a certain stage, commit those actions which Jaspers calls 'crimes of nostalgia'. They kill the sons of the families in whose service they work. They end up in psychiatric clinics. They are deemed foolish, but what matters to Jaspers is not this judgemental sentence: it is not the diagnosis, the taxonomy, the inscription into one of the codified spaces of current nosography. It is rather their story, their provenance context, the clash with an alien environment, the experience of an unknown solitude, the tragic and violent way out experienced by whoever sees herself trapped in a dead-end street. We find again all the inspiring ideas of the first Jaspersian formation: the sociological sensibility, fed on Weber alongside Simmel; the attention for the story of a singular life, in which we find recapitulated the tensions of a whole era and the 'constants of sense' of a biographical adventure, understood in terms of the Diltheyan reflections on biography as a literary genre and as a litmus test for the historiographical work; the upsurge of experiences from one another, in accordance with the 'nexus of sense' which the *Allgemeine Psychopathologie* will describe by stating that the psychical raises out of the psychical, so disagreeing with the mainstream psychiatry, which endeavoured to derive symptoms from a set of organic causes.

We are confronted, in this case, with an essential point of contact which represents, all the same, also a point of divergence, with the figure of Emil Kraepelin, who in Heidelberg had premised his psychiatric practice upon a fresh attention for the patients' life-stories, still without ever disjoining it from the idea that a physician should, at the last resort, mainly classify symptoms and syndromes, instead of giving priority to the reconstruction of the meanings of a gesture or the overall sense of a biography. Jaspers has not acquired a method of his own yet, but, at the same time, he is drenched in the atmosphere of what at the time was targeted as the *Methodenstreit*, the 'conflict on methods', whose core lay in the contraposition between the champions of *Naturwissenschaften*, the sciences of nature, and the supporters of the *Geisteswissenschaften*, the sciences of spirit (or mind, or culture ...). It is clear to him that psychiatry, as well as, more generally, medical science, are sciences of complexity, that is, sciences which address composite and multi-faceted realities, realities that lend themselves to different, complementary outlooks. None of these outlooks exhausts that ultimate, irreducible reality which is—in Diltheyan terms—the individual; none of these outlooks can dispense with one another, given that what is precisely at stake here is not faithfulness to a method, but faithfulness to the 'object' one deals with. And if, in the field of psychiatry, a great organicistic tradition flourished at the time, what was still missing was a systematic and thoughtful endeavour to build up a parallel tradition, oriented to the other side of the human, the one which the *Geisteswissenschaften* had entrusted themselves with the task of describing and understanding. That is the task which Jaspers charges himself with, from the start of his new life as physician and thinker.

Jaspers and Dilthey

The aforementioned tradition, from Binwsanger onwards, has identified its roots in the *Allgemeine Psychopathologie* (1913), in which this first stage of Jaspersian investigations finds a synthesis.

It is well known that, in the *Allgemeine Psychopathologie*, what assumes a central relevance is the distinction, typically and rigorously Diltheyan, between explaining and understanding, *Erklaeren* and *Verstehen*. To explain means to causally explain, by individuating heterogeneous elements in the examined phenomena, by interweaving those elements in a discrete temporal series, by making the ones the cause of others. To explain means, in other terms, to observe from outside, and, just in virtue of this, analytically. To understand, instead, means to understand from within, having direct access to that phenomenon that we 'are', and not simply the one which we 'encounter' outside ourselves; for the very same reason, to understand from within means to understand not through de-composition and re-composition of parts, but according to that unity which is more primeval than the parts into which it is always possible to de-compose the unity itself. It means to rediscover ourselves in the phenomenon, to some extent, and to rediscover the phenomenon in ourselves.

If we get back to the roots of those formulations, it will be easy to reconstruct, in the indications provided by Jaspers himself, the genealogy of that theme which was doomed to great fortune in psychiatry and in the twentieth-century human sciences. In an article entitled 'Kausale und verständliche Zusammenhänge' (1913/1990a: 329–412), Jaspers ascribes a similar distinction between fields to Simmel (whose essay 'Die Probleme der Geschichtsphilosophie' he recalls in the earlier mentioned work) and to Weber (the essay quoted by Jaspers is 'Roscher und Knies und die logische Probleme der historischen Nationaloekonomie'). Notably, if in the first edition of the *Allgemeine Psychopathologie* the indications upon such a genealogy are more generic, in the fourth edition they are made richer and remarkably more articulated. Now Jaspers refers to Droysen, Dilthey, Spranger. Once again, it is outside the sphere of psychiatry that Jaspers tracks down the essential core of the method he is setting up.

But the triad Droysen, Dilthey, Spranger, gets more precisely to the point, particularly in the direction of the reflections of German historians and philosophers of history of the second half of the nineteenth century. This can hardly surprise us. Back to the times of his juvenile work on the crimes committed out of nostalgia, Jaspers chooses to place at the very centre of his concern the patient's life instead of the sum of her symptoms, the nexuses of sense which tie the phases and the events of that life instead of the correspondence between the symptoms present in the patient and the nosographic pictures of nineteenth-century psychopathology. Right from the beginning, Jaspers reflects within the dimension of time, within the domain of becoming. He therefore interrogates himself upon the unity of that becoming, upon its constituting a life which is always, instead of its multifaceted expression, 'one' life, one 'story'. Jaspers is, in this respect, a thinker of the 'continuum'. It is a Diltheyan legacy, besides its being ultimately a Goethian heritage. It is Dilthey himself who thinks that at the beginning there is the continuum, that our experience is first of all a continuity having no caesurae, a 'unity of life', as he writes in the *Einleitung in die Geisteswissenschaften* (1914/1979: 329–412), within which it is always possible, but only at a second and subsequent time, to carve out some 'objects', 'aspects', 'items', trying then to account for their reciprocal ties, and maybe even for their reciprocal causality relationships (Dilthey 1894/1976: 139–140). Psychopathologists of the time, by contrast, expunge from their observational horizon both time and the compound of the nexuses of sense which sustain it diachronically, in order to reflect within the dimension of space, within the order of a pure synchrony, by looking at the simple concomitance of specific events, signs, manifestations. They work by symptoms and syndromes, not in terms of stories and becoming concatenations of meanings.

So, the reason why Jaspers, aiming to refine and systematize this sensitivity of his, addresses historians in particular, appears, once again, more than logical, although by all means audacious on a methodological ground for the young physician he is at the time. It is historians who, in the panorama of nineteenth-century German culture, find themselves faced with a series of 'facts', just like the scientist, although they have to suppose, as 'scientists of spirit', that those facts or events are the outcome not of a clash among blind forces, but of an interaction between actors being endowed with projects, fears, intentions, desires, besides being subjected to all those material, social, economical constraints which every project and every desire must cope with. From Hegel to Dilthey, this is the question to which the historian and the philosopher of history get committed: notably, that of reconstructing 'a story' where an inhabitant of planet Mars might detect a simple compresence of disentangled traces. Were a historian uncommitted to such a task, were he uncommitted to the idea of recollecting 'one' story within the heterogeneous material he finds on the field, he would shirk a crucial task required of his discipline, one which, remarkably, concerns the understanding of a complex game, made by material conditions that, nevertheless, might have been exploited in many different fashions, interpreted in many possible directions; in short, revived within different, but undeniable margins of intentionality by its actors.

What is at stake in this discourse, in other words, is just the scientific nature of the path progressively walked through by the historian and, more generally, by the scientist of spirit. The founding fathers of modern sciences, like Descartes, have expunged any observation that might possibly proceed over and above pure matter, as they carved out the object of their science as nothing but matter, extension, *partes extra partes*. Proceeding 'scientifically', however, does not mean to proceed in any domain of inquiry just as Descartes did. It means, rather, to proceed as required time by time by the peculiar object of one's own science. And the object of the historian presents different requirements from the object studied by the physicist; it demands a specific outlook, it poses problems, and offers solutions all of its own. As Dilthey writes: 'We do not show ourselves genuine disciples of the great scientific thinkers simply by transferring their methods to our sphere; we must adjust our knowledge to the nature of our subject matter and thus treat it as the scientists treated theirs' (Dilthey 1894/1976: 89).

Much more might be said, on the other hand, on properly philosophical, and not simply methodological grounds. It is just because it is never an inhabitant of planet Mars who reads those traces, that the traces themselves are never truly unrelated; by contrast, they suggest, over and over again, possible nexuses and meanings which prove themselves to be more or less plausible depending on the circumstances. In other words, one understands what one has done or might have done at the first person, as Vico was the first to notice in the *Scienza Nuova*. That is the methodological meaning of Vico's saying: *Verum et factum convertuntu*. Dilthey would probably gloss this Vichian claim by observing that, if we understand those men who made history, this happens so simply because we are, as historians, men who in their turn act within history and make history. Whoever understands and whoever gets understood share the same stuff, i.e. one whose plot is textured by sense besides being textured by facts.

Jaspers and Kant

This is an issue which is far more profound and radical than Jaspers (and maybe Dilthey himself) seem to realize when they enounce it. For if one follows the argument through, one might not so much derive the following dualistic stance: being is divided into two regions, that of nature and that of spirit, and each of them requires, if we want to describe it faithfully, that is, scientifically, a peculiar method. Rather, it is a monistic viewpoint that might be drawn from the argument: that is, the view that being is just one; it is the spirit's being, the being of its operations of understanding of the real; and one of the inner specifications and forms of this understanding activity is explanation, i.e. the objectivation of that stuff according to exterior (causal) instead of interior (sense) nexuses. Understanding and explaining are not, in sum, two parallel ways; they respectively constitute a central trunk and a collateral ramification of that trunk.

This is what Dilthey continuously sees and continuously removes out of his sight. He sees it with absolute clarity in his youth: when he declares, in his *Diaries*, that it is not so much a matter of elaborating a 'critique of the historical reason'(this will be the project he will pursue throughout the years of his maturity) as a matter of elaborating a 'historical critique of reason' (as we would say nowadays, a culturalistic, constructivist, hermeneutical or narrativistic critique of human reason in all its expressions, inclusive of its more technical, and, at a face value, less historically affected, expressions, such as the so called hard sciences, and the hardest science of all, mathematics) (Dilthey 1960: 81–83).[1]

In the following years, Dilthey will gradually leave this turn of his discourse to the background, as an unavoidable consequence of the given premises, but also as an implication of his discourse which would not be, after all, too prudent to put under everybody's eyes in the social arena. In one word, while gradually getting into his intellectual path, Dilthey steers more focus to the necessity to carve out, in the context of a fierce positivism, a range field of legitimacy for the rank of the sciences of spirit, than to the more radical possibility

1 See once again his dedication to Yorck von Wartenbug in the *Einleitung in die Geisteswissenschaften* (Dilthey 1914/1979).

of showing that the operation through which the sciences of nature take shape are still and always operations of the spirit. That is to say, to show, as Kant—the ultimate backdrop of all the Diltheyan labour—would have said and as the old Husserl would one day have confirmed in the *Krisis der europaeischen Wissenschaften*, that there are by no means sciences of nature and sciences of spirit: there are only sciences of spirit, which speak about spirit itself either in a direct way (the *Geisteswissenschaften*), or in an indirect, unaware, unwitting way (the *Naturwissenschaften*, nature being for them a mirror, more than an object). In the case at issue, Husserl makes it explicit that the causal nexus is nothing but a reduction of the motivational nexus, of the originally qualitative stuff in which the 'thematic' motives of experience get reciprocally intertwined according to their specific nexuses of sense. Even more expressly, in the *Kritik der reinen Vernunft* Kant states that causality is nothing but one of the categories according to which the intellect reads and reconstructs experience, the latter originally taking place outside the categories, then outside causality. So that in Kant or Husserl nothing lends itself to a psychologistical misunderstanding of the transcendentalist thesis.

In Dilthey's case, it is difficult to establish whether, in his discourse, such a shift, such a bracketing of certain themes in favour of others depends either on a 'strategic' choice (as we already said, that of venturing oneself into the discussion of time through the most efficacious way, even if a less profound one from a philosophical standpoint), or on a gradual eclipse of the properly speculative issue in favour of another kind of reflection (i.e. a merely pragmatical distinction of methodological dimensions, marked by relativistically-oriented and 'pluralistic' outcomes). But for our purposes it might be more interesting to reflect on the underlying speculative problem which a Diltheyan or a Husserlian approach poses. That is, a problem which might ultimately be traced back to a scheme of such a kind. The scientist 'of nature' does not by any means think that his nature sits 'next to' the other nature in which the spirit would consist. He simply thinks that spirit is a piece of nature that has not been not explained yet, that is, one that has not yet been reduced to nature itself. The impressive force of modern science lies—much more than in its methods of verification or experimental falsification—in the properly metaphysical reach of this totally monistic assumption. Symmetrically, at the peak of the phenomenological-hermeneutic tradition, the battle seems to assume the traits not of a compounded dualism or of a tolerant methodological pluralism, but those of a radical monistic claim. Everything is spirit, as Husserl would say in the *Krisis*, or symbolical forms, as Cassirer would say in the *Philosophie der symbolischen Formen*, or cultural construction, Nelson Goodman would say.

With regard to this, one might wonder to what extent the phenomenological-hermeneutic psychiatry has confronted itself with his erupting implication, and to what extent it got satisfied with a 'weak'—*à la Jaspers*—or ambiguous—*à la Dilthey*—declination of the problem, by carving itself a task in the last analysis 'descriptive', and thus barring itself from both the way of the critique of organicism (i.e. an organicism which, as a matter of fact, it frequently leaves totally intact and master of the theoretical situation as well as of the concretely therapeutic one) and the road of an autonomous elaboration of a specific therapeutic approach of its own (which it never comes to think through and elaborate as something more than a mere complement, i.e. one whose relationships with the other side of the therapeutic approach, i.e. the pharmacological, turn out to be often indeterminate and, nevertheless, for unexplained as well as symptomatic reasons, subordinated).

Jaspers and Husserl

The big fight between explaining and understanding outlines the first interpretive line which Jaspers undertakes in the *Allgemeine Psychopathologie*. The core of a second decisive line, strictly intertwined with the first and more apparent, and perhaps more 'ancient' in Jaspers' intellectual biography, is the idea that what is to be understood, rather than to be explained, is an illness and, more precisely, the story of an illness, and the story of a life. But a third interpretive line of the Jaspersian project should be remembered, a third debt held by the *Allgemeine Psychopathologie* towards its own time: on Jaspers' view, what the psychiatrist ought to identify, for each form of psychopathological life described in his work, is just a form, or, as he says, a 'typicality'.

In this case, the debt is twofold, according to what emerges since the time of a juvenile writing like the one Jaspers devotes to the relationship between psychosis and life context, notably by investigating a series of 'typical' connections, that is, connections distinctive and meaningful not simply at the level of their statistical recurrence, but also and especially at the level of their sense and understandability in a Diltheyan sense (Jaspers 1913/1990a: 329–412). A twofold debt, in a philosophical respect towards Husserl's phenomenology, in a sociological respect towards Weber's research.

On Husserl's influences on Jaspers a lot of ink has been shed, starting from those commonplaces in which his name is expressly quoted in the text of the *Allgemeine Psychopathologie* as well as from those utterances of admiration repeatedly addressed by Jaspers to the one who has been, by all means, one of the most influential thinkers of the early, and even the whole, twentieth century. Reference to the 'typicality' in a Husserlian sense is, without doubt, compelling and elucidative in more than one direction. It is well known that for Husserl each experience has a 'typical' course, a series of gaits and developments which carry forward, by varying but also confirming, a certain form, one in which they had found themselves commencing, or better stated, re-commencing, in that unceasing tangle of transformations which is experience in its wholeness. Experience does not make jumps, this is the sentence that Husserl might replace, from his transcendentalistic peak position, to the traditionally naturalistic motto according to which it is nature that does not to make jumps.

If I find myself in a room, I gradually explore it, I turn right, then left, I walk it through, moving toward a window or a writing desk, and what happens is an unceasing renewal of the scene, but also a minute and extremely gradual transformation of what was given at a first time, as it gives itself to my present and in my present time. My experience continues always according to one and the same configuration 'style', Husserl says. It is in part the datum that provides a given theme to my variations, in part the structure that underlies the constitution of experience, to act as guide-theme for those variations which will be the single 'contents' of my experience. To do phenomenology means, in this sense, to train oneself to recognize these typicalities, to pick up what distinctive feature lies in a certain experience or in a certain way of structuring the experience. The perceptive experience has certain typicalities which are not those of either the imaginative or the anamnestic experience. A frightened individual's perceptual experience presents certain typicalities which are not the same as those held by whoever perceives the world in a *Stimmung* of serenity, of love passion, of melancholic abandonment. Every experience has its own typicality, and phenomenology's vocation is that of exploring and classifying its stylistic characters, of targeting the *eidos* of these different contents. And this, from the microcosm of a single individual's perception to the macrocosm of the overall style of a culture or an epoch[2] (Husserl 1950).

The same holds true for the personal experience of a patient who, in her turn, experiences the world according to a certain 'typicality', that is, according to a certain distinctive and recurring modality. It will be the case of the typicality of a patient, related to her illness and life story. And, in other respects, if we broaden our gaze similarly to widening concentric circles, it will be the case of the typicality of a certain psychopathological form of life and of experiencing. A certain kind of delusion will have its own typicality, another typology of delusion will correspondingly have another typicality. And, in the overall sense, a certain general form of existence we can name schizophrenia will have a typicality which the melancholic form of existence will ignore. The Jaspersian gaze is the gaze which aims to set up a unity out of multiplicity, to group the fragments and the innumerable expressions of a psychopathological experience according to certain lines of possible congruence, synchronic and diachronic. In other words, to find within that experience a sort of law, at the same time eidetic and genetic. It is this first juvenile insight, which will come to constitute the project of the *Allgemeine Psychopatologie*, the project, simply stated, of rewriting under the profile of the 'typicality' what was the simple generality and abstractness of the categories of nineteenth-century nosography.

Jaspers and Weber

Still, it cannot be denied that much of the Jaspersian phenomenology is only indirectly and in specific places generically Husserlian.

For instance, we can catch no glimpse of the transcendentalist Husserl, who will exert a very powerful influence on the phenomenological movement after 1913 (the year of *Allgemeine Psychopathologie*), but also the year of that Husserlian monument represented by the first book of the *Ideen zu einer reinen Phänomenologie und phänomenologische Philosophie*, although it announces itself overwhelmingly already in the first decade of the century. Many themes which subsequent history might, in retrospect, induce us to assess as properly Husserlian are in fact Diltheyan themes, and only the neat Husserlian turn that Binswanger will carry out, at the threshold of the 1920s, upon a psychiatry which he will anyhow keep on considering within a Jaspersian framework, will manage to fade away the contours of Jaspers' debt towards the *Lebensphilosophie* by imposing on it the appearance of a thoroughly phenomenological vocation.

With regard to the 'typicality', Max Weber, as much as, or more than Husserl, is the author to which Jaspers seems to have appealed so as to equip himself with the tools required to reconstruct in 'comprehensive' terms the majestic taxonomic and descriptive project which nineteenth-century psychopathology had undertaken. And about German sociology of the beginning of twentieth century, one must repeat what has been said about historians and historicism. Even sociology is an eminently nineteenth-century undertaking, a profoundly positivistic invention, at least in its first big systematic and 'scientific' formulation, i.e. the one worked out by Comte. And even German sociology, at the end of the nineteenth century, can be understood, in many respects, as a response to Comte's sociological positivism. That is, as the attempt to think over and get through the enigma of human sociality, not

[2] Husserl (*Cartesianische Meditationen* (1950)); see in particular the 'Fifth Meditation'.

from the standpoint (in the last analysis Hobbesian) of a physics of the social body, but from that of an interaction between single and collective bodies governed by principles and rules of vital and intentional order.

Nevertheless, it should be pointed out that a decisive implication of Weber's undertaking aims to defend at all costs the possibility, for the sociological outlook, to reach a specific but rigorous objectivity of its own, so staying true to the vocation of each science to draw out of the variety and the mobility of a given observed phenomenon the indication of a line of stability, of a consistency plan that proves univocal and verifiable. This is actually what Weber identifies in his concept of *Idealtypus*, the one to which Jaspers explicitly refers for the first time in his already quoted 'Kausale und verständliche Zusammenhänge', and in a more or less direct but pervasive way in the *Allgemeine Psychopathologie.*[3] From this point of view, Jaspers holds that insight, empathy, immediate understanding are just some of the tools which the psychiatrist finds at their disposal, tools which make available an initial material—the contents of the patient's experience—on which it is possible and actually necessary to subsequently exert a series of operations (confrontations, critical analysis, comparative elaborations) which are the same which the historian or the sociologist perform on the materials they work with (see for instance, Weber's essay on 'Die Objektivität sozialwissenschaftlicher und sozialpolitiker Erkenntnis', recalled by Jaspers in the aforementioned pages).

The insight of the great—Weberian—sociologist establishes a connection with a wide range of phenomena which have to be 'typified', that is, sifted through, by expunging from the picture those items which will be assigned to other forms and other logics, the mixture traces which will point to other pictures and styles of experiencing, accidental and transient elements in relation to the nucleus which in this way the researcher will have both recognized and forged by their own gaze. But this is ultimately what the great clinician must do, and in a certain way has always done in his clinical activity, behind the veil of the 'Cartesian' discourse he holds in the academic arena. The great clinician is not the great biologist, he is not frontally confronted with that universal object called 'life', or with the anonymous process of 'living'. And he is not a physiopathologist, i.e. one who reflects on the universal alterations of that function, in itself universal, which is the physiology of a living being. On the contrary, he is faced with a singularity which he is able to disentwine from the generalizations of scientific knowledge. He undoes the aggregates of symptoms and 'observable' items which the tradition hands over to him as correspondingly empty forms, so as to assemble given symptoms of an old syndrome together with certain observable data pertaining to another syndrome; so as to rediscover in this new constellation that form and, all the same, that content which is the singular event of the experience, or the illness, in which the clinician, etymologically speaking, 're-clines' himself.

Something which was situated at the centre of the field will become marginal, something which used to appear as marginal will now be the core of the phenomenon. The Weberian ideal type is in this respect a Goethian form, a form which is also content, a generalization

3 Among Weber's writings, those which Jaspers takes into account are 'Die Objeltivität sozialwissenschaftlicher und sozialpolitischer Erkenntnis' (now in *Gesammelte Aufsaetze zur Wissenschaftslehre* (1904/1973a)), and 'Roscher und Knies und die logische Probleme der historischen Nationaloekonomie' (also in *Gesammelte Aufsaetze zur Wissenschaftslehre* (1903–1906/1973b)).

which is also in a state of tension with its particularity. The great clinician sees, in one word, something new where the knowledge of his colleagues used to see old things only. He gives his own name to an illness that might coincide with that single patient in which it was found. Or, in other respects, with his own gaze, that is, the gaze proper not to a 'discoverer' but to an 'inventor'. Once again, does not the great sociologist do the same, when he partitions a society according to new ranks and affinities of which the population itself was unaware, or when he recognizes incipient tendency lines, which turn upside down the way in which a collective story was expected to evolve?

Jaspers and Nietzsche

It is not possible to speak about Jaspers in his time without taking issue with the relationship between Jaspers and Nietzsche. Nietzsche is the other seminal backdrop, alongside Goethe, of the *Lebensphilosophie* and the nineteenth-century German hermeneutic seasons. But Nietzsche also stands out as a figure of burning topicality in early twentieth century Germany, an inescapable touchstone for any theoretical undertaking set up in the German land before and after the tragic adventure of Nazism.

The adversaries as much as the supporters of Nazism have ultimately found in Nietzsche the germs of degeneration of the present time as well as the premises and promises of an antidote and a way out. Alfred Baeumler characterizes him as the theorist of a biologizing will to power, a direct instrument of legitimation of any plan of conquest of the *Lebensraum* necessary to the German population. Heidegger, in a series of memorable courses, published as a book at the beginning of the 1960s (*Nietzsche*, 1961), renders him the great thinker of Nihilism and the last great, double-faced Nihilist thinker of the history of Western metaphysics. And Jaspers, who deals with him in different ways and moments of his career, by devoting to him lesson courses, a wide volume of comprehensive reconstruction, and also by drawing inspiration from him with respect to some remarkable reflections on the health-sickness nexus, reflections that will appear for the first time in the second edition of the *Allgemeine Psychopathologie* (1920) and find an ampler and decisive formulation in the fourth (released in 1946: a date even more symptomatical with regard to Jaspers' confrontation with Nietzsche: the war has already ended, the ruins of Nazi Germany are still smoking, Jaspers gave his text licence from his exile in the—Nietzschean—town of Basel).

Already in the pages of the second edition of the *Allgemeine Psychopathologie* (1920) we read that man is a 'sick being' because of his own incompleteness, and that what hands man over to liberty and his peculiar creativity is precisely the same thing which marks his imperfection, his structural incompleteness, his fundamental deficiencies.[4] In the fourth edition, Jaspers deals with the same problem more extensively by observing that human life is inhabited by an inescapable form of 'danger', which is at the same time his creative overture and the constant possibility of failure, of misdirection, of delusion *latu sensu*. And it is by thinking of these relatively belated pages of Jaspers that one might grasp something profoundly Nietzschean in the vision of the *Allgemeine Psychopathologie* or, to put it better, of the anthropology which acts as its backdrop. Jaspers' anthropology is an anthropology of vulnerability, to borrow an expression used by Jakob Wyrsch and happily taken up in more

4 Jaspers (*Allgemeine Psychopathologie*, 2nd edn: 4; *Allgemeine Psychopathologie*, 8th edn: 656–657). On Nietzsche see his posthumous fragments, from 1880 onwards (Nietzsche 1887–1889/1967).

recent times (Stanghellini 1997[5]). And vice versa the focalization of such an inflection in the Nietzschean speech represents the specific feature of Jaspers' Nietzsche, a point of no return in the critical adventure of Nietzsche in the second half of the twentieth century, besides Heidegger's Nietzsche, or Bataille's, or Deleuze's.

To read in the thought of the will to power a thought of impotence or, to use a Pauline formula, the thought of a power which accomplishes itself in impotence, in misdirection, in failure, is in some respects a hermeneutical tour de force, especially at the time in which Jaspers makes it as an absolute forerunner; but in other respects it is an inescapable necessity in the light of the texts themselves. The key issue, naturally, is what one should understand by 'power' (*Wille*) in Nietzsche. If we read the posthumous fragments, from the early 1980s onwards, it is totally clear, in fact, that Nietzsche thinks that, among two beings, 'powerful' is the one who is more open, more capable of assimilating, more prone to encompass whatever is far from and possibly extraneous to him. But this also means that the most powerful is that being who is less able or less inclined to defend and preserve himself, who less can keep himself within the boundaries of his own prudent measure, of his own acquired identity.

If we think that the Nietzsche of these years is a formidable reader of biology, physiology, embryology (the authors that most frequently recur in his fragments about these issues are Roux, Rolph, Haeckel), one might say that, if Nietzsche is trying to outline a physiology of power, this physiology is structurally a physiopathology. *Qua* physiology of a living being, that is, of a being in a state of constant transformation, of a being who is never totally 'given' but continuously 'becomes', instability is the only form of stability which this physiology can get acquainted with. But this 'biological' issue becomes all the more thumping for the profoundly sick man who Nietzsche has been. What does 'to do well' mean, for a living being as for an existing being? What does 'to be in good health' mean? The question on the good can no longer find any answer in a law that cautiously distinguishes the assimilable from the inassimilable, the tolerable from the intolerable. The possibility of a similar law is swept away by acknowledgement that the inassimilable is actually the only object of assimilation, that the intolerable is the only thing that the living being ought to ever tolerate. Those that defend themselves from the new and react to an unexpected event are in fact the 'reactive' characters, the weaker organisms, the men of resentment, as the *Genealogy of Morals* used to call them. A 'powerful' being has, first and foremost, the power of opening himself to what happens to him, to the new, the unexpected, the limits of his own possibilities, the boundaries of his own conditions of survival and preservation.

At the end of the 1880s, Nietzsche hardly tolerates such a conclusion, which, as a matter of fact, is simply Dionysian, that is, Nietzschean in its quintessence. He hardly bears, in other words, the fact that power has to do with de-potentiation and failure. It is an exceedingly Christian thought, for a thinker who intended himself as an antichristian par excellence. A Pauline thought, so to speak. It is in the Second Letter to the Corinthians (2 *Cor.* 12, 9) that Paul writes that 'power accomplishes itself in weakness (*dynamis en astheneia teleitai*)', and notices: 'when I am weak, I am powerful'. On the other hand, Nietzsche cannot recede from this threshold which is by now irrefutable, within the system of his premises and his

[5] To some extent, an effect similar to the one I am identifying in Jaspers will be brought about by Nietzsche's 'anthropology' on thinkers like Helmut Plessner and Arnold Gehlen.

philosophical project. If to assimilate is to assimilate what is not assimilable, the formula of living is the same formula of dying. Health cannot any longer take the shape of 'possession' of a given optimal state, of coincidence of the organism with a certain normalized functioning, of execution of an assured and pre-established programme. To do 'well' means to inhabit the openness, the excess, the wound which warrant the distinctive power of a living being by handing it over every moment to impotence and deviation.

The Kierkegaardian eye of Jaspers will be able to put these Nietzschean insights into profitable use, by turning psychopathology into an anthropology, and this in two main senses. First, his psychopathology would be a psychopathology 'aware' of those philosophical premises which, even if silenced, would anyhow guide the thought of psychiatry, although simply in the fashion of a removed and unconscious instance. Secondly, and more profoundly, the anthropology of the Jaspersian man cannot be anything but an anthropo-pathology. According to a well-known Jaspersian formula, madness is a pathology of liberty, inasmuch as it mortifies freedom itself, locks the subject into a repetition with no variation, in a cage which rewrites any experience according to the modules of anguish and loss, in a grip which forces one to relive the experience which others will have lived in our place, or to think the thoughts that others will have thought and injected into our minds. But madness is the pathology of freedom even in another, more profound acception, precisely a Nietzschean one. It is just because he is free that man is foolish. Man is structurally enfranchised from the repetition of a 'datum', however one may conceive it, either in terms of adaptation to a given environment, execution of a genetic programme, of full-fledged faithfulness to a given original environment. And this is why man finds himself naked when confronted with his own becoming, short of habits and customs, lacking in the mechanisms and automatisms which would preserve him from the risk of the (Kierkegaardian, once again) possible. The necessary is the only guarantee in the vast sea of the possibles, and even more in the vortex of creation of the possibles; and the nudity of madness is, in this way, a figure of the new, the chance of a date without veils with the world and the others.

References

Dilthey, W. (1960). *Der junge Dilthey. Ein Lebensbild in Briefen und Tagebüchern 1852–1870.* Stuttgart-Göttingen: Vanderhoeck und Ruprecht.

Dilthey, W. (1976). 'Ideas for a Descriptive and Analytic Psychology', in H.P. Rickman (ed), *Dilthey, Selected Writings*. Cambridge: Cambridge University Press, 87–97. (Original work published in 1894.)

Dilthey, W. (1979). *Einleitung in die Geisteswissenschaften. Versuch einer Grundlegung für das Studium der Gesellschaft und der Geschichte*. Stuttgart-Göttingen: Vanderhoeck und Ruprecht. (Original work published in 1914.)

Husserl, E. (1950). *Cartesianische Meditationen*. Den Haag: Nijhoff. (Original work published in 1929.)

Jaspers, K. (1913). *Allgemeine Psychopathologie* (1st edn). Berlin: Springer.

Jaspers, K. (1920). *Allgemeine Psychopahologie* (2nd edn). Berlin: Springer.

Jaspers, K. (1946). *Allgemeine Psychopathologie* (4th edn). Berlin: Springer.

Jaspers, K. (1990a). 'Kausale und verständliche Zusammenhänge', in *Gesammelte Schriften zur Psychopathologie*. Berlin: Springer, 329–412. (Original work published in 1913.)

Jaspers , K. (1990b). 'Heimweh und Verbrechen', in *Gesammelte Schriften zur Psychopathologie*. Berlin: Springer, 1–84. (Original work published in 1909.)

Jaspers, K. (1997). *General Psychopathology* (7th edn) (J. Hoenig, M.W. Hamilton, trans.). Baltimore, MD: Johns Hopkins University Press.

Nietzsche, F. (1967). 'Nachgelassene Fragmente', in G. Colli and M. Montinari (eds), *Kritische Studienausgabe*. Berlin: De Gruyter, BD XIII. (Original work published in 1887–1889.)

Stanghellini, G. (1997). *Antropologia della Vulnerabilità*. Milano: Feltrinelli.

Weber, M. (1973a). 'Die "Objektivität" Sozialwissenschaftlicher und Sozialpolitischer Erkenntnis', in J. Winckelmann (ed), *Gesammelte Aufsätze zur Wissenschaftslehre*. Tübingen: Mohr, 146–214. (Original work published in 1904.)

Weber, M. (1973b). 'Roscher und Knies und die Logische Probleme der Historischen Nationalökonomie', in J. Winckelmann (ed), *Gesammelte Aufsätze zur Wissenschaftslehre*. Tübingen: Mohr, 1–145. (Original work published in 1903–1906.)

Chapter 2

Phenomenology and psychopathology: in search of a method

Osborne P. Wiggins and Michael Alan Schwartz

Introduction: towards a method for psychopathology as a science

Karl Jaspers was always occupied with the topic of method. Much of his great *General Psychopathology* is devoted to delineating the various methods that provide access to different aspects of mental disorder (Jaspers 1965, 1997). Jaspers thought it crucial to specify both the proper subject matter of any given method and to demarcate the limits beyond which a method could not legitimately go (Jaspers 1963, 1968). We share Jaspers' concern that the methods for psychopathology be developed and well founded. Hence method in psychopathology is the main focus of this chapter.

Psychopathology is no longer the robust discipline it previously was in the field of psychiatry. By 'psychopathology' we mean the scientific study of abnormal psychological processes. If we take psychopathology in this sense, however, we must recognize that today this discipline has been replaced by lists of the signs and symptoms of mental disorders, such as we find in the *Diagnostic and Statistical Manual of Mental Disorders* (fourth edition, text revision; DSM-IV-TR) published by the American Psychiatric Association (American Psychiatric Association 2000). Psychopathology has been replaced by these lists of syndromes because they are more useful for the practical purpose of uniform diagnosis, both for therapy and research. Utilizing such lists is said to provide a more 'reliable' diagnosis than one based on detailed descriptions of abnormal mental states. And once reliability has been firmly achieved through the progressive perfecting of the lists, psychiatry can move on to seeking 'validity' in diagnosis and eventually even in the specification of underlying causes. We see then that there is a longer-term project guiding the substitution of lists of syndromes for what was previously the thriving discipline of psychopathology. This project has gone by the name of 'the medicalization of psychiatry'. Psychiatry seeks to show that it can progress in basically the same manner that medicine in general has been able to progress in its reliable procedures of diagnosis and its evidence-based research into the aetiologies of diseases. From such progress in medicine, as we know, treatments and therapies have arisen that could hardly have been conceived only half a century ago.

Underlying this substitution is also a 'scepticism' regarding the very possibility of psychopathology as a science. The scepticism consists in the profound doubt that the abnormal mental processes that psychopathology seeks to describe are accessible to a truly scientific cognition. In other words, it is the conviction that abnormal mental states cannot really be studied by scientific methods capable of yielding the intersubjective confirmation of findings and claims. The scepticism, then, is directed towards the scientific status of the method of psychopathology. This essay is devoted to addressing this problem of a scientific method for psychopathology.

In this chapter we shall concern ourselves with psychopathology as a 'pure science'. That is, we shall consider psychopathology as the scientific search for knowledge of abnormal mental states for its own sake. A fully developed pure science of psychopathology could indeed furnish a knowledge base for psychiatry as a practical discipline (McHugh and Slavney 1983). But we shall not restrict the interests of psychopathology to its function in informing the therapeutic and research aims of psychiatry. Psychopathology in our view should be pursued for the sole purpose of understanding a wide variety of psychological phenomena, the ones we now consider 'pathological' phenomena. For this reason it deserves development for its own sake, just as psychology as the pure science of psychological phenomena in general deserves—and is undergoing—development.

We shall follow Edmund Husserl in his characterization of the essential components of a scientific method (Husserl 1973a). We shall adopt some of the central contributions of Karl Jaspers in his depictions of the scientific method of psychopathology (Jaspers 1963, 1965, 1968, 1997). Joining Husserl and Jaspers on the question of psychopathology as a science, however, will require that we supplement what both said with some—we hope, phenomenological—descriptions of our own.

Some phenomenological concepts and the experiencing of other people

Before we launch into the methodological discussion, we must first define and clarify some fundamental phenomenological terms. The first phenomenological concept that requires clarification is that of 'intentionality' (Husserl 1982: 211–307). This term refers to the inseparable correlation between an experiencing mental process and the 'object' that is experienced, the intending process and the intended object. It is crucial to note that in phenomenology the phrase 'intended object' is used in the broadest conceivable sense of 'object'. This is the sense in which anything whatsoever can be an 'object'. For example, a physical thing, another person, a mythological figure (Zeus), an angel, a universe without living beings, a round square, etc., could be an 'object' in the phenomenological sense. In this essay we are concerned with this correlation between the experiencing subject and the world that he or she experiences. Hence when we speak of pathological experiences, we shall also refer to the world that is 'meant' through these experiences, a pathological world.

Martin Heidegger and Maurice Merleau-Ponty capture the reality we wish to depict when they speak of 'being-in-the-world' (Heidegger 2010; Merleau-Ponty 2000). This phrase too denotes the correlation between intending subject and intended object, between experiencing subject and experienced world. For purposes of brevity we may refer to the patient's mental life; but when we do so, we also mean the world as he experiences it as well as his experiences of it.

Now we can employ this concept to emphasize a fundamental standpoint of phenomenological psychopathology: when I am aware of another person, I am to some extent aware of 'what' that person is aware of. When this person speaks to me about his dream of the night before, I am aware of his experiences; but I am also aware of those aspects of the dream about which he speaks. I am aware of 'what' he is intending, the intended object of his mental life. Hence I am aware of the 'intentionality' of his experience. For example, if a patient tells me about a dream in which she was pursued by three menacing, inhuman forces, I am aware of her experience of fear, but I am also aware of the three forces that she experienced. I am aware of her fearful feeling, but I am also aware of the three forces she was fearful of.

Towards a method for psychopathology

As we indicated, the topic of a scientific method for psychopathology shall be addressed here from the perspective of the phenomenology of Edmund Husserl. Issues of scientific method fall for Husserl under the more general title of 'the phenomenology of reason' (Husserl 1973a: 56–64; 1982: 326–349). From this point of view, reason always aims at 'direct evidence', towards the 'self-giving', the 'self-presentation', of the state of affairs one seeks to know. Not every mental process, however, does directly present the state of affairs that it intends. Some mental processes intend objects or aspects of objects that are not directly given. These intendings do intend the 'sense' of their objects but only 'emptily'. For example, we are now aware that the university extends beyond the room in which we are gathered, but those aspects of the university are aspects that we are only emptily intending. Therefore, Husserl distinguishes between evidential and non-evidential awarenesses. And his conception of reason is that it always aims at the evidential intending of the object under investigation even when that object is only emptily intended (Husserl 1973a: 11–17, 56–64; 1982: 326–349). We shall use this Husserlian conception of reason in developing our methodology for psychopathology.

It is now crucial to recognize that ontologically different kinds of objects evidentially present themselves in different ways. For instance, mathematical formulae evidentially present themselves to consciousness in ways very different from the ways in which musical performances present themselves. Likewise, the experiences of other people evidentially present themselves to us in manners quite different from the manners in which gene structures directly present themselves.

Because of these different categories of evidence based on the ontological differences between the kinds of objects in question, there can be no single 'scientific' method. For years a positivistic philosophy of science contended that there was only one genuinely scientific method, and accordingly they sought to require that all disciplines that aspired to be truly scientific adhere to that unitary method. Husserl's stance fundamentally differs from this (Husserl 1982: 171–181). For Husserl, different kinds of objects require different kinds of methods depending on the ways in which those objects evidentially present themselves. In short, there are different scientific methods for different kinds of objects. As Husserl himself expresses this idea:

> A method … is nothing which is or which can be brought in from outside … a determinate method … is a norm which arises from the fundamental regional specificity and the universal structures of the province (of objects) in question, so that knowledge of a method depends essentially on knowledge of these structures. (Husserl 1982: 173)

Jaspers too, of course, underlines the fallacy in positing a single 'method'. As he writes, 'The goal of knowledge in understanding is not to be oriented to the criteria of the natural sciences or to the formal logic of mathematics. Truth in understanding has other criteria' (Jaspers 1965: 299, our translation; 1997: 358–359).

So let us briefly restate Husserl's argument. Scientific methods are paths for gaining evidentially grounded claims about objects. Consequently, these methods depend upon the various ways in which we can secure the direct givenness of the objects under study. Moreover, different kinds of objects evidentially present themselves in different kinds of ways. Accordingly, there must be a plurality of methods, each of which must be geared to obtaining the best evidence for the kind of objects in question.

One important qualification should be added. Because evidences differ, different methods provide 'different degrees of credibility' for the claims made. In other words, with regard to certain kinds of objects much evidence can be obtained while with regard to other kinds of objects less evidence can be secured. As a result, objects of the first kind can be interpreted with a higher degree of believability than can objects of the second kind. Lesser degrees of believability in the claims, however, do not disqualify a method as 'unscientific'. Methods are 'scientific' if they secure access to 'the best evidence available' for the kind of object under study.

The best evidence for psychopathology is in the clinical encounter

One of the first implications of Husserl's view for the methodology for psychopathology is this: descriptions of pathological experiences require a 'direct clinical encounter between the psychopathologist and a patient' in order for those descriptions to have the firmest possible evidential basis. Only with the direct givenness of the patient as he fully relates his experiences in their complex detail, i.e. only in the 'clinical' situation, can the psychopathologist gather the evidence needed for an adequately grounded interpretation of those experiences. In the clinical encounter, psychopathologist and patient can carry on a dialogue in which the psychopathologist can carefully ask questions and otherwise prompt the patient to elaborate on his experiences. Of course, written reports of patients' experiences (especially by patients themselves) can also qualify as evidence in the Husserlian sense. But written reports always point back to the original situation in which they were written or spoken, and this situation is the true basis for any interpretation that utilizes them.

Evidence in the experiencing of other people

In any direct encounter with another person I am 'immediately' aware of the 'entire' person. In phenomenological terms, I intend the 'whole' human being, all of his or her aspects and constituents. It is not the case that I am merely aware of that 'side' of the person that is directly turned towards me and that I must 'infer' that he or she is also having mental experiences and that there are other 'unseen' sides of him or her. No inference or other 'additional' operation must be performed in order to be immediately aware of the whole human being who confronts me.

Although, however, the whole person is intended by me, he is intended with 'inadequate evidence', to use a Husserlian concept (Husserl 1973a: 14–15). The distinction we made earlier regarding the difference between evidential and non-evidential intendings is relevant here. This distinction is always operative in our awareness of other persons. In the intending of other people there are some of their aspects that are 'self-given' to me and some of their aspects that are only 'emptily intended' by me. That is to say, the emptily intended aspects of the other person are intended together with the other aspects (hence I intend the whole person), but the emptily intended aspects are not directly self-given. In Husserlian terms, these other aspects are 'appresented' to my mental life, but they are not directly 'presented' to it. Nevertheless, I am aware of the 'whole' person, some of whose aspects are directly presented and some only appresented.

If we, as phenomenological methodologists, are concerned with specifying the 'evidence' on which claims about a patient are based, we must concentrate on those aspects of other people that are self-given, directly presented, and distinguish these from those aspects that are only emptily intended. Wilhelm Dilthey, in his studies on hermeneutics, has made a distinction that we shall adopt here since we believe it to be phenomenologically well founded. Dilthey places all of these evidentially given aspects of human life into the encompassing category of 'expressions' (*Aüsserungen*). The specific members of this category are facial expressions, bodily gestures, linguistic utterances, and other written, painted, or sculpted symbols. The least ambiguous of these are, of course, linguistic utterances, expressions of language. This point was, of course, also made by Jaspers in several places. Here we quote only one sentence from *General Psychopathology:* '"The understood" attains empirical reality only to the extent that it appears in objective, meaningful facts of expression, action, and works' (Jaspers 1965: 296–297, our translation; 1997: 356).

The indirect givenness of the mental lives of others

However, it is only these expressions, actions, and works of other people that are directly presented, self-given, to us. The mental lives of other people can never be directly presented to us (Jaspers 1968). And correlated with this are the experienced worlds of other people. These worlds can never be directly given to us. In other words, the mental lives of other people as well as the worlds experienced by them can be only 'appresented' to us, never directly presented.

We therefore have arrived at a more complete picture of the methodological problem posed for a phenomenological psychopathology. In order to describe the mental life and the world as experienced by a person suffering from a mental disorder, we realize that the psychopathologist must take into account and make use of the 'expressions, actions, and works' of the mentally ill person to make sense of that person's experiences and experienced world (Jaspers 1968). The patient is intended by the psychopathologist in his entirety: the whole person is intended. However, precisely those aspects of this person that the psychopathologist seeks to know are only emptily intended by her. The patient's mental life and his experienced world can be only 'appresented' to the psychopathologist.

It would be a mistake to assume that what must be done now in order to secure this distinction between the directly presented and the emptily appresented is to 'abstract from' the whole in which the two are co-intended in order to conceptually isolate a 'stratum' of the evidentially presented and disregard for the moment the emptily appresented aspects. It would be a mistake because it is impossible to separate into two different strata the evidentially given and the emptily intended in order to isolate the former from the latter. The directly presented and the emptily appresented play inseparable roles in constituting our awareness of other people. No separation is conceivable without deforming and distorting the sense of the reality of others.

Indirect evidence and hermeneutic interpretation

How then does the psychopathologist attempt to describe the patient's mental life and his experienced world if it is precisely these realities that are not directly given? The psychopathologist must follow the path of indirection, namely, the path of 'hermeneutic interpretation'. Jaspers develops his conception of hermeneutics in the section of *General Psychopathology* entitled 'The Basic Laws of Psychological Understanding and of Meaningfulness' (Jaspers 1997: 355–363). There he states that understanding is 'governed by certain general basic principles' (Jaspers 1997: 355), and he explicates those six principles. It is crucial parts of those principles that we are reformulating here.

The facial expressions, bodily movements, and linguistic utterances—the entire spectrum of 'expressions'—of the patient must be interpreted as evidence 'expressing' his experiences and experienced world (Jaspers 1965). This hermeneutics should be, however, a 'hermeneutics of suspicion', to appropriate Paul Ricoeur's useful phrase (Ricoeur 1970). Ricoeur is concerned with the multiplicity of meanings that can inhabit a seemly singular meaning: Ricoeur is concerned with the multiplicity of meanings that can inhabit a seemly singular meaning. The task of his hermeneutics of suspicion is to penetrate the apparently singular meaning in order to render explicit the underlying multiplicity. In other words, it is necessary to interpret the 'overt' meaning of the patient's expressions in such a way as to unearth the layers of 'covert' experiences that underlie them (Ricoeur 1974). The psychopathologist should penetrate 'behind' or 'inside' what the patient 'explicitly' says in order to try to decipher what he is 'implicitly' intending. This 'suspicious' strategy must be employed for two reasons: (1) the patient may not accurately understand and consequently not be able to accurately report what he is experiencing, and (2) even if the patient accurately understands, he may not be willing to accurately report his experiences; he may seek to dissemble before the psychopathologist. Hence a doubly suspicious attempt must be made to penetrate the strata of meaning here.

Hermeneutic interpretation in need of psychiatric expertise

An accurate interpretation of the patient's mental life is possible, however, only if the interpreter, the psychopathologist, has acquired the expertise of a highly experienced psychiatrist. We shall characterize the basic nature of this psychiatric expertise because it is frequently overlooked when writers discuss issues in psychiatry and psychopathology.

To acquire the expert skills of a psychiatrist one must be enculturated or socialized into the culture of psychiatry. As Harry Collins expresses this idea in *Rethinking Expertise*, 'Acquiring expertise is ... a social process—a matter of socialization into the practices of an expert group—and expertise can be lost if time is spent away from the group' (Collins 2007: 3). Such a social group is composed of many persons who are already familiar with and behave in accordance with the norms, ways of perceiving, thinking, and acting of the group. These ways of perceiving, thinking, and acting constitute the group's culture. In addition, a culture is composed of the literature, meetings, councils, and other ways in which the participants are involved in the group experiences and share information and knowledge.

The culture of psychiatry is actually a 'subculture', i.e. a culture within a larger, more encompassing culture. One of the larger cultures of which psychiatry is a part is, of course, the culture of medical practice. Thus the historically developed knowledge and practice of both psychiatry and medicine constitute parts of the psychopathologist's awareness.

A culture is passed on from generation to generation by preserving and passing on a 'tradition' (Polanyi 1964: 53–54). 'Tradition' is the continuing and changing collective realm of thought and action in which people live and participate. Modern-day traditions are transmitted from generation to generation by a combination of an initially uncritical apprenticeship to teachers and by subsequent critical reflection on the validity of the various constituents of the tradition. An important and even defining feature of modern-day psychiatry, as of other modern scientific and professional fields, is that it is self-critical. Psychiatry is open to questioning, modification, and improvement through appeals to increasing data, research, and practice. As a result, the 'tradition' of psychiatry is not simply passed on from generation to generation but is rather critically revised, corrected, and better grounded. Accordingly, crucial ingredients of the culture of psychiatry are the scholarly journals, academic conferences, research reports, and debates that come forth regularly.

Skills are first developed through examining individual patients while following the explanations of a teacher-mentor, i.e. someone who is already an expert in this area. In order for learning to occur with a mentor the student-novice must attend directly to what the mentor points out in the case under examination. The student must attend in this manner because he or she is striving to 'come to see' what the mentor 'already does see'. Since the student cannot yet interpret the telling characteristics of the patient's condition, he or she must be instructed by a mentor-expert who can already interpret them. Because learning here involves the student coming eventually to directly see these characteristics, it can take place only when the patient is directly given to both student and teacher. Student and mentor must be able to directly attend together to what in the patient the mentor points out although the student cannot yet interpret what the teacher already can (Polanyi 1964: 123–137).

Coming to possess such expert skills involves coming to see several aspects of patients as disclosing a meaningful pattern. These various aspects must come to 'fit together' in such a way as to reveal the overall significance of the whole. Some of the aspects that are so noticed and that contribute to the recognition of the whole are only implicitly noticed. In other words, they are not explicitly apprehended. Although they are only tacitly noted, recognition of the whole would fail without them. Michael Polanyi thus speaks of the 'tacit knowledge' of the scientist: because the items are only implicitly registered in the scientist's mind, he or she is not consciously aware of how they do contribute to recognition of the whole (Polanyi 1964). As Collins says, 'tacit knowledge [is] things you just know how to do without being able to explain the rules for how you do them' (Collins 2007: 13). Similarly Polanyi points to 'the unspecifiability' of our implicit knowledge: we have trouble articulating this knowledge in language (Polanyi 1964: 62–63).

Such tacit learning can occur only by apprenticing oneself to someone who is already an expert, i.e. only by becoming socialized into psychiatric culture. Again Collins expresses the point well, '"Enculturation" is the only way to master an expertise which is deeply laden with tacit knowledge because it is only through common practice with others that the rules that cannot be written down can come to be understood' (Collins 2007: 24).

Expert skills are guided by what Husserl calls 'typifications' (Husserl 1973b: 331–337): ways of seeing something in which the parts of the whole form a recognizable and familiar pattern, a *Gestalt:* one sees the thing as a 'typical' such-and-such. To see something as a 'typical such-and-such' is to see it as embodying a generic type of thing: it is seen as 'another one of those', the 'those' being a generic kind of thing.

Typifications are already operative in our pre-scientific, common-sensical understandings of and dealings with people (Husserl 1973b: 331–337; Wiggins and Schwartz 2004: 480–482). We see the individuals we encounter in the everyday lifeworld as typical kinds of persons, as postmen, policemen, teachers, clerks, bus drivers, etc. In fact such common-sensical typifications inform not only everyday understanding but psychiatric knowledge as well: our understanding of people in the lifeworld continues to inform our understanding of people at more sophisticated, expert levels. However, psychiatrists through the development of increasing expertise also acquire expert ways of typifying their patients. In other words, they develop a subtle array of expert psychiatric typifications that tacitly organize and give meaning to their perception of patients and their behaviours (Schwartz and Wiggins 1987; Wiggins and Schwartz 2004: 480–481).

Explicitly defined psychiatric classifications presuppose such implicit typifying perceptions (Husserl 1973b: 331–337). Explicitly defined features enumerated in classifications are ones that expert psychiatrists can to a significant extent already directly see in what their patients do and say. Because this expert ability to typify patients has been acquired the way expertise is acquired, they constitute a 'personal knowledge'. They are part and parcel of the individual psychiatrist's way of making sense of patients although this knowledge may be difficult—if not impossible—to impart to others who have not undergone the period of training under a mentor which alone is the path to genuine expertise.

Concluding our discussion of the expertise necessary for developing a well-founded psychopathology, we note that expertise connotes 'being fully capable' or 'being able to perform one's task well', at least in a particular area or field. In our sense, then, expertise will mean being fully qualified to exercise the skills we have described. Or, more formally, expertise consists in the skills to perceive and interpret without distortion the realities with which a particular area is concerned. It should be noted that an element of innate talent may also assist the acquisition of expertise. Some people become better experts than others because they simply possess 'natural gifts' in this area. Hence we again return to our basic proposition that psychopathology, even as a 'science', can be developed only if it depends upon and utilizes the vast learning of the clinical psychiatrist.

Reliving the patient's experience

However, more than expertise in discerning the patient's experiences is required if full understanding of these experiences is to be obtained. In order to comprehend adequately the patient's mental life, the psychopathologist must take up the point of view of the patient. In other words, the psychopathologist must seek to empathically put herself in the patient's place and 'relive' (*Nachleben*) the experiences of the patient in which he intends his world. The notion that fully understanding another person requires the re-experiencing (*Nacherleben*) of that person's world is found not only in Dilthey and Jaspers. It also appears at least twice in Husserl's published writings, in *Cartesian Meditations* (Husserl 1973a: 9) and in *Formal and Transcendental Logic* (Husserl 1969: 9–11). From the Husserlian point of view, the requirement of such a self-transposal arises from a demand for evidence. For Husserl, the optimal kind of the evidence of mental life is self-reflection. Self-reflection consists in the phenomenologist directly reflecting on her own ongoing mental experiences and the world intended in those experiences (Husserl 1982: 171–210). That is, self-reflection consists in directly observing the noetic and the noematic poles of one's own mental life. This requirement of best evidence entails that the psychopathologist relives the patient's experiences and thereby re-experience the patient's world while at the same time directly reflecting on these experiences and experienced world. Hence the need for empathic self-transposal into the mental life of the patient in order to relive it and reflect directly upon it (Wiggins and Schwartz 1997).

Of course, this methodological requirement does not imply that the psychopathologist actually become the patient. This identification with the patient is only an imagined identification, a phantasized identification. Husserl contends that the human imagination can replicate in phantasy various kinds of intentional processes, and he calls this kind of experience an 'as-if awareness' or 'presentification' (*Vergegenwärtigen*). Dorion Cairns translates it as a 'feigned awareness'. Accordingly, my mental life can imagine itself having the same sorts of experiences that another person has although that other person is quite different from me (Wiggins and Schwartz 1997).

As Jaspers has emphasized, any psychiatrist or psychopathologist who seeks to understand the patient's experiences to this extent should remain aware that the extent is limited (Jaspers 1965: 253–254, 302; Jaspers 1997: 305, 363). Unfortunately, however, the limits of such reliving are not easily detected. One can believe that one is understanding the patient when in fact one is simply constructing illusions—meaningful illusions but illusions nonetheless. Here Jaspers seems to be endorsing a central tenet of Kant's critical philosophy: we can transgress the limits of true knowledge without realizing that we have transgressed them. We think we are making constant headway in our understanding of the patient's highly unusual experiences when we are in fact only fooling ourselves. Hence the Kantian warning: knowledge has its limits, difficult though these limits may be to detect in any particular case. Jaspers is especially aware of how applicable this warning is to psychopathology. Crucial to the expertise that one must develop as a psychopathologist is the skill to recognize that there are facets of the ill person's mental life that psychopathologists will never be able to understand. The limit of the 'un-understandable' remains a necessary component of the wisdom of the psychopathologist.

Jaspers' position here is clearly seen in his criticism of Freudian psychoanalysis' failure to respect these limits. Jaspers writes, 'The limits of every psychology of meaningful connections must necessarily remain the same for psychoanalysis in so far as the latter is meaningful'. He mentions three reasons for such limits: (1) 'the innateness of empirical characteristics'; (2) 'organic illness and psychosis': and (3) 'Existence itself', that which the individual really is in himself (Jaspers 1997: 363). Especially with regard to the latter Jaspers charges:

> The illumination of psychoanalysis proves here to be a pseudo-illumination. Though Existence itself is not directly there for psychological understanding, its influence is felt in the limits it sets for psychological understanding at the point where something is which only shows itself in the inconclusiveness of the meaningful. Psychoanalysis has always 'shut its eyes' to the limitations and has 'wanted to understand everything'. (Jaspers 1997: 363; on this point see also Rossi Monti, Chapter 3, this volume)

Concept formation

Having carried out such imaginative re-experiencing herself, the psychopathologist can then reflect carefully on her own phantasized experiences and carefully analyse their features.

For the purposes of the science of psychopathology, one is seeking to describe the general structural features of the different kinds of mental disorder. Particular details do not matter. Only the 'general' is of interest. Phenomenological descriptions thus seek to depict general structural properties of the imagined pathological processes that one reflectively finds in one's own imagined pathological life.

'General' features can be reliably discerned, of course, only if one reflectively examines many different instances of such pathological experiences. Accordingly, the psychopathologist must imagine a variety of examples of experiences of, say, auditory hallucinations in schizophrenia. This surveying of various exemplifications of the same general kind of experience is closely allied with Husserl's method of 'variation in free phantasy'. Husserl's method, too, considers 'many phantasized cases' of the kind of intentionality under investigation. Hence we endorse Husserl's method of reflecting on imagined experiences and their intended objects, varying these experiences and objects, and then discerning the general, invariant features that remain the same throughout the variation of particulars.

These invariant features can then be conceptualized as empirical generalizations. Notice that we say 'empirical' generalizations and not essential universals. Husserl's phenomenology aims at essential universal concepts. Psychopathology, however, can seek only 'general empirical' concepts. Jaspers was determined to make clear his own divergence from Husserl's essentialist method on this point (Jaspers 1965, 1997; Wiggins and Schwartz 1997). We, too, wish to emphasize that this difference between eidetic and empirical methods signals the difference between Husserl's free variation in phantasy and the procedures we have outlined.

Conclusion

Our main concern in this chapter has been to delineate a methodology for the science of psychopathology. We have drawn on the thoughts of Karl Jaspers and Edmund Husserl in performing this task. The method we have outlined consists of several components: the quest for direct evidence, expert hermeneutic interpretation, re-living and re-experiencing the intentional processes of mentally ill patients, reflecting on these imagined intentional processes, and varying them in an attempt to bring out what remains invariant, namely, the general features of pathological mental processes. We contend, however, that this many-step method is what is required for a methodologically strict phenomenological psychopathology. Only thus can we answer the critics who persist in maintaining that the pathological mental lives of patients are inaccessible to science.

Jaspers, as we have interpreted him in another essay (Wiggins and Schwartz 1997), recognized the methodological features of re-living and re-experiencing the experiences of mentally ill patients, reflecting on these imagined mental processes, and varying them in order to specify what remains invariant. We have focused on implications of the Husserlian theory of evidence and reason in order to emphasize how a methodology that demands the grounding of all claims in the evidence appropriate to the subject matter could adopt these Jaspersian theses. In his *General Psychopathology* Jaspers made fruitful use of what he knew of Husserl's phenomenology. We seek to bring Jaspers and Husserl together again in order to restore psychopathology to a respected place in the general study of the human mind.

References

American Psychiatric Association. (2000). *Diagnostic and Statistical Manual of Mental Disorders, Fourth Edition, Text Revision, DSM-IV-TR*. Washington, DC: American Psychiatric Association.

Collins, H., Evans, R. (2007). *Rethinking Expertise*. Chicago, IL: The University of Chicago Press.

Heidegger, M. (2010). *Being and Time*. Albany, NY: The State University of New York Press.

Husserl, E. (1969). *Formal and Transcendental Logic*. The Hague: Martinus Nijhoff Publishers.

Husserl, E. (1973a). *Cartesian Meditations: An Introduction to Phenomenology*. The Hague: Martinus Nijhoff.

Husserl, E. (1973b). *Experience and Judgment: Investigations in a Genealogy of Logic*. Evanston, IL: Northwestern University Press.

Husserl, E. (1982). *Ideas Pertaining to a Pure Phenomenology and to a Phenomenological Philosophy, First Book*. The Hague: Martinus Nijhoff.

Jaspers, K. (1963). *Gesammelte Schriften zur Psychopathologie*. Berlin: Springer-Verlag.

Jaspers, K. (1965). *Allgemeine Psychopathologie* (8th edn). Berlin: Springer-Verlag.

Jaspers, K. (1968). 'The Phenomenological Approach in Psychopathology', *British Journal of Psychiatry*, **114**: 1313–1323.

Jaspers, K. (1997). *General Psychopathology* (7th edn) (J. Hoenig, M.W. Hamilton, trans.). Baltimore, MD: Johns Hopkins University Press.

McHugh, P.R., Slavney, P.R. (1983). *The Perspectives of Psychiatry*. Baltimore, MD: Johns Hopkins University Press.

Merleau-Ponty, M. (2000). *Phenomenology of Perception*. New York, NY: Routledge.

Polanyi, M. (1964). *Personal Knowledge: Towards a Post-Critical Philosophy*. New York, NY: Harper Torchbook.

Ricoeur, P. (1970). *Freud and Philosophy: An Essay on Interpretation*. New Haven, CT: Yale University Press.

Ricoeur, P. (1974). *The Conflict of Interpretations: Essays in Hermeneutics*. Evanston, IL: Northwestern University Press.

Schutz, A. (1966). *Collected Papers, III: Studies in Phenomenological Philosophy*. The Hague: Martinus Nijhoff.

Schwartz, M.A., Wiggins, O.P. (1987). 'Typifications: The First Step for Clinical Diagnosis in Psychiatry', *Journal of Nervous and Mental Disorders*, **175**(2): 65–77.

Wiggins, O.P., Schwartz, M.A. (1997). 'Edmund Husserl's Influence on Karl Jaspers's Phenomenology', *Philosophy, Psychiatry, & Psychology*, **4**(1): 15–36.

Wiggins, O.P., Schwartz, M.A. (2004). 'Philosophical Issues in Psychiatry', in G. Khushf (ed), *Handbook of Bioethics: Taking Stock of the Field from a Philosophical Perspective*. Dordrecht: Kluwer Academic Publishers, 473–487.

Chapter 3

Jaspers' 'Critique of Psychoanalysis': between past and future

Mario Rossi Monti

Karl Jaspers published his 'Critique of Psychoanalysis' (*Zur Kritik der Psychoanalyse*') in 1950. This contribution represented the culmination of a journey begun many years before with the publication of *General Psychopathology* in 1913. Jaspers' initial attitude towards psychoanalysis was extremely cautious. Over the years Jaspers radically changed his position, both on the basis of a theoretical reflection and in relation to some particular events that concerned the position of psychoanalysis within the academic field. His 1950 essay is characterized by a severe and radical criticism of psychoanalysis: it is a judgement without appeal, in which he sums up all the criticism he had elaborated over the years. What are the developmental stages of Jaspers' observations on psychoanalysis? What are the key targets of his sometimes fierce criticism? Matthias Bormuth (2006) has dedicated a significant volume to the topic (*Life Conduct in Modern Times. Karl Jaspers and Psychoanalysis*), in which he offers a detailed historical reconstruction of the conditions which induced Karl Jaspers to adopt such a radical and critical view of psychoanalysis. In order to better understand the culmination of Jaspers' journey I will take the following points into consideration: the stages that marked the history of Jaspers' critical thought, the historical context, the tone of his criticism, and, finally, its content. The final part of this essay attempts to show how some of Jaspers' critical observations on psychoanalysis should not be considered as a thing of the past, because they were and still are a fundamental topic of discussion and debate within the Freudian psychoanalytic movement.

The history of criticism

The historical evolution of Jaspers' criticism of psychoanalysis can be briefly schematized in three stages (these stages correspond to the development of his existential understanding of psychotherapy—see Schlimme, Chapter 11, this volume). The first stage is represented by the first edition of *General Psychopathology* in 1913. Here Jaspers shows interest and tolerance towards the psychoanalytic perspective, and especially towards that minor section of the psychoanalytic thought which is concerned with the clinical setting closer to his own interests, namely the psychoses and particularly the schizophrenic psychosis. In fact, although Freud conducted much of his clinical and theoretical work in the vicinity of one of the largest asylums of the time, his interest in institutional psychiatry was close to zero. Freud was not interested in psychiatric institutions and probably ignored what was going on inside them. Terms like 'asylum' or 'psychiatric hospital', apart from very few exceptions, are not present in his works. One of these exceptions is the case of Mrs Emmy von N., described in *Studies on Hysteria* (1893–1895), where we can see evidence of how Freud's idea about a psychiatric institution was distant from reality:

> Since she talked so often about asylums in her waking state, I interrupted her and asked on what other occasions she had been concerned with insanity. She told me that her mother had herself been in an asylum for some time. They had once had a maid-servant one of whose previous mistresses had spent a long time in an asylum and who used to tell her horrifying stories of how the patients were tied to chairs, beaten, and so on. As she told me this she clenched her hands in horror; she saw all this before her eyes. I endeavored to correct her ideas about insane asylums. (Freud 1893–1895: 55)
>
> She brought out new fears about asylums—that people in them were treated with douches of ice-cold water on the head and put into an apparatus which turned them round and round till they were quiet. When, three days ago, she had first complained about her fear of asylums, I had interrupted her after her first story, that the patients were tied on to chairs. I now saw that I had gained nothing by this interruption and that I cannot evade listening to her stories in every detail to the very end. After these arrears had been made up, I took this fresh crop of fears from her as well. I appealed to her good sense and told her she really ought to believe me more than the silly girl from whom she had had the gruesome stories about the way in which asylums are run. (Freud 1893–1895: 61)

In 1911, Jaspers starts working on his *General Psychopathology* in order to give an account of the kind of research work developed by institutional psychiatry when dealing with the world of psychosis. From this point of view, the area of the psychoanalytic thought that interests Jaspers the most is represented by that minor part of psychoanalysis that grapples with the great problems of clinical psychiatry within the asylum institutions. The Zurich School, born inside one of the most prestigious clinics in Europe (Burghölzli), represents the privileged area of Jaspers' interests. At Burghölzli, in fact, besides Eugen Bleuler, Carl Gustav Jung and Karl Abraham were also working. They are two of the few psychoanalysts who immediately show a deep interest in the area of serious pathologies and their institutional treatment. In that context, the concept of 'schizophrenia' was born, on the basis of a pathogenetic interpretation founded on the theoretical and clinical concepts that Freud had developed while studying the neuroses. In his work *Dementia Praecox oder Gruppe der Schizophrenien*, Bleuler (1911) shows gratitude towards his colleagues (particularly Jung and Abraham) and includes his contribution in the area of psychoanalysis, declaring that his essay is nothing but the application of Freud's ideas on what Kraepelin had called *dementia praecox*. The pathogenetic interpretation of schizophrenia proposed by Bleuler and Jung and based on Freudian psychoanalysis represents a contribution which Jaspers judges worthy of discussion, even if it is based on the transposition of the theoretical and clinical concepts derived from the analysis of the neurotic mental pathology in the field of schizophrenia. However, according to Jaspers, one of the major credits of Freudian psychoanalysis lies in its tendency to direct the maximum amount of attention to even the smallest details, showing that comprehensive psychology can be usefully extended even to this level. Around 1910—Jaspers recalls in his philosophical autobiography—psychiatry was firmly dominated by somatic medicine, and psychological studies were considered subjective, unscientific, and basically useless.

The second stage is represented by the second edition of *General Psychopathology* in 1920. In this edition, Jaspers gradually shifts the focus of attention from the clinical and psychopathological level to the philosophical one, introducing certain philosophical elements that go in the direction of his philosophy of existence. In this phase, the knowledge and the theories developed by psychoanalysis are to be rejected *in toto*: first of all, this is due to the asymmetric features of the setting of the psychoanalytic work. Such a setting gives the medical analyst an authority that undermines any possible authentic and open communication. Secondly—and here Jaspers is referring to one of the strongest points of the anti-Freudian criticism—this is due to the excessive importance given to the infantile sexual life. Only the psychoanalytic therapy practice as defined by Freud in *Studies on Hysteria* (1893–1895) remains as a possible object of interest.

The third stage is represented by the fourth edition of *General Psychopathology* in 1946. In the first edition Jaspers' attitude towards psychoanalysis is characterized by a certain tolerance and interest with respect to some aspects of the psychoanalytic thinking applied to psychosis. In the 1920 edition, psychoanalysis was portrayed as a psychology of understanding that had had its day. However, it is only while reviewing the fourth edition of his work that Jaspers develops the systematic criticism of psychoanalysis that will find its full expression in the 1950 essay. While dealing with the general problem of psychotherapy in the medical field, Jaspers identifies psychoanalysis as an arch enemy. In reality, the object of this criticism is the first part of Freud's work. In fact, Jaspers—as he himself declares—had quit reading psychoanalytical texts long before (both Freud's and his followers' ones).

Therefore, the accentuation of the critical tone has little to do with the evolution of psychoanalytic thought and much more to do with Jaspers' rethinking of the role of psychotherapy within the cultural scenario of the end of the 1940s. This way, Jaspers' criticism reaches radical tones: he underlines the cold or even filled-with-hate atmosphere in which Freud's clinical investigations were developed and even reaches the point of wishing the extinction of psychoanalysis as an obstacle to human freedom. One underlying idea, formulated in a letter to Carl Friedrich von Weizsäcker in 1953, survives: 'The devil is at the root of this. For this reason there can only be complete rejection' (Jaspers 1953a, quoted in Bormuth 2006: 2). As Jaspers' thought gains some of the philosophical implications which lie at the basis of his existential philosophy, psychoanalysis increasingly becomes in his eyes a paradigmatic example of the degeneration of psychotherapy. On the one hand, the development of Jaspers' existential philosophy leads him to collide with psychoanalysis, and, on the other, moves him away from clinical psychiatry. It is well known—as Bormuth reports—that Kurt Schneider harshly criticized the 'overgrowth of the philosophical aspect' or what Hans Gruhle had called 'the philosophical saturation' of the fourth edition of *General Psychopathology*—so much so that he recommended to his staff the reading of the 1913 edition instead of the new edition, which in his eyes was too oriented toward existentialism (Bormuth 2006: 80).

The context of Jaspers' criticism

The context within which Jaspers directs his criticisms against psychoanalysis is an articulated and complex one. It is, at the same time, both a cultural and an institutional context. Also and above all, it is a personal context in the sense that the criticism of psychoanalysis is rooted in the troubled relationship between Jaspers, Viktor von Weizsäcker, and Alexander Mitscherlisch. Weizsäcker and Mitscherlisch represent the spearhead of the rebirth of psychoanalysis in Germany after the Second World War and are guided by the intention to create a space within the University of Heidelberg dedicated to the study of psychosomatics.

As a potential medical discipline, psychosomatics could also work as a true bridgehead for psychoanalysis within the university. The goal is to develop a discipline that, without losing its relationship with clinical medicine, can, at the same time, be based on psychoanalysis. This way, from the status of a 'science of the catacombs', psychoanalysis aspired to rise to the status of an officially recognized academic discipline (Pohlen 2000). The context within which Jaspers builds his criticism of psychoanalysis can be divided into two main aspects: the first one concerns in general the diffusion and popularity of psychoanalysis in post-war Germany; the second one is more specific and local, and concerns the foundation of an institute of psychosomatic psychoanalysis at the University of Heidelberg.

As for the first aspect, the condition of psychoanalysis in post-war Germany is of a particular kind. In the first place, at the end of the war and with the fall of Nazism, Jaspers is forced to admit that his prediction of a rapid obsolescence of psychoanalysis had been disproved by the facts. Psychoanalysis had not been wiped away by history and was not an historical phenomenon that had its day. On the contrary, psychoanalysis, reborn from the ashes of Nazi persecution, is very much alive and in full shape. This revival is not only a cultural phenomenon but also an institutional phenomenon.

While Jaspers in Germany witnesses such a revival of psychoanalysis from its own ashes, Hannah Arendt informs him that in the United States psychoanalysis is becoming more and more popular, spreading rapidly through society and culture. In fact, since the late 1940s psychoanalysis had begun to spread in American culture with the speed and progression typical of a true 'contagion', a contagion that recalls Freud's prophetic words spoken at the end of August 1909, when arriving in New York for a series of conferences aboard an ocean liner. He seems to have said: 'They do not know that we bring them the plague'. Jaspers' fear is that such plague" will take roots in Germany as well, will become a mass phenomenon (Bormuth 2006: 112), and will infect young people, especially the new governing class, on which rests the task of rebuilding Germany. Jaspers fears that the new generation, which had been dominated and made passive by the Nazi dictatorship and propaganda, could be infected by the fascination with the abyss promoted by depth psychology without having valid antibodies to counteract an uncritical acceptance. Jaspers is certainly among those who came out of the catastrophe of Nazism with his head held up high. Von Weizsäcker and Mitscherlisch enjoy great respect as well. Therefore, it is not easy, not even from a political point of view, to address a harsh criticism to psychoanalysis, a discipline that had paid such a high price in its confrontation with Nazism. The ambition of von Weizsäcker and Mitscherlisch to find a space for psychoanalysis within the German university is also supported by arguments of this type. Thus, it is not easy to oppose von Weizsäcker's arguments, according to which it is necessary to make amends to psychoanalysis because of its persecution as a Jewish science (Bormuth 2006: 99).

The risk glimpsed by Jaspers with respect to von Weizsäcker and Mitscherlisch's psychoanalytically founded psychosomatics consists in a distortion of the traditional conception of the physician: this distortion would imply an attack on the foundations of the concept of the physician and a strong limitation of his freedom, by which the physician would turn into a shepherd of souls. Furthermore, the interest of psychoanalysis in psychosomatics, developed by von Weizsäcker and Mitscherlisch, is seen by Jaspers as a real Trojan horse designed to unhinge the foundations of medicine: using psychosomatics, psychoanalysis tries to extend its field of application and intervention well beyond the specific area of the neuroses (within which it was born), with the intention to export the 'revolution' well into the field of medicine. In fact, von Weizsäcker presents himself as the promoter of a true 'medical anthropology' based on the systematic investigation of the relationship between the physician and the patient and on the use of psychoanalytic tools. Actually, the essential contribution of psychoanalysis to medicine would consist in regarding the physician–patient relationship as a privileged field of knowledge, research, and therapy. In this sense, it is not so much a matter of promoting an integration or engagement of psychoanalysis with the medical culture, but more of developing a global project that goes beyond the limits of psychology: the goal is to humanize the whole medicine in order to learn to consider the morbid somatic event as a phenomenon that carries a meaning and modulates the identity of the subject. Inside the 'interpersonal laboratory' created by Freud, von Weizsäcker is able to create a situation where the physical functions of the sick person can begin to talk and can be heard as an expression of a valid self-perception of one's life processes.

The second important aspect of Jaspers' criticism concerns the foundation of a university institute for psychosomatic psychoanalysis at the University of Heidelberg. In January 1946, Viktor von Weizsäcker obtains the chair of Clinical General Medicine at the University of Heidelberg. Encouraged by this first success, von Weizsäcker and Mitscherlisch strongly request the creation of an institutional space for psychosomatics and psychoanalysis within the Faculty of Medicine. Von Weizsäcker's approach, focused on the patient–physician relationship, is strongly supported by Mitscherlich. Von Weizsäcker had been awarded the honorary presidency of the German Society for Psychotherapy and Depth Psychology. The Society had been founded in 1949 after the collapse of Nazism, in an attempt to rebuild the professional community of psychotherapists which, during the Third Reich, had gathered under the wing of the Göring Institute. Two years earlier, in 1947, Mitscherlisch had founded the journal *Psyche* in which psychoanalysis was presented as a discipline belonging to the humanities, with particular interest in political and social aspects. The project of founding an institute of psychosomatic psychoanalysis at the University of Heidelberg is based on the ambition to rely on the discoveries of psychoanalysis in order to revolutionize the whole medical discipline, starting with psychosomatics. According to von Weizsäcker and Mitscherlisch, medicine was relying on methods of study that were too objectifying and impersonal.

Of course this project immediately collides with the complexity of the institutional relationships within the academic community, and also with the conservative positions of most of the academics, both those belonging strictly to the medical field and those belonging to the psychiatric field. Ernst Kretschmer, in particular, representing the influential General Medical Society for Psychotherapy (founded in Marburg in 1948), strongly opposes any type of psychological therapy as proposed by the schools of depth psychology or psychoanalysis (Cocks 1985). Besides that, Kretschmer shows hostility towards the creation of special institutes for the teaching of psychotherapy and especially towards the assignment to psychologists of therapeutic tasks which are not subject to medical authority. According to Kretschmer, psychotherapy should be practised only by physicians. As with Kretschmer, the majority of the psychiatric academic community is not only highly critical of Freudian psychoanalysis, but is also distrustful of the possibility that any psychotherapy can be practised and taught by those who are not qualified as physicians and psychiatrists (Cocks 1985). Even Kurt Schneider, professor of psychiatry at the University of Heidelberg, firmly stands out against the creation of a space for psychoanalysis within the academic field. As a condition for a favourable vote, Schneider asks for a formal commitment to limit the activity of the future institute to the counselling and treatment of non-psychiatric conditions (Bormuth 2006: 101). In essence, the psychiatric academic community is trying to contain the impact of the proposal made by von Weizsäcker and Mitscherlisch and to defuse a mechanism that would turn the new institute into a means to disrupt the traditional structure of medical disciplines. According to the psychiatric community, the new institute should limit itself to the sole practice of counselling and should be still subject to the close supervision of the medical authority, without relying too much on the ideas of Freudian psychoanalysis. In this context, Jaspers appears to be the best candidate for attempting a mediation. Despite Jaspers' strong reservations toward psychoanalysis, Mitscherlisch appears to him as the only person capable of containing the psychoanalytic approach within the boundaries of science, while avoiding a drifting-away scenario.

Jaspers seems to hope for a transformation of psychoanalysis into a codified procedure whose results can be recognized as scientifically valid or, in other words, into a scientific form of psychotherapy. Relying on this hope, founded on the respect and trust he has for Mitscherlisch, Jaspers reaches the following conclusion: the evaluation of the psychoanalytic perspective does not justify by itself the foundation of an institute. On the other hand, Mitscherlisch's commitment to contain psychoanalysis within the limits of traditional medicine and to promote a scientifically-oriented evolution of it is a valid justification for the foundation of the new institute. In substance, Jaspers' favourable opinion is not based on the legitimacy of the discipline, but on Mitscherlisch's personal and professional qualities: Mitscherlisch represents the guarantee of a medically and scientifically oriented transformation of psychoanalysis in its application to psychosomatics.

In September 1946 the Faculty of Medicine votes for a measure of compromise. There is no decision regarding the establishment of an independent institute of psychoanalytic psychosomatics, but a new working environment is created where Mitscherlisch is free to practise his method under the supervision of the Clinical General Medicine chair, headed by von Weizsäcker. Two years later, thanks to the direct support of the Ministry of Justice—which sees Mitscherlisch as one of the few academics who have acted in an exemplary manner during the Nazi period—such a new working environment becomes the Psychosomatic Clinic of the University of Heidelberg. This is the place where German psychosomatics was born, known to history as the 'Heidelberg School' of psychosomatics (Ammon 1974).

After the foundation of the Psychosomatic Clinic the situation changes and the relationship among Jaspers, Weizsäcker, and Mitscherlisch becomes more complicated. Jaspers' 1950 criticism of psychoanalysis finds its place in a polemical discussion triggered by the reading of the reports, published in *Psyche* in 1949, presented by Weizsäcker and Mitscherlisch at the Wiesbaden conference. Jaspers sees the content of these reports as a real provocation, as an attack on the objectivity of science accompanied by the claim to reform medicine on the basis of a psychoanalytic psychosomatics. Mitscherlisch's grappling with the problem is already evident in the title of his report: 'The Scope of Psychosomatic Thought in Medicine'. Illness is seen in terms of an existential crisis: therefore, the course of treatment should not be focused only on the symptoms but should promote a growth of the whole personality. This way, according to Jaspers, psychoanalysis presents itself as a guiding star and takes the form of a fideistic thought or salvific doctrine which claims to possess a total knowledge about man. Mitscherlisch's view represents for Jaspers a true betrayal of the confidence he had put in him. Shortly after the foundation of the Psychosomatic Clinic, Mitscherlisch takes a radical position, forgetting the importance of a scientific approach and promoting a subversive psychoanalytically based psychosomatics. According to Jaspers, instead, such a fideistic declension of psychoanalysis relies on fanaticism and ends up—precisely because of its fideistic nature—hindering an authentic knowledge of man. In order to stem the risk deriving from a psychoanalytically based psychotherapy by means of his philosophy of existence, in 1950 Jaspers starts publishing a series of essays concerning the relationship between psychotherapy and medicine. With this, he gives a final form to his radical criticism of psychoanalysis as a kind of faith and sect.

The tone of Jaspers' criticism

The tone of Jaspers' criticism of psychoanalysis is extremely hard, bitter, sometimes ironic, aggressive, and openly hostile. Jaspers does not tone down his words. In fact, he even exacerbates the issues at stake. He accuses Freud of being cold, of deliberately obscuring and even hating knowledge. He also accuses him of being a victim of his own rambling thoughts, which he always tries to overcome with new bright ideas. This, on the one hand, shows how some aspects of psychoanalysis that were so different from Jaspers' existential philosophy were really bothering him, and, on the other hand, reveals the extent of Jaspers' personal involvement.

Mitscherlisch's turnaround must have hurt Jaspers badly; nonetheless, Jaspers was convinced of playing a crucial battle, contrasting the diffusion of psychoanalysis in Germany. In particular, Jaspers' concern with the psychoanalytic training system, against which he is strongly polemical, reflects his anxiety about the spread of a psychoanalysis centred around an authority principle within a society and a culture incapable (due to their recent history) of a sufficiently critical assessment. Vanna Berlincioni and Fausto Petrella (2000) properly described the 'arrogant tone' with which Jaspers conducted 'a concise liquidation of psychoanalysis', in a 'violently critical and intolerant' essay, aimed at a radical rejection of psychoanalysis. The authors attribute such a style to Jaspers' narrow view of psychoanalysis. Of course—they write—Jaspers was exceedingly bothered by the psychoanalytic chattering and naive expectations. Psychoanalysis seems to him like an ill-founded faith, as a vision of the world. It is not science; it is not philosophy, it is neither authentic psychology nor a true religion. This is probably right, but, as Bormuth writes (2006: 113), 'only within this context is the polemical acerbity of the two articles "Critique of Psychoanalysis" and "Physician and Patient" understandable'. The analysis of the historical context helps to explain the motives of so much hatred and intolerance and allows one to see the split between the tone and the content of Jaspers' criticism, in such a way that the discomfort felt in front of the form of this criticism does not prevent one from grasping the nature of its content.

The contents of Jaspers' criticism

Beyond its often provocative tone, Jaspers' criticism focuses on a limited number of problems that I will try to list in the following sections.

Psychoanalysis as 'pseudoscience'

Jaspers' first accusation towards psychoanalysis regards the adoption of a pseudo-scientific method, based on some 'objective errors'. Among those errors, Jaspers mentions the confusion between the comprehension of meaning and the causal explanation. While the first is achieved by reciprocal communication, the second is alien to meaning and can be recognized only from distance. While the first relies on freedom and does not have any effect on the events, the second enables one to intervene on the events in a rationally predictable manner. From the confusion between the comprehension of meaning and the causal explanation derives a mortification of freedom. According to Jaspers, psychoanalysis is a comprehensive psychology that, however, has the tendency to present itself as a causal explanation. Freud's fallacious idea that everything in psychic life is comprehensible is due to this confusion between comprehensible relationships and causal relationships.

From this first error—argues Jaspers—a second error derives: Freud builds causal theories of psychic life on the grounds of comprehensible relationships regarding psychic life. But comprehension cannot lead to theories which are the outcome of causal explanations. In addition, the theories that can be elaborated by following the path proposed by Freud are oversimplified and reductive. This way, the infinite multiformity of understanding is missed. Freud's 'understanding' is often conceived as an 'understand as if', by means of which Freud enters the unobserved psychological life raising it to the level of consciousness. The second error concerns the claim to assess the effectiveness of the psychoanalytic procedure without keeping in mind the fact that, for thousands of years, all of the psychotherapeutic methods were successful when in the hands of skilful personalities. The patient's personal satisfaction cannot be considered as a sufficient criteria when the effectiveness of the procedure or the recovery of the patient are concerned.

The third mistake lies in the fact that the neuroses are not characterized on the basis of their comprehensible content but rather of a translation of the mental into the physical (apparently meaningless somatic events) or into psychological mechanisms. Only few people fall victim to this kind of freedom loss; the most part remove, forget, leave in suspense, suffer, and tolerate heavy situations, without ever transposing their pain into a somatic or psychic symptom.

The totalitarian characteristic: psychoanalysis as faith

Like all human undertakings, even psychotherapy has its risks and may undergo degeneration. Many psychotherapeutic movements, despite being founded on medical grounds, have gradually abandoned the field of science and have become faith movements (Jaspers 1953b). Psychotherapists often succumb to the temptation of turning their theories into religious movements and their schools into some kind of sects. According to Jaspers, the specific risk run by psychotherapy is to be transformed into a substitute for metaphysics or into a sort of religion, similar to the one professed by the Gnostic sects. The risk is much higher in an era marked by the crisis and confusion of the post-war Germany. The freedom of the individual therapist is often put at risk by the demands of the group which, by transforming a theory into a faith, seeks total cohesion in order to achieve the illusion of an absolute knowledge and superiority over other rival groups. But the risk of this transformation should not turn into a destiny. To avoid this degeneration, psychotherapy must take care of its scientific and philosophical presuppositions in order not to be seduced by totalitarianism and sectarianism. Jaspers claims that psychoanalysis was not able to contain this risk within acceptable boundaries. From the moment when Freud hurled his anathema against his infidel students, psychoanalysis has turned into a faith movement wearing scientific 'clothes'. Such an evolution of psychoanalysis proves that the psychotherapeutic sects become a substitute for religion, that their theories become a doctrine of salvation, and their therapy becomes a form of redemption. In this sense, the psychotherapeutic sects are located at the antipodes of medical science, at the antipodes of love for freedom and of spirituality and true philosophy. Jaspers' arguments, indicating psychoanalysis as 'pseudoscience' and as comparable to a religious faith, can also claim to be founded on methodological reasonings (Schlimme et al. 2012, Chapter 11, this volume). As is well known, Jaspers, especially in his late works, was extraordinarily critical with respect to epistemological limitations of every kind of scientific method. But what are the essential characteristics of the psychoanalytic faith? They can be schematically represented by the fact that:

- *All that happens to the human beings and inside them is endowed with sense and therefore understandable*: from the psychoanalytic perspective the process of signification is absolutized; this leads to a worldview where everything becomes a symbol. The interpretation can be extended without limits. New and infinite possibilities for interpretation, over-interpretation, and re-interpretation constantly emerge and eventually any opportunity to distinguish the truth from the false is lost: this way, what is knowable is immersed in the endless flow of the interpretations and ceases to be knowable.
- Psychoanalysis claims to be able to develop *a complete knowledge of the human being* and grasp its true essence: since everything is 'determined', everything is governed by causality. Besides being scientifically impossible, this concept of the human being has strong analogies with totalitarianism in a socio-historical sense and is based on the confusion between knowability and freedom: a freedom reduced to an object is no longer freedom.
- An illness reduced to its causes tends to be seen as *guilt*: one of the many possible viewpoints is now unduly extended to all pathological conditions.
- Psychoanalysis evokes a representation of human *perfection* and calls it health.
- Psychoanalysis has an *occult, fanatical, and destructive tendency* which is rarely expressed in an explicit way—as when von Weizsäcker openly describes the subversive nature of psychosomatic medicine.

According to Jaspers, this totalitarian and fideistic feature of psychoanalysis finds its best expression in the training analysis.

The problem of the training analysis

Jaspers identifies the didactic or training analysis as a particularly critical aspect of psychoanalysis. According to him, the training analysis is the best possible subject for a true *experimentum crucis* where the totalitarian and fideistic nature of psychoanalysis can be fully revealed. Actually, Jaspers has nothing to object to the training analysis itself. In *General Psychopathology* he refers to a long quote from Jung in order to show how and when the need for training analysis was born in psychoanalysis. The reason for this training—although this is often an opinion hard or unpopular to sustain—has to do with the fact that the physician, in order to practise as a psychotherapist, has to go through a process of self-clarification. The critical point on which Jaspers insists is not the training analysis itself but rather the way in which the training process fits into the process of becoming a psychoanalyst.

What Jaspers criticizes is the choice of giving a rigid and predetermined form to such a need for personal clarification, which thus becomes a mandatory procedure without which it is impossible to practise as a professional psychoanalyst. According to Jaspers, this choice is a choice of unfreedom and offends the spirit of the scientific enterprise, for the sake of which Jaspers claims the necessity of a personal choice. For Jaspers, to prescribe such a mandatory procedure means crossing the line: those who are willing to go through it can certainly benefit from such a personal clarification, but when the training analysis becomes a precondition for becoming a psychoanalyst, this means that science is denied.

As a negation of individual freedom, the training analysis shows—in Jaspers' eyes—clear evidence of the totalitarian and sectarian features of psychoanalysis and puts the freedom and health of the soul in serious danger: the mandatory training analysis does harm to the physician's true nature. This way, the therapist's justified need for self-clarification gets twisted and bent to the needs of a sectarian institution. How can one use the psychoanalytic method without becoming enslaved to it? The mandatory training analysis is the main road to slavery. But what are the goals of this requirement? According to Jaspers, there are at least four of them.

The first goal is to develop a firm solidarity within the movement. Such solidarity does not rely on scientific dialogue, but on a total, fluid, and constantly changing conception on the basis of which one feels authorized to award diplomas that certificate the student's affiliation to a sect. The second goal is to encourage obedience: the knowledge instilled during the long psychoanalytic training gradually turns into a faith. Whoever is obedient enough to let himself be instructed becomes a fully recognized member of the community. The obedience is never openly discussed, but, as Jaspers writes, it is the real hidden requirement. The third goal is to promote orthodoxy: Freud's excommunications of the students who did not adhere to his doctrine clearly showed how the aim of the psychoanalytic training is to raise psychoanalytically orthodox students. Finally, the fourth goal is indoctrination, which is the privileged tool in order to shape the minds of the new analysts. The training analysis represents the moment when a faith is skilfully instilled and systematically reinforced by repeated spiritual exercises (Jaspers 1958). These spiritual exercises do not lead to a truth by developing a shared and universally valid knowledge, but by training oneself to modify one's own conscience. This way—Jaspers concludes—the didactic analysis imprints a faith deeply in the student's mind, a faith which tends to settle and turn him into a coreligionist of a congregation (Jaspers 1958: 78).

The topicality of Jaspers' criticism

Beyond its tone and determined historical context, Jaspers' criticism of psychoanalysis touches on some fundamental elements regarding the psychoanalytical training and identity. Much of Jaspers' criticism went together with the contemporaneous debate about psychoanalytic training, a debate that already concerned the proper denomination of it: education or training? Ekstein (1969) shows how the two terms are by no means synonymous. The first one has more to do with a training passed from above, the second one with a student-centred perspective that empowers the candidates to make decisions and to assume responsibility for their own learning. As described with great clarity by Jaspers, already at this level it is evident how the debate about the training regards exactly the theme of freedom. Within the psychoanalytic community that recognizes itself as part of the International Psychoanalytical Association founded by Sigmund Freud, the debate about the training issue revives periodically. In order to show how harsh Jaspers' criticism is, in this last paragraph I will briefly refer to some aspects of this debate.

Although driven by the desire to promote his philosophy of existence and to prevent the possibility of the diffusion of psychoanalysis, Jaspers, however, rubbed salt in the wound of psychoanalysis by identifying some of its extremely vulnerable aspects. Beyond the contingency of the polemic and the prejudicial hostility towards psychoanalysis, Jaspers' criticism identifies with great lucidity and foresight some highly critical and potentially destructive aspects involved in the transmission of knowledge and training of the new analysts.

To sum up Jaspers' thought: the ferocious polemic against the training analysis was essentially linked to the rigid, predetermined, and mandatory form in which a justified need for of self-clarification was put: this was an imposed and un-free choice that contrasted with the climate of freedom that should characterize any scientific enterprise and revealed the authoritarian and sectarian face of psychoanalysis. In this sense, the transmission of the psychoanalytic knowledge required a sectarian solidarity, an obedience to a faith, a maintenance of the orthodoxy and an indoctrination reinforced through the continuous repetition of spiritual exercises. In reality, many of the themes discussed by Jaspers in 1950 had already emerged in the debate within the psychoanalytical movement. It is sufficient to read what Michael Balint writes in 1948 regarding the atmosphere that characterized the training:

> The whole atmosphere is strongly reminiscent of the primitive initiation ceremonies. On the part of the initiators—the training committee and the training analysts—we observe secretiveness about our esoteric knowledge, dogmatic announcements of our demands and the use of authoritative techniques. On the part of the candidates, i.e. those to be initiated, we observe the willing acceptance of the exoteric fables, submissiveness to dogmatic and authoritative treatment without much protest and too respectful behaviour. (Balint 1948: 167)

Many influential analysts have also developed a severe criticism towards the psychoanalytic training and the mechanisms of transmission of psychoanalytic knowledge, showing their antithetic character with respect to psychoanalytic thought and their tendency to 'infantilization' (Bernfeld 1962: 480), to 'factionalism, parochialism' (Bass 2000), to absolutism (the belief that 'we have found the way and all others are in error'), to conformity (an intolerance of diversity) and fanaticism (Sorenson 2000: 853). As Jaspers wrote, psychotherapists as a group are exposed to a number of dangers: for example, they can turn their theories into a religious faith and their school into a kind of sect. Casement (2002) shows that currently some serious deviations in the training practices are taking place: too much ideology, too much phase certainty, too many false selves in psychoanalytic candidates and their teacher. Teachers frequently function as the priesthood of the institute to which they belong. This way, their teachings easily become dogmatic and tend to maintain the status quo. Therefore, comments Raubolt, it is important to take account of 'the destructive power of groups where indoctrination replaces training and narcissistic, charismatic leadership turns candidates into disciples' (Newcombe 2011: 114). Together with Kenneth Eisold (1994, 1998, 2004), Otto Kernberg is one of the bitterest critics of the system of transmission of knowledge in psychoanalysis. Kernberg is a prestigious psychiatrist and psychoanalyst, past-president of the International Psychoanalytical Association (1997–2001). Kernberg's journey started a long time ago and led to a battle aimed at introducing radical changes in the organizational structure of psychoanalytic Institutes. In this context, Kernberg has recently stated that the training analysis is extremely harmful and represents one of the aspects of psychoanalysis which mostly contribute to its ossification (Kernberg 2011: 464). Much of the criticism directed to the current system of training organization agrees on this point. (Casement 2002, 2005; Kernberg 1996, 2000, 2006, 2010; Reeder 2004; Wallerstein 1993, 2007; Ward 2010).

One of the paragraphs of Kernberg's 2010 work has a very significant title: 'Abolishing the training analysis system'. One of the important aspects of his criticism is represented by the stultifying nature of psychoanalytic education: the training, as it is conceived, due to its authoritarian structure, tends not only to infantilize students, but also results in a real inhibition of the growing process.

It is Kernberg in particular (1996) who tried to bring into focus the exact mechanisms of this process. He identified 'Thirty Methods to Destroy The Creativity Of Psychoanalytic Candidates'. I will quote only a few: strengthen the graduation rituals by whatever intelligent means you find (number 9); candidates should be discouraged from premature visits to other societies or institutes, from participating in congresses and meetings or in analytic work in other institutions (number 12); always have the least experienced candidates present cases in the presence of more experienced ones and of the faculty (number 17); make sure that some unusually critical or rebellious candidates who threaten the atmosphere of harmony at seminars, challenge their senior instructors or dare to talk publicly against training analysts in the presence of their analysands … are gently kept back or stimulated to resign (number 18); a certain degree of paranoid fear, the counterpart of the idealization processes fostered by the training analysis, permeates most psychoanalytic institutions (number 22); above all, maintain discretion, secrecy, and uncertainty about what is required to become a training analyst, how these decisions are made, where and by whom (number 29); keep in mind that the main objective of psychoanalytic education is to acquire well-proven knowledge regarding psychoanalysis to avoid its dilution, distortion, deterioration and misuse (number 30).

After all, Kernberg had already taken a medical perspective in 1986, when he directed his attention towards a series of institutional problems in psychoanalytic training, namely diagnosing the symptoms, identifying their cause, and establishing a treatment plan. We can start with the analysis of the causes that concern the training models. Which is the model adopted by the psychoanalytic institutes? Is it the model of an academy of art or a school of business and technology? Or the one typical of religious education? Or perhaps the model of university colleges? Kernberg concludes that, altogether, the psychoanalytic training is a mixture between a school of technology and a religious seminary, although it would be more appropriate for it to adopt a model that combines the features of an academy of art with those of a university college. As for the diagnosis of the symptoms, Kernberg's conclusions are remarkably similar to what Jaspers had predicted. The symptoms of 'disease' that afflict the training process can be grouped into four areas:

- Infantilization of the candidate, indoctrination, stultifying effect on the candidate, fostering a quasi-religious attitude.
- Scientific isolation and ignorance: narrowness of mind with respect to scientific exploration, disinterest and ignorance towards any other psychotherapeutic approach (based on the belief of having found 'the way'). For this reason 'psychoanalytic institutes remain highly reluctant to introduce relevant information from sciences bordering on our field into seminars and discussion groups' (Kernberg 2000: 108). Systematic neglect of empirical research and methodology, distrust of university and of clinical psychiatry and clinical psychology are other side effects: 'psychiatrists and psychologists who spend

significant time in academic endeavors are suspected of not being true psychoanalysts' (Kernberg 2000: 109).

- Authoritarianism and arbitrariness founded on an idealization of the training analysis and the training analyst himself. When authoritarianism, dogmatism, and rigidity are prevailing, a paranoiagenic atmosphere spreads within the institutes. This atmosphere is encouraged by the absence of explicit and public criteria for the treatment of information, knowledge, and criteria that regulate career progressions. For example, there is an 'offensive vagueness and perceived arbitrariness of the selection of those in charge of analysing psychoanalytic candidates' (Kernberg 2010: 1007). The decision-making processes are often shrouded by mist. The consequences of this are servility, flattery, and discouragement of any original thought. The final effect is a decline, flattening, and impoverishment of the psychoanalytic work.
- Denial of external social reality: institutes of psychoanalysis are likely to turn into more and more closed systems that become immune to external challenge.

In conclusion: Jaspers' criticism of psychoanalysis focuses on a paradox. On the one hand, there are methodological reasons fuelling Jaspers' critique of psychoanalysis, but the virulence of his criticism comes from personal, contingent, and local reasons. This perhaps explains the tone of his criticism. Jaspers' personal reasons are related to the sense of betrayal experienced in his relationship with von Weizsäcker; the contingent reasons are related to the particular situation of post-war Germany; the local reasons, finally, have to do with the academic policy adopted by the University of Heidelberg, especially regarding the relationship between psychoanalysis, psychosomatics, and medicine. From this point of view, one might wonder to what extent Jaspers' attack on psychoanalysis was an attack on psychoanalysis *tout-court*, or vice versa, on that particular form of psychoanalysis he saw unfolding before his eyes—a psychoanalysis so evidently aimed at gaining credit in the medical and academic world.

On the other hand, however, Jaspers detects in the psychoanalytic training the evidence of the authoritarian and sectarian trait of psychoanalysis (a trait hostile to freedom and science), and carries the attack to the heart of psychoanalysis, targeting its vital centres and reproductive system. These considerations transcend local and contingent issues, but, at the same time, they identify a critical point in the transmission of psychoanalytic knowledge that has much to do with the future of psychoanalysis. More than half a century later, the problems mercilessly identified by Jaspers are still located, so to say, in the eye of the storm.

References

Ammon, G. (1974). *Psychoanalyse und Psychosomatik*. München: Piper & Co.

Balint, M. (1948). 'On the Psychoanalytic Training System', *International Journal of Psycho-Analysis*, **26**: 163–173.

Bass, A. (2000). 'Psychoanalysis in a New Key: Commentary on Paper by Randall Lehmann Sorenson', *Psychoanalytic Dialogues*, **10**: 875–888.

Berlincioni, V., Petrella, F. (2000). 'Note su "Per la critica della psicoanalisi" di Karl Jaspers', *Atque*, **22**: 151–164.

Bernfeld, S. (1962). 'On Psychoanalytic Training', *The Psychoanalytic Quarterly*, **31**: 453–482.

Bleuler, E. (1911). *Dementia praceox oder Gruppe der Schizophrenien*. Leipzig: Franz Deuticke.

Bormuth, M. (2006). *Life Conduct in Modern Times. Karl Jaspers and Psychoanalysis*. Dordrecht: Springer.

Casement, P. (2002). *Learning From our Mistakes: Beyond Dogma in Psychoanalysis and Psychotherapy: Psychoanalysis and Beyond*. London: Routledge.

Casement, P. (2005). 'The Emperor's Clothes: Some Serious Problems in Psychoanalytic Training', *International Journal of Psycho-Analysis*, **86**: 1143–1160.

Cocks, G. (1985). *Psychotherapy in the Third Reich. The Göring Institute*. Oxford: Oxford University.

Ekstein, R. (1969). 'Concerning the Teaching and Learning of Psychoanalysis', *Journal of the American Psychoanalytic Association*, **17**: 312–332.

Eisold, K. (1994). 'The Intolerance of Diversity in Psychoanalytic Institutes', *International Journal of Psycho-Analysis*, **75**: 785–798.

Eisold, K. (1998). 'The Splitting of the New York Psychoanalytic Society and the Construction of Psychoanalytic Authority', *International Journal of Psycho-Analysis*, **79**: 871–885.

Eisold, K. (2004). 'Psychoanalytic Training: The "Faculty System"', *Psychoanalytic Inquiry*, **24**(1): 51–70.

Freud, S. (1893–1895). *Studies on Hysteria*. S.E., vol. 2.

Jaspers, K. (1913). *Allgemeine Psychopathologie* (1st edn). Heidelberg and Berlin: Springer.

Jaspers, K. (1920). *Allgemeine Psychopathologie* (2nd edn). Heidelberg and Berlin: Springer.

Jaspers, K. (1946). *Allgemeine Psychopathologie* (4th edn). Heidelberg: Springer.

Jaspers, K. (1950). 'Zur Kritik der Psychoanalyse', *Der Nervenarzt*, **21**: 465–468.

Jaspers, K. (1953a). *Correspondence with Viktor v. Weizsäcker*. Marbach: Germany Literary Archives.

Jaspers, K. (1953b). 'Die Idee des Arztes', Schweizerische Ärztezeitung, **34**(27): 253–257.

Jaspers, K. (1958). 'Der Artz im techischen Zeitalter', *Klinische Wochenschrift*, **36**: 1037–1143.

Kernberg, O. (1986). 'Institutional Problems of Psychoanalytic Education', *Journal of the American Psychoanalytic Association*, **34**: 799–834.

Kernberg, O. (1996). 'Thirty Methods to Destroy the Creativity of Psychoanalytic Education', *International Journal of Psycho-Analysis*, **77** (5): 1031–1040.

Kernberg, O. (2000). 'A Concerned Critique of Psychoanalytic Education', *International Journal of Psycho-Analysis*, **81**: 97–120.

Kernberg, O. (2006). 'The Coming Changes in Psychoanalytic Education: Part I. Educational and Professional Issues', *International Journal of Psycho-Analysis*, **87**: 1649–1673.

Kernberg, O. (2010). 'A new organization of psychoanalytic education', *Psychoanalytic Review*, **97**(6): 997–1020.

Kernberg, O. (2011). 'La formazione in psicoanalisi e psicoterapia dinamica oggi: conflitti e sfide', *Psicoterapia e Scienze Umane*, **XLV**(4): 457–471.

Newcombe, R. (2011). 'Book Review: Richard Raubolt (ed), Power games: Influence, Persuasion, and Indocrination in Psychotherapy Training', *Clinical Social Work Journal*, **39**: 113–115.

Pohlen, M. (2000). 'Organizzazione della psicoanalisi evoluzione, retrospettiva e prospettiva dei più importanti psicoanalisti della generazione successiva al 1945 in Germania', *Psicoterapia e Scienze Umane*, **XXXIV**(1): 61–71.

Reeder, J. (2004). *Hate and Love in Psychoanalytical Institutions. The Dilemma of Profession*. New York: Other Press.

Schlimme, J.E., Paprotny, T., Brückner, B. (2012). 'Karl Jaspers: Aufgaben und Grenzen der Psychotherapie', *Der Nervenarzt*, 83(1): 84–91.

Sorenson, R.L. (2000). 'Psychoanalytic Institutes as Religious Denominations: Fundamentalism, Progeny, and Ongoing Reformation', *Psychoanalytic Dialogues*, **10**: 847–874.

Wallerstein, R.S. (1993). 'Between Chaos and Petrification: A Summary of the Fifth IPA Conference of Training Analysts', *International Journal of Psycho-Analysis*, **74**: 165–178.

Wallerstein, R.S. (2007). 'The Optimal Structure for Psychoanalytic Education Today: A Feasible Proposal?', *Journal of the American Psychoanalytic Association*, **55**: 953–984.

Ward, A., Gibson, W., Miqueu-Baz, C. (2010). 'Between Paranoia and Creativity: Candidates' Experience of Psychoanalytic Training', *Journal of the American Psychoanalytic Association*, **58**: 891–926.

Chapter 4

Impact of Karl Jaspers' *General Psychopathology*: the range of appraisal

Christoph Mundt

Introduction

Jaspers' epochal textbook *General Psychopathology* caused great interest when it was first published in 1913 by the 30-year-old psychiatrist to be. When he was expelled from his chair of psychology much later in 1941, he entirely rewrote *General Psychopathology* during the subsequent two years. The ensuing fourth edition became the 'classical' one with hardly any further changes up to the ninth final edition. For this overview, the eighth edition of 1965 was used.

There is now a flood of publications about Jaspers' work on *General Psychopathology* on behalf of the 100th anniversary of its first publication in 1913. The renaissance of this monumental monograph happened not only because of the anniversary but also, and probably predominantly, due to a growing unease in the scientific community with the empirical reductionism of the Hempel–Oppenheim schema underlying the third edition of the *Diagnostic and Statistical Manual of Mental Disorders* (DSM-III; American Psychiatric Association, 1980) and its subsequent editions. The more the DSM categories turned out to appear unsatisfactory to validly separate clinical syndromes given their obvious transitions, the more the call for a reconsideration of the classical authors came up. However, even more important for reconsidering DSM is its methodological sway to a radical objectivism which neglects the importance of a view from inside the patient based on empathy and a concerned relationship as part of diagnosis and psychotherapy. Jaspers' systematized and philosophically established the dual methodology approach to psychopathology (Mundt 2013) which offered a solution for the conundrum of how to get best access to the patient's subjective experience. Hence, Jaspers' *General Psychopathology* reached an unexpected timeliness now reflected by a great number of publications on methodology, philosophical reflections about the access to and the nature of psychopathology, and its potential to elucidate human nature in general. This article will review recent publications which specifically refer to and work on Jaspers' methodological considerations, his clinical psychopathological concepts, and their contrast to the present categories of classification. A special aspect in his work is the mutual reference between psychopathology and philosophy, distinct to the respective combination in anthropological phenomenology. The latter may be considered as content-related with respect to understanding mental and emotional processes whereas philosophy in Jaspers' work is mostly focused on methodology, supporting the split in 'understanding' and 'objective' empirical methods. It was a novel approach as simple as it was audacious to accept the methodological dichotomy as essential to human cognition instead of trying to overcome it. Reflecting upon the very roots of the methodological scope to get information about the psychopathology of a person and its context of cause and consequences makes *General Psychopathology* fundamental, and of lasting interest. Reports of novel approaches often use Jaspers' *General Psychopathology* as a point of departure for their argument. The deep impact of *General Psychopathology* on almost any psychopathological field cannot be exhaustively discussed here. Seven sections shall comprise the most influential topics.

Timeliness after 100 years: Jaspers, an authority and stepping stone for conceptual discussion

The introduction to the German version of DSM-III by Koehler and Saß (1984: ix–xvi) emphasized that this manual rests with European psychiatry. They particularly mention experiential symptoms as specifically referring to the phenomenology of Jaspers. In contrast, psychodynamic aspects are not taken into consideration for the manual. However, the subsequent passage on Schneider and Kraepelin rather suggests a methodology dedicated to objectivity standards, not to a multi-method approach as in Jaspers' *General Psychopathology*. Instead, the editors of the German version of DSM-III speak of a renaissance of Kraepelinian and Schneiderian concepts, not of Jaspersian ones. The authors feel supported by the French psychopathologist Pichot, who takes interest in the forthcoming objective methodology of DSM. In a foreword to DSM-III, Janzarik writes that he hesitates to believe in the compatibility of Jaspers' *General Psychopathology* with DSM-III. However, he acknowledges that DSM-III is a remarkable advance for objectivity free of prejudice: more data but fewer presuppositions, he believes. More recent evaluations have cast doubt about such statements (Jäger et al. 2008) despite the introduction of the Hempel–Oppenheim schema of logical empiricism which clearly confesses to a rigid objectification of psychic phenomena (Schwartz and Wiggins 1986).

Although Jaspers never has been directly involved in the development of operational psychiatric diagnosing, his concepts have reached DSM indirectly through Kurt Schneider's first-rank symptoms of schizophrenia (Kraus 2009). Jaspers and Schneider kept close contact and exchanged ideas throughout their lifetimes.

Many psychopathologically oriented publications start off with quotations from *General Psychopathology* and lean on Jaspers' authority. So did Bürgy (2009) when he started his analysis of schizophrenic self-disorders (there is no differentiation in the English version between self and the German 'ego') by quoting Jaspers extensively on the activity, unity, identity, and awareness of the self before going on to describe the first-rank symptoms as defined by Kurt Schneider and their evaluation by Klosterkötter. Jaspers' descriptions are also the point of departure for Schneider's first-rank symptoms and Klosterkötter's ten most predictive basic symptoms of the risk of imminent psychosis to manifest. Other authors who started off with Jaspers' description of minute disturbances of the self are Parnas and his group who worked out a schedule for the assessment of these subjective symptoms (EASE; Parnas et al. 2005).

Some authors quote Jaspers to justify the topic as worth concentrating on, as a sort of primordial authority having figured out an aporia, i.e. how to assess subjective symptoms objectively. Once the topic is set by briefly quoting Jaspers, the authors often leave him without content-related reference for other literature more relevant today for their respective paper. This suggests roots which are not really effective any more. There are, however, more sincere references which seriously try to adapt and reinstate Jaspers' terms and concepts to present debates. Two examples may be mentioned:

1. In an essay about psychiatry as a science belonging to the humanities, Bormuth (2010) starts off with Jaspers for an analysis of the inevitable methodological dualism in psychiatry being disregarded today. Janzarik and Heimann are mentioned as opposing the prevailing positivism in biological psychiatry using Max Weber's ideal type approach to characterize psychopathological phenomena whereas the dualistic methodology appeared less intriguing to them. Interestingly, Jaspers was not biased towards one side of his methodological dualism although it was adopted as reference for the humanities in psychiatry. Jaspers rejected Viktor von Weizsäcker's amalgamation of psychosomatics with psychoanalysis and he also considered Viktor Frankl's constituting of meaning as too predominant—entailing 'too little Socratic attitude'.
2. One of the early critics of DSM-III was Gary Tucker (1998). He thought it deplorable that none of the promises of DSM-III had been fulfilled. He accused DSM-III of failing to make diagnoses more reliable and precise, instead losing the individual patient and his story. As a remediation Jaspers was quoted to rely on a more subtle and methodologically more open psychopathology.

Methodological pluralism

There are several authors, psychiatrists and philosophers, who resumed Jaspers' debate about plural methodology. However, the term plural methodology is actually misleading because Jaspers adopted a dual methodology paradigm, not a randomly selected plurality. He took over the dual methodology from Dilthey and Weber and adapted it to the specific demands of exploring psychopathological symptoms. Taking the splitting of access to psychopathology into objective measurement and empathic understanding as necessarily given and not possibly to overcome was cutting the Gordian knot of the methodological fallacies of psychopathology. A multi-method approach, however, was actually adopted by the DSM philosophy assuming that all fields of psychiatry may contribute to the definition of syndromes including biological and social data. Jaspers' dual methodology is restricted to understanding versus measuring, empathy versus objectifying.

Ghaemi (2007) refers to the understanding–explaining dichotomy as taken over by Jaspers from Dilthey and Weber. He relates this dichotomy to a number of presently influential philosophers, in particular to Popper's philosophy of science and Pierce's pragmatic philosophy of science. Popper, Ghaemi says, relies on Hume, who showed that with the inductive method empirical findings can be refuted but not proven, thus pointing at the problem of lack of positive evidence. Popper does not tell us which theory is proven, he says. Hence he ultimately did not solve the 'human riddle'. Ghaemi further quotes Patricia Churchland's polemics against 'folk psychology', the utility of which she denies. Several more philosophers are discussed, some of them representing mostly inductive philosophy of mind, as, for example, Charles Peirce. He, at least, concedes that consensual findings gained from several investigators by empathy, may corroborate results generated by not blinded methods.

Ghaemi adopted Jaspers from Pepper and Ehrlich's translation of *General Psychopathology*. In his view Jaspers' perspectives were: (1) readiness to adopt any method (this is not correct and a contradiction to a later statement), (2) general validity, (3) provable insights, (4) clarity of method, and (5) meaningful scission. While relying on Pepper, Ghaemi attributes features of a modern methodologically versatile approach to Jaspers. The main features are characterized by Pepper as follows: self-limiting in method, cogently certain, universally valid, unlimited in scope, endless in development, theoretically expansive, as well as precise and concrete in explanation, never final in its categories, anti-dogmatic. All categories characterize modern scientific undertaking. The ideal type breaches the Kantian gap. Understandable and non-understandable should be the only distinction between the dichotic endogenous diseases. This statement is further emphasized by a critique of the diagnostic manuals as creating too many invalid categories which blur natural boundaries between disorders: 'nosologomania'.

The phenomenological method

A particular problem is posed with clinicians' use of the term phenomenology (cf. Sass et al. 2011). The term 'phenomenology' has been used in American psychopathology in an ambiguous way for European readers: the American meaning of this term signifies concrete symptoms as they appear in clinical context, systematically collected and laid down in textbooks. They are subject to tuition and examination of medical students. Also the standardized symptom checklists for medication studies with highest inter-rater reliability are referred to as phenomenology. The term is used, however, in a different way in European psychiatry, rather opposite to the American way: in European psychopathology it refers to philosophical phenomenology as represented by Edmund Husserl and his technique of epoché or 'bracketing', i.e. to deprive an observation of all common sense meanings, intruding perceptions, and evaluations in order to get through to the very essential features of it, the 'essencies'. Jaspers doubted as did many other psychiatrists that this method can be applied in a reliable way with a high degree of congruence between investigators. And yet it is necessarily practised in a way by clinical psychiatrists when they try to open their mind to the most unusual ideas of a patient, for example, a deluded one, without declaring it as a formalized teachable technique. As an example: Mezzich (2003) writes about symptoms but means signs. Hence he confuses empathy and observation (Gupta and Kay 2002: 77). His definition of phenomenology as resting with both objective observation and aetiological inferences on one hand and empathic understanding on the other hand) misses the point of reconciling the methodological dualism referred to by Jaspers. Like authors, Mezzich (2003) just uses Jaspers' authority to lend credibility to his suggestions of a standardized systematic and comprehensive psychiatric assessment.

It appears that despite his rejection of the procedure according to phenomenological psychopathology sensu stricto, Jaspers practised a sort of epoché in many instances without declaring it as such. It can be grasped in many of his clinical descriptions and it is most obvious in his work about delusion. He elucidates differences between error and delusion, psychopathic and psychotic delusion. And, most importantly, he describes a specific nature of psychotic delusion and its relation to the personality when he claims that the psychotic delusion 'comes from the depth' of the personality. Such a statement inevitably needs 'bracketing' since common-sense understanding would focus on the absurdity of delusion; incidentally, a criterion of delusion in DSM-IV is bizarreness enriched by a quantitative component, namely the extent of common-sense absurdity.

As a consequence of his critical view on Husserl's method of 'epoché', Jaspers took a critical stance towards phenomenologists, i.e. the application of Husserl's philosophy to psychopathological phenomena and the ensuing holistic view on person, life, 'situation', and relationships of patients. What impact emerged from this rejection?

Jaspers' critique of the phenomenological perceptual methodology did not really weaken the upsurge of psychiatric phenomenology and its impact for several decades up to the present. There was some sympathy on Jaspers' side with Viktor von Weizsäcker's work which to a certain degree was inspired by phenomenology. This lasted, however, just as long as Jaspers could assume that von Weizsäcker held against psychoanalysis. When an amalgamation of both was looming, Jaspers withdrew. Hence his impact in this case was not a positive one but induced a lasting antagonistic relationship between psychoanalysis and mainstream psychiatry, as well as between mainstream psychiatry based on his psychopathology and phenomenology. Nevertheless, some psychiatric centres and single outstanding personalities in Germany, France, Italy, Switzerland, and Japan focused on phenomenology for some time in the 1950s to the end of the 1960s until the turn to biological paradigms in 1972 pushed it to the background (Spiegelberg 1972). There is, however, an unexpected happy return now with experimental neuropsychology taking an increasing interest in phenomenology.

An extensive description of the reception of phenomenology has been given by Gupta and Kay (2002): the overlap with and delineation from mainstream psychopathology with particular reference to Karl Jaspers is part of it. He asserts that current North American literature defines the method of diagnostic assessment as phenomenological. However, none of the major philosophical and psychiatric definitions of this term are reflected in North American theorizing of psychopathological assessment. Instead the term has taken on an idiosyncratic, clinical meaning of signs and symptoms. Nevertheless, phenomenology has made major contributions, mainly to self-psychology and to psychotherapy in general even in the United States. Thus, the concept of empathy within psychotherapy evidences the continuous influence of philosophical phenomenology on psychiatry. Hence phenomenology may be seen as an important complementation to the dominant North American paradigms. The author reconfirms that the term phenomenology as used by North American psychiatry does not really refer to Husserl or Jaspers who are considered as the main reference for it with regard to its application to psychiatry and psychotherapy. Husserl's 'bracketing' is not compatible with explanations relying on psychological interpretation, or on brain function.

Gupta and Kay (2002) go into details of Husserl's way of exploring essences, i.e. the essential properties of conscious phenomena: (1) investigate their core attributes, (2) determine how essences of different phenomena relate to each other, (3) determine how they appear in our consciousness. Husserl wanted, Gupta and Kay claim, to find out how we experience being in a state of consciousness and thus how consciousness itself is structured. According to Gupta and Kay, it was, paradoxically, this phenomenological method that was adapted and applied to psychopathology through Jaspers' concept of 'understanding': 'One immerses oneself, so to speak, in the patients' gestures, behaviour, expressive movements … and by accounts which they, under our guidance, give of their own experiences or of written self-experiences' (Gupta and Kay 2002: 75). Hence there are three routes to understanding (Schwartz and Wiggins 1997): The psychiatrist must transpose himself into the mental life of the patient and 'co-experience' it. These transpositions and co-experiencing constitute empathy and open access to the patient's mental state. This method necessitates in turn the elimination of any presuppositions, as regarding, for example, the cause of mental symptoms. The authors of DSM-III-R do state that the manual is 'phenomenologically descriptive'. However, 'they increasingly rely on behavioural signs since they are more reliable'. This has the 'effect of collapsing the total experience of mental disorder into specific observable behaviours'. Such a procedure excludes presuppositionlessness (Schwartz and Wiggins 1997).

The extent to which Jaspers' phenomenology is related to Husserl's is a pertaining matter of dispute. Neither the purpose nor the phenomena being investigated by Jaspers' phenomenology were similar to Husserl's. Critics claim that Husserl's phenomenology could only reveal one's own consciousness, not that of others (Gupta and Kay 2002). To Jaspers, phenomenology was defined by the process of creating a 'representation, description, definition, differentiation, and classification of individual patients experienced by means of empathy and understanding' (C. Walker, cited in Gupta and Kay 1995; 2002: 85). Jaspers believed that empathy was an imperfect but indispensable route to others' mental states. Both Husserl and Jaspers attempted to study consciousness without an explanatory model of mental contents, however, by eschewing presuppositions. It was a 'protest against reductionism' (Spiegelberg 1972, cit. in Gupta and Kay 2002: 85). It is, so to speak, the opposite of Occam's razor, namely grasping the contextual meaning of a mental phenomenon. Gupta and Kay also highlight the subtle differences in the meaning of phenomenology depending of the psychoanalytic and Kraepelinian tradition.

Ellenberger (quoted in Gupta and Kay 2002) outlined two different phenomenological methods derived from Jaspers: genetic structural and categorical phenomenology. The genetic structural method postulates a fundamental unity of factors in consciousness as common denominator or 'genetic factor', very similar to Argelander's formulation of the psychoanalytic 'core conflict', Minkowski's *trouble generateur*, Ellenberger's 'categorical analysis': a system of phenomenological coordinates referring to temporality, spatiality, causality. It is to be investigated how the patient's 'inner universe of experience' is structured. It could be argued that although derived from the patient's exploration, it is 'one step removed' from him. The authors claim that these methods deviate from Jaspers. They are abstractions of the mental state. These ideas were brought to the United States grossly by European emigrants. Spiegelberg (1972) claims that in the United States some of those ideas independently rose through Roger's teachings.

Nevertheless, according to Gupta and Kay, North American psychiatry retains some commitment to presupposition-lessness. In order to assess patients' subjective symptoms, Jaspers had suggested his 'putting oneself into the mind of the patient'. But empathy is neither an essential part of the data gathering of psychiatric assessment nor of phenomenology. In fact, the manuals attempt to sort out subjective symptoms as far as possible (Gupta and Kay 2002: 79). Therefore Gupta and Kay state that the 'phenomenological approach' to psychiatric assessment as described in US textbooks does not correspond to Jaspers' phenomenology. The dictionary definitions are somewhat broader and include subjective experiences as determinants of behaviour.

Jaspers concepts of 'putting oneself into the position of the patient' and reconstructing their state of mind has been interesting to phenomenologists as being akin to Husserl's epoché, if more simple. Kraus emphasizes the different way of talking with the patient in manual-based versus phenomenological approaches: in the former, the experience of a disorder is predefined; there is a selection by attention according to the match of criteria. Kohut, the psychoanalyst of the self, quotes Jaspers with regard to empathy: 'There is no psychological assessment without introspection and empathy' (Gupta and Kay 2002: 84). He claims that observation and empathy are achieved by 'vicarious introspection' of patient and therapist. It generates descriptive data rather than explanation, a statement close to that of Jaspers. Putting the collected information into an order is crucial. The diagnostic and psychotherapeutic process is ever intertwined and never concluded. Vicarious introspection made a genuine attempt to blend phenomenology and psychoanalysis on one side with existential phenomenology on the other side—Atwood, Mezzich, Kraus, Ellenberger, Kohut, Spiegelberg, cf. Gupta and Kay (2002).

Summing up Jaspers' impact on phenomenology and psychoanalysis it can be stated that despite his repudiation and fierce fighting against their clinical applications he himself included many of their features in his own practice and his writings (Schlimme et al. 2012). This, however, did not preclude a rather hostile relationship to both directions within the realm of psychiatry.

Limit situations

Jaspers' concept of limit situations was appealing both to existential philosophy (Kaegi 2009) and to psychiatrists (Cesana 2009). Although considered by Jaspers as not belonging to psychiatry but as being a philosophical topic of existence, it was briefly mentioned in *General Psychopathology*. The actual elaboration of the concept though was worked out in Jaspers' *Psychologie der Weltanschauungen* and *Philosophie*. The clinical application was particularly appealing to psychiatrists in the 1970s when the medical model of psychiatric illness was complemented by the elaboration of the concept of 'crisis' in order to get 'crisis-intervention' financed by health insurance companies after an attempted suicide, although an attempt of suicide was not considered a medical disease at those times. Jaspers defined limit situations as antinomies inevitably given in human existence: fight, guilt, haphazard, finality, suffer. There may be attempts for auto-protection, for example, by adopting a *Weltanschauung* or by joining a religious community. Jaspers used a metaphor to characterize this autoprotection: The 'edifice', a nut shell or oyster shell as a shelter against limit situations, however, never reliable.

The concept of limit situation induced several elaborations and adaptations to psychiatric and psychotherapeutic purposes (Mundt 2013). The most elaborate dynamic model of limit situation was presented by Kick and Dietz (Dietz and Kick 2005; Kick and Dietz 2008). They discriminate three phases: In the first one the challenge of novel ways of behaviour is still buffered by convention or repression, evading, and symptoms. In the second phase the actual crisis intensifies ambivalences and despair. Retreat, reactive down-regulation of feelings, or engagement may give relief and some security. The so-called life serving barriers—pain, shame, despair, and morale or conscientiousness—guide the transition to the third phase of either manifest psychopathology or restructuring with new values. This sequence has been exemplified by the authors by referring to ancient Greek myths. Fuchs (2008) has used the limit situation concept to elaborate 'existential vulnerability' and 'limit situation competency', for example, with the 'engagement calamity', i.e. engagement without knowing whether it will prevent, resolve, or precipitate a limit situation.

A critical stance to limit situations as prompting maturation and growth is taken by Segev (2009). In a bitter report extracted from diaries and reminiscences of Jean Amery's experience of torture in a Nazi concentration camp the incommensurability of annihilation of existence with any other of Jaspers' limit situations was asserted. In case of survival of the victim the sequelae go beyond the common concept of trauma. Von Baeyer has used the term annihilation if the person was tortured. In particular the combination of extremes of pain, humiliation, and the perspective of anonymity, being excluded and lost from human memories as an individual with personal identity, was considered as beyond a limit situation in the sense of Jaspers. In case of survival, lifelong change of personality would remain instead of a crisis instigating development.

Delusion

The diagnosis of delusion in the operationalized diagnostic manuals has readily incorporated Jaspers' three diagnostic criteria for delusion: subjective experience of unrivalled certainty, unchangeable by experience, impossibility of content. These and other aspects of delusion worked out by Jaspers suggest a view from outside the deluded assertions of a person, opposite to an empathic position, rather than contrasting the delusion with the way of thinking acceptable to common-sense beliefs. Given the striving for objectivity, assessment of symptoms determinable with high inter-rater reliability were welcome. Subjective experiential qualities of delusion, however, were less intriguing to the manuals although they are needed to establish a therapeutic relationship to the patient.

There is an obvious difference of criteria for the diagnosis of delusion in operational diagnostic manuals and Jaspers' more complex descriptions of delusion underneath those formal criteria. These variegated perspectives were recently evaluated by Brückner (2009) and Kraus (2008). Several authors contrast the definition of delusion in the manuals, for example, the criteria of false content or lack of understandability, with Jaspers' empathy in the nature of delusion as deeply rooted in the personality, emerging before reason and judgement become effective. Brückner discriminates four aspects of research on delusion: functioning, genetic understanding, phenomenological understanding, and the 'meaningful comprehensive gestalt'. The aspect of functioning refers to the instrumental emotional, intellectual, and social competencies of patients which can be trained and addressed by Socratic dialogue.

Within his second passage on phenomenological understanding, Brückner raises the interesting question whether Husserl's epoché can be used at all to examine a deluded person since a non-deluded subject is needed to delineate delusion from common-sense meaning, i.e. an external criterion is needed. However, external criteria may fail to determine delusion in cases where delusional ideas become common-sense beliefs among group members (Bell et al. 2005) or refer to cross-cultural or religious beliefs not familiar in Western countries. As a third topic, Brückner mentions Jaspers' concept of primary delusion or delusion proper and secondary delusion. Primary delusion emerges from the very roots of the personality and needs to be embedded in the personality while the secondary delusion may be a variant of real experiences confined to a specific realm of the patient's relationships or ambitions. The primary delusion needs embedding in the personality otherwise the personality would be able to cope with it. In the fourth section of his account of research topics of delusion, Brückner addresses the content and anthropological topics which give the content of delusion a certain trans-individual repetitiveness and even conformity. It may gain an archetypal quality which is embedded in artefacts as is the case with those of the Prinzhorn Collection in Heidelberg. Jaspers has acknowledged it but not without valuing (Mundt 2007).

Kraus (2008, 2009) uses Jaspers' definition of delusion to criticize the DSM and International Classification of Diseases (ICD) manuals, specifically the restriction to negative connotations as bizarre, not plausible, not understandable, not connected with usual life experience. Kraus misses the 'exhaustive inner comprehension of the psychic condition of the deluded patient' as expected by Jaspers. Also, most important but missing in the manuals, the 'encompassing whole of the personality' and life situation needs to be understood. Kraus argues for the phenomenological approach to delusion because it can define delusion positively by existential criteria.

Another application of Jaspers' concept of delusion is the rejection of the extent and confirmation of the pathological belief as particularly reliable for diagnosing. Tenacity in keeping and defending a delusion is decisive even if doubts are expressed on and off about the delusional content. Kraus combines Jaspers' descriptions and determinants of delusion with approaches from existential philosophy and psychiatry (mainly Heidegger and Binswanger), to delineate psychotic from psychopathic delusion and the latter from overvalued ideas.

To sum up the section on delusion: it is obvious that this topic is one of the most controversial ones among empirical approaches on one hand and interpretative and phenomenological ones on the other hand. Recurring to Jaspers implicitly suggests that classification restraint to measurement and objective assessment misses the actual access to the phenomena of delusion as an inner space in its own rights only accessible by reconstructing the subjective world of the patient. Jaspers seems to be particularly timely in this special field of psychopathology due to his very clear and determined statements on delusion.

Jaspers and the fine arts

Several philosophers, psychiatrists, and art historians have referred to Jaspers for comparing and analysing specific styles and thinking in modern times with psychopathological states. Louis Sass (1992) hinges his treatise on modern relativism on a statement of a schizophrenia patient quoted by Jaspers. This statement reveals alienation from common-sense meanings of language and ciphers. In modernism, Sass says, the mode of experiencing the world, the multiplicity of the self in different contexts of the lifeworld of a person may be compared with the dissolution of coherence and unity of the self in the experiences of schizophrenic patients. Sass relates typical schizophrenia symptoms such as disorders of identity, perspectivity, distance, and participation to the phenomena of alienation in modern art: the 'triumph of the sign over the object, … the affirmation of a world of signs without fault, without truth, and without active interpretation, … ephemeral concepts linked to limited contingencies' (Sass 1992: 151). John Cage and Jacques Derrida are quoted as representatives of this relativism in modern art. The analogy to schizophrenia misses, of course, the fact that diseased patients are forced into alienation, whereas the artist uses it as technique, as a play with symbols for the hidden truth still invisible and yet effective. To document this parallel Sass uses an example of a narrative of a schizophrenic patient: a partly incoherent and eventually concretistic statement of a patient who interprets the drawing of a couple (Sass 1992: 155). Sass compares this statement with some of the 'most sophisticated narratives (or anti-narratives) of our time'.

A volume edited on behalf of the late Reiner Wiehl (Hügli et al. 2009) contains several essays on art and Jaspers' concept of limit situations. Art may anticipate limit situations as in Oedipus when the chorus says 'life is a delusion, destruction of delusion is perish' (Saner 2009). According to Jaspers, art is a message which is conveyed by representation, not by speculation and thought. The ciphers for it are taken from nature. They tell a message beyond the effigy. A piece of art becomes a metaphor beyond language. It is not to be exhausted by reason (Pieper 2009; Saner 2009: 23). Nevertheless, Jaspers has indulged in pathographies about Strindberg, van Gogh, and Hölderlin. Although his interpretations of the artists' work and life history go to the very roots of their existence and perhaps also to the emergence of their art, relating art and illness as Jaspers has done with Hölderlin's phases of his illness has been abolished today by art historians (Mundt 2007). A canonical measure of assessing sneaks into the interpretation which appears as not doing justice to work and person. A similar fate could be observed with the Prinzhorn Collection which having been overlooked for decades lately received an adequate acknowledgement in its own rights without external criteria of valuing.

Critique on Jaspers and misperceptions

Clear-cut critique on Jaspers' *General Psychopathology* is rare. Some authors connect positive assessment with critical remarks. Trimble (1996) acknowledges methodological distinction between what is meaningful and what is causal. In contrast to Kraepelin, he says, Jaspers was more interested in psychopathology than in diseases. So far his statements are correct and positive. However, he then goes on that both Jaspers and Kurt Schneider favoured statistical methods for differentiating types of personality, not ideal types. Schneider, he says, continued Jaspers work. John Wing's Present State Examination was based on him. He contends that personality disorders are not understandable in Jaspers' view. It is amazing that in the section on psychoses then only Bleuler, Jung, and Kurt Schneider are mentioned, Jaspers is not even in the passage on delusion, instead Lewis is, although Jaspers' descriptive part of his work on delusion has been used for the DSM. Trimble objects to the opinion of Jaspers that neuroses encompass personality disorders and obviously misperceives the allocation of 'non-understandability' as meaning all personality disorders. McMillan et al. (2002) suggest a selection of psychopathological assessments which is based on utility instead on validity, the latter attributed to Jaspers and claiming lasting duration although swaying according to shifted paradigms.

The sharpest critic of Jaspers is Berrios (1996). In his superbly knowledgeable work on descriptive psychopathology since the nineteenth century, he quotes Jaspers 44 times, few with positive, many with critical connotations. The main dissatisfaction to Berrios with Jaspers' *General Psychopathology* is its negligence of European psychiatrists of other languages who in many instances had published similar findings and conceptualizations as Jaspers had done, often just one or two years before the publication of *General Psychopathology*. Moreover, it is reported with some disapproving connotation towards Jaspers that German emigrants brought concepts similar to his to the English-speaking countries suggesting that they had a primacy with them. Also some minor psychopathological differentiations which should be allocated to other authors were reprimanded for not being quoted with the first publishing author although Jaspers probably would not have claimed first authorship.

Berrios also casts doubt on Jaspers' competence since he was only 28 years old when writing *General Psychopathology* and had little experience with patients due to his disease, whereas Chaslin could use his stock of over 200 cases collected over 20 years of clinical work. This is certainly a point but the fair assessment of the result should count. All aspects of delusion Jaspers had described have been discussed in English psychiatry before, Berrios says. There are two faulty biographical notes (Berrios 1996: 136), one saying that Jaspers was a philosopher who started to write about psychopathology; and another one that he left revision of the subsequent editions after the third edition to Kurt Schneider. In fact, Jaspers was a physician who started his postgraduate psychiatric training as young medical doctor and clinical assistant at the psychiatric hospital of the University of Heidelberg. He revised all editions of *General Psychopathology* himself, certainly at times with fruitful exchange with Kurt Schneider, and this intensified after the Second World War. The decisive fourth edition with its enlargement and more elaborated concepts and positions was worked out over two years from 1941 to 1943, after Jaspers had been suspended from his chair by the Nazi regime. Later editions did not have significant changes.

Summary and conclusion

Growing unease in the scientific community with the philosophy of the DSM has stimulated the renewed reception of classical authors, among them Karl Jaspers. *General Psychopathology* serves as a quarry where suitable material can be gained for widening the methodological scope of psychiatry at least to a dual methodological approach and soothing the battles for the exclusively correct position. By drawing on existential philosophy Jaspers has given *General Psychopathology* a depth and background which allows reflection upon the methodological premises of the access to psychopathological information. Also the very nature of man is reflected with limit situations intrinsic to human life, as is man's open nature given the ability to transcend, an equivalent to religion.

With regard to anthropological phenomenology in the sense of Edmund Husserl, the scientific community of this field of psychopathology received only transient support from Jaspers if at all. His attitude was ambivalent at the beginning. Later, however, the school of Viktor von Weizsäcker and Mitscherlich's psychoanalysis were established with chairs at the University of Heidelberg, rigorously objected by Jaspers. Nevertheless, mainstream psychopathology returned to Jaspers for elaborating some syndromes both in understanding their nature as well as defining them by his very precise criteria apt for diagnostic manuals. Delusion is an example of it, psychotic symptoms of the self another one. The method of 'putting oneself in the position of the patient' and 'vicarious representation of the patient's self-presentation' as well as the psychiatrist's representation of it gained increasing acceptance despite its rejection for a long time due to expected low reliability.

Substantial critique on *General Psychopathology* is rare. There are some debates with phenomenologists who consider Jaspers as ephemeral. However, Jaspers declined any mingling of philosophy and psychopathology although he did not strictly stick to it given his brief remarks about limit situations in *General Psychopathology*. There are some petty remarks about his omission of quoting mainly French authors who had published similar thoughts as Jaspers a few years before. The comprehensiveness and structuring of the material is the strength and merit of *General Psychopathology* not the actual first presentation of single parts.

It is amazing that in times when concepts and perspectives in medicine are short lived a book published 100 years ago exerts such a steady influence on the scientific community. This steady interest may be an indication that *General Psychopathology* touches upon the very roots of mental life and, perhaps, with its last chapter, upon the soul as a never decipherable enigma man keeps to himself.

References

American Psychiatric Association. (1980). *Diagnostic and Statistical Manual of Mental Disorders, Third Edition.* Washington, DC: American Psychiatric Association.

Berrios, G.E. (1996). *The History of Mental Symptoms.* Cambridge: Cambridge University Press.

Bell, V., Grech, E., Maiden, C., Halligan, P.W., Ellis, H.D. (2005). '"Internet Delusions": A Case Series and Theoretical Integration', *Psychopathology*, 38: 144–150.

Bormuth, M. (2010). 'Psychiatrie als Kulturwissenschaft. Überlegungen nach Max Weber', *Nervenarzt*, **81**: 1346–1353.

Brückner, B. (2009). 'Geschichtlichkeit und Aktualität der Theorie des Wahns in der Allgemeinen Psychopathologie von Karl Jaspers', *Journal für Philosophie & Psychiatrie*, (2)3.

Bürgy, M. (2009). 'Zur Geschichte und Phänomenologie des Psychose-Begriffs. Eine Heidelberger Perspektive', *Nervenarzt*, **80**: 584–592.

Cesana, A. (2009). 'Selbstsein. Jaspers' Philosophie der Existenz und der Prozess der Subjektivierung', in A. Hügli, D. Kaegi, B. Weidmann (eds), *Existenz und Sinn. Karl Jaspers im Kontext.* Heidelberg: Winter, 73–94.

Dietz, G., Kick, H. (eds) (2005). *Grenzsituationen und neues Ethos. Von Homers Weitsicht zum modernen Weltbild.* Heidelberg: Universitätsverlag Winter.

Fuchs, T. (2008). 'Existenzielle Vulnerabilität. Ansätze zu einer Psychopathologie der Grenzsituationen', in S. Rinofner-Kreidl, H. Wiltsche (eds), *Karl Jaspers' Allgemeine Psychopathologie zwischen Wissenschaft, Philosophie und Praxis.* Würzburg: Königshausen & Neumann, 95–104.

Ghaemi, N. (2007). 'Pluralism in Psychiatry: Karl Jaspers on Science', *Philosophy, Psychiatry & Psychology*, **14**(1): 57–66.

Gupta, M., Kay, L.R. (2002). 'The Impact of "Phenomenology" on North American Psychiatric Assessment', *Philosophy, Psychiatry, & Psychology*, **9**(1): 73–85.

Hügli, A., Kaegi, D., Weidmann, B. (eds) (2009). *Existenz und Sinn: Karl Jaspers im Kontext. Festschrift für Reiner Wiehl.* Heidelberg: Verlag Winter.

Jäger, M., Frasch, K., Becker, T. (2008). 'Die Krise der operationalen Diagnostik in der Psychiatrie', *Nervenarzt*, **79**: 288–294.

Kaegi, D. (2009). 'Leiden als Grenzsituation', in A. Hügli, D. Kaegi, B. Weidmann (eds), *Existenz und Sinn. Karl Jaspers im Kontext.* Heidelberg: Winter, 57–71.

Kick, H., Dietz, G. (eds) (2008). *Verzweiflung als kreative Herausforderung: Psychopathologie, Psychotherapie und künstlerische Lösungsgestalt in Literatur, Musik und Film.* Berlin: Lit Verlag.

Koehler, H., Saß, H. (1984). *Diagnostisches und Statistisches Manual Psychischer Störungen DSM III.* Basel: Weinheim, Basel.

Kraus, A. (2008). 'Der Wahn bei Karl Jaspers im Vergleich mit der Operationalen Diagnostic (ICD-10 Kapitel V(F) und DSM-IV-Tr) sowie neueren psychopathologischen Ansätzen', in

S. Rinofer-Kreidl, H. A. Wiltsche (eds), *Karl Jaspers Allgemeine Psychopathologie zwischen Wissenschaft, Philosophie und Praxis*. Würzburg: Königshausen & Neumann, 127–145.

Kraus, A. (2009). 'Die neue Glossardiagnostik und die Allgemeine Psychopathologie von Karl Jaspers', in D. von Engelhardt, H.-J. Gerigk (eds), *Karl Jaspers im Schnittpunkt von Zeitgeschichte, Psychopathologie, Literatur und Film*. Heidelberg: Mattes, 129–136.

McMillan, J. (2002). 'Jaspers and Defining Phenomenology', *Philosophy, Psychiatry, & Psychology*, **9**(1): 91–93.

Mezzich, J.E. (2003). 'Classification of Mental Disorders: International Perspectives on Psychiatric Diagnosis', in H. I. Kaplan, B. J. Sadock (eds), *Comprehensive Textbook of Psychiatry VI* (6th edn). Baltimore, MD: Williams and Wilkins, 692–702.

Mundt, C. (2007). 'Zum Verhältnis von Kunst und Psychiatrie in Jaspers' Hölderlin-Pathographie und heute', in K. Eming, T. Fuchs (eds), *Jaspers in Moskau*. Heidelberg: Universitätsverlag Winter, 185–196.

Mundt, C. (2013). *Karl Jaspers's Concept of Limit Situations: Extensions and Applications*. Berlin: Springer.

Parnas, J., Møller, P., Kircher, T., Thalbitzer, J., Jansson, L., Handest, P., *et al.* (2005). 'EASE: Examination of Anomalous Self-Experience', *Psychopathology*, **38**: 236–258.

Pieper, A. (2009). '"Grenzen und Ursprünge." Jaspers liest Nietzsche', in A. Hügli, D. Kaegi, B. Weidmann (eds), *Existenz und Sinn. Karl Jaspers im Kontext*. Heidelberg: Winter, 120–137.

Saner, H. (2009). 'Kunst als Antizipation von der Grenzsituation', in A. Hügli, D. Kaegi, B. Weidmann (eds), *Existenz und Sinn. Karl Jaspers im Kontext*. Heidelberg: Winter, 23–36.

Sass, L. (1992). *Madness and Modernism: Insanity in the Light of Modern Art, Literature, and Thought*. New York, NY: Basic Books.

Sass, L., Parnas, J., Zahavi, D. (2011). 'Phenomenological Psychopathology and Schizophrenia: Contemporary Approaches and Misunderstandings', *Philosophy, Psychiatry, & Psychology*, **18**(1): 1–23.

Schlimme, J.E., Paprotny, T., Brückner, B. (2012). 'Karl Jaspers. Aufgaben und Grenzen der Psychotherapie', *Nervenarzt*, **83**: 84–91.

Schwartz, M.A., Wiggins, O.P. (1986). 'Logical Empirism and Psychiatric Classification', *Comprehensive Psychiatry*, **27**(2): 101–114.

Schwartz, M.A., Wiggins, O.P. (1997). 'Edmund Husserl's influence on Karl Jaspers's phenomenology', *Philosophy, Psychiatry, & Psychology*, **4**: 15–36.

Segev, A. (2009). 'Die Wut der Existenz – ein phänomenologisches Experiment im KZ', in A. Hügli, D., Kaegi, B. Weidmann (eds), *Existenz und Sinn. Karl Jaspers im Kontext*. Heidelberg: Winter, 229–237.

Spiegelberg, H. (1972). *Phenomenology in Psychology and Psychiatry. A Historical Introduction*. Evanston, IL: Northwestern University Press.

Trimble, M.R. (1996). *Biological Psychiatry* (2nd edn). New York, NY: John Wiley & Sons, 24–40.

Tucker, G. (1998). 'Putting DSM-IV in Perspective' (Editorial), *American Journal of Psychiatry*, 155: 159–161.

Weidmann, B. (2009). 'Der philosophische Glaube in der postsäkularen Gesellschaft', in A. Hügli, D. Kaegi, B. Weidmann (eds), *Existenz und Sinn. Karl Jaspers im Kontext*. Heidelberg: Winter, 239–278.

Section 2

Methodological issues and concepts

Chapter 5

Karl Jaspers' *General Psychopathology* in the framework of clinical practice

Otto Doerr-Zegers and Héctor Pelegrina-Cetrán

Karl Jaspers' *General Psychopathology* is a monumental work. It encompasses all areas of psychiatry and delves intelligently and deeply into psychology and philosophy. Its influence in the German speaking world was immediate and remains so today. There is practically no work of psychopathology or even of general psychiatry written by a German author that is not inspired in its analyses or which criticizes Jaspers. Its impact on the rest of the world has been directly dependent on the translations. The first one was into French, in 1933, the Spanish one appeared in 1955, and the Italian in 1964. The knowledge of his work in the English-speaking world had to wait for the excellent translation by Hoenig and Hamilton of 1963. However, its influence has been rather scarce, being limited in the United States to only some names, such as Paul McHugh (McHugh and Slavney 1983; Slavney and McHugh 1987), Michael Schwartz (Schwartz and Wiggins 1985, 1987a, 1987b; Wiggins and Schwartz 1988) and Nassir Ghaemi (2003), and in England, to the trace left by the German immigrant Wilhelm Mayer-Gross (1954/1974), who was a member of the so-called Heidelberg School until 1933. In Spain, the case we know best, Jaspers' influence was felt prior to the translation, since the great masters of Spanish psychiatry of the first half of the twentieth century had studied in Germany and knew Jaspers' work from their first editions. Examples of renowned Spanish psychiatrists with extensive training in Germany and who taught *General Psychopathology* in their universities are Juan José López-Ibor Sr. (1966), from Madrid and Ramón Sarró (1987), from Barcelona. In Latin America his influence began to be noted as soon as the translation appeared, with the exception of Peru, where the doctor who was professor of generations of Peruvian psychiatrists, Honorio Delgado (1966), had been trained in Germany before the Second World War, and knew Jaspers' work extensively.

Jaspers' greatest achievement was to establish psychopathology as a hard science, the basis of psychiatry as professional practice. And he did this from a strictly methodological perspective, looking for the rigorous exploration and categorization of psychic disturbances to replace the pre-existing semiologies operating according to the model of medicine of that time. 'Nobody before him was able to establish the relationship between the peculiarities of a methodology and the field of reality opened through it' (Blankenburg 1984: 448). Now, in order to give psychopathology a scientific character, Jaspers structured it adopting a deeply critical attitude, coinciding with modern epistemology, according to which what distinguishes these two types of knowledge—scientific and common—is not so much rigour of scientific methods and submission to the epistemological rules, as the critical attitude of science faced with the naivety of common knowledge (see Bunge, 1980: 43–45). But Jaspers goes beyond methodological criticism replacing the analytical attitude—proper for the science of that time—with a synthetic one, which is the paradigm at present. He always considers the patient and his psychopathological manifestations within the horizon of the totality of existence:

> Whenever the object studied is Man and not man as a species of animal, we find that psychopathology comes to be not only a kind of biology, but also one of the Humanities. With psychiatry the doctor enters a world which lies outside the other disciplines with which he is already familiar. The fundamentals of his education generally consist of chemistry, physics and physiology, but here he is in need of a different basic training […] the psychopathologist, who is concerned with the human being as a whole and more especially the human being in times of sickness. (Jaspers 1997: 36)

But our present question is about the effects of Jaspers' psychopathology on clinical practice in the last 100 years. Let us consider that this topic is so broad and deep that it would be practically impossible to summarize it in a few pages. The only way will be to focus on some of his contributions, such as, for example, the introduction of phenomenology and of the method of understanding, the concepts of process and development, the concept of situation, and the dialectic perspective in psychopathology.

The introduction of phenomenology in psychopathology and in clinical practice

Conditioned by his time, Jaspers introduced the phenomenological method for grasping 'the subjective manifestations of ill psychic life' (Jaspers 1997: 55). As is well known, he accepted only the first step of phenomenology, the descriptive moment, and he declined to take the next step, in search for essences, considering it of a philosophical or metaphysical character and consequently, not scientific:

> The term phenomenology was used by Hegel for the whole field of mental phenomena as revealed in consciousness, history and conceptual thought. We use it only for the much narrower field of individual psychic experience. Husserl used the term initially in the sense of 'a descriptive psychology' in connection with the phenomenon of consciousness; in this sense it holds for our own investigations also, but later on he used it in the sense of 'the appearance of things' (*Wesensschau*) which is not a term we use in this book. Phenomenology is for us purely an empirical method of inquiry. (Jaspers 1997: 55).

In a very striking study, Berrios goes beyond Jaspers himself, postulating that his phenomenology has little to do with that of Husserl: 'It would seem, therefore that there is little evidence that Husserlian phenomenology had a major influence on Jaspers' (Berrios 1992: 320). We don't completely share Berrios' conclusions. We rather think that Jaspers' philosophical intuition of Husserl's phenomenological way opened the doors, in psychopathology, to overcoming both idealism of conscience on the one hand and sensorial empiricism on the other. Furthermore, several of Jaspers statements show proximity with respect to the intuition of essences. Thus, for example, he states: 'Phenomenology, then, deals with what is actually experienced. It views psychic events "as from within," and brings them into immediate realization'[1] (Jaspers 1912/1968: 1322). Also in the phenomenological procedure of delimiting psychopathological phenomena and isolating them, Jaspers established them 'in order': 'an order[2] which will arrange psychic phenomena according to their phenomenological affinities with each other, somewhat in the way that infinite numbers of colours are arranged in the spectrum in a manner which is phenomenologically satisfying' (Jaspers 1912/1968: 1320). Such order cannot but allude to a vision of the essence of what is observed. Other statements by Jaspers which show us how he, in spite of his prejudice faced with this transcendental moment of Husserl's phenomenology, was quite close to his method, include the following: 'Phenomenology only makes known to us the different forms in which all our experiences, psychic reality, take place' (Jaspers 1912/1968: 1323). Or: 'Close contemplation of an individual case often teaches us of phenomena common to countless others' (Jaspers 1963/1997: 56). These forms, as well as this 'common', surely do not correspond to inductive generalizations of empirical findings, starting from the observation of a multiplicity of cases, but to the intuitive grasping of the eidos in the sense of Husserl.

Now, why was Jaspers' introduction of phenomenology to psychopathology and to psychiatric practice so important? First, because he introduced into the empirical study of psychopathological phenomena the subjective experiences of the patients without objectifying them in sensorially perceivable data, that is to say, without converting them into mere signs to be grasped by a semiologist. This was all the more significant, as the scientific attitude of that time consisted of eliminating the patient as observer and as subject of judgements about his own psychic phenomena; an intention to discard symptoms and be guided only by signs. Jaspers tells us: 'An experience is best described by the person who has undergone it. Detached psychiatric observation with its own formulation of what the patient is suffering is not any substitute for this'. And shortly afterwards, he says: 'The patients themselves are the observers' (Jaspers 1997: 55). This is very much in accordance with Husserl's phenomenological attitude and, on the other hand, is very much in accordance with the new paradigm of science, as, for example, with the transition from classical ethnology to cultural anthropology, which distinguishes between a primary observer, a member of the observed culture, and a secondary observer, who participates in the cultural world being studied so that he can grasp the real sense of the behavioural features in the life of 'that' culture.

The phenomenological approach to patients, introduced by Jaspers, became established in clinical practice as a new general operating framework. Clinical psychiatrists could no longer ignore a patient's subjective experiences because they were not scientifically reliable, as in the previous semiology. Moreover, these experiences became the fundamental object of phenomenological investigation both in the field of endogenous psychoses and of neuroses. From the feeling of threat in the phobic situation and the formal obsessions

1 Michael Schwartz has proposed 'representation' for the German word *Vergegenwärtigung*, with which we completely agree.

2 In the English version which appeared in the *British Journal of Psychiatry* (1968), the word '*Ordnung*' is translated as 'classification'. We widely prefer the word 'order', because it fits much better the sense of the German word.

of an obsessive–compulsive disorder up to the experience of destruction of the world in catatonia or of loss of natural evidence in some schizophrenias (Blankenburg 1971), all of these fields deal with subjective experiences. Thus, all clinicians, in order to be able to differentiate a psychopathological structure from another and these from normality, study the personal and intimate way in which patients constructed their forms of relationship with objects and with other persons. The personal forms of intentionality—the intimate way of affecting or being affected by life situations—are what determine the specific pathological character of each symptom.

This reciprocal respectivity between the human individual and his situation constitutes precisely the central concept of Husserl's phenomenological intentionality, which inaugurated the replacement of the gnoseological objectivist vision for a dialectic-communicational one. Jaspers introduced it explicitly in his work: 'In all developed psychic life we find the confrontation of a subject with an object and the orientation of a self towards a content as an absolutely basic phenomenon' (Jaspers 1997: 57). This is a bi-univocal relationship:

> But the state of self-awareness and the objective aspects of that 'other,' to which the self directs itself, interlock in a mutual movement whereby the 'self' is caught up by what is given externally and is at the same time driven internally to grasp at what is there. Description of what is objective leads on to the meaning of this for the self and a description of the states of the self (emotional states, moods, drives) turns into a description of the objective aspects under which these states become apparent. (Jaspers 1997: 57–58)

Here 'the self' and 'the object' are not entities 'in themselves', constituted prior to the ulterior relationship between them. Rather, the form of interaction subject/object, 'intentionality', is the one that constitutes the way of being of the comprehensive phenomenon of experience.

Psychiatric phenomenology introduced by Jaspers opened the way, in the second half of the twentieth century, for some notable psychopathologists, who incorporated elements from the late Husserl, that of the lifeworld, from Heidegger and from Merleau-Ponty, and applied a hermeneutic phenomenology. This meant an advance from the subjective experiences of the patient up to the essential structures underlying psychopathological manifestations. In the phenomenological-anthropological and/or phenomenological-existential orientation, authors such as L. Binswanger (1947, 1957), E. Straus (1960), von Gebsattel (1954), H. Tellenbach (1961), and W. Blankenburg (1971) stand out. In a previous paper (Doerr-Zegers 2000) we showed in detail some of the extraordinary contributions these authors have made to psychopathology and to psychiatry. But none of this would have been possible without the fundamental change launched by Jaspers when he introduced into psychopathological sciences both the subject of the patient and the subject of the explorer. His psychopathology introduced a dialogic, interactive way, in the exploration as well as in the conception of psychopathological structures. The symptoms are structures of the meaning of life built and interpreted by the patient (Pelegrina 2006: 55–62). However, Jaspers could not overcome some prejudices of his time. Thus, he insists, for example, on differentiating 'form' from 'content' too strictly. And he adds that 'phenomenologically we are interested only in forms', while 'the psychologist who looks for meaning will find content essential and the form at times unimportant' (Jaspers 1997: 59). This distinction has tended to disappear and thus, investigations into the perception of *Gestalt* psychology have showed the intimate relationship and the mutual influence of content (or meaning) over perceptual forms and of forms over content. Something similar occurs in *Phenomenology of Perception* by Merleau-Ponty (1945). Other works of phenomenological-anthropological orientation have also demonstrated the intimate relationship existing between the content and the form. Thus, Häfner and Wieser (1953) could show the formal conditions under which a given theme ceases being experienced as desire, thought, or representation and is transformed into a hallucination (change of form), which would be conceived as a perception separated from the Self. For his part, Kisker (1960), through psychotherapeutic experiences with schizophrenics, was able to prove in an almost experimental way how through the recovery process the hallucination began to be transformed into thought hearing, then into forced thinking, finally ending as normal and fully accepted representations.

In any case, Jaspers' phenomenology, for the reasons stated earlier, is much closer to the modern developments of ontology and epistemology of the life sciences, from biology itself (Jonas 2001; Luisi 2006) up to the cognitive (Varela 1991) passing through ethology (Lorenz 1978) and linguistics (Apel 2003). His phenomenology also coincides with contemporary philosophy, which does not happen with the prevailing psychiatry of pragmatic-empiricist orientation. Under the sway of the later, 'logical positivistic' constructs predominate, with each symptom objectified and transformed into a sign caused by a supposed brain disease or dysfunction. The consequence is a blurring of the profile of the nosological unities or entities and an inordinate increase of comorbidities (Cole et al. 2008; Farmer and McGuffin 1989; Kessler et al. 1996; Parker 2006). In psychopathology it is impossible to know what the structures of the symptoms of a particular patient mean without exploring the entire situation in which the symptom appears. Only from the totality of sense of behaviour is it possible to unveil and to discover the processes of the genesis of psychopathological structures, be these of a biological, psychological, or sociological nature. This perspective, which starts from the 'self-constructive (*autopoietic*) unity of life' (Pelegrina 2006: 157), as a general system and behaviour generator, can today represent Jaspers' key concept of the totality of human being and his life, as the horizon of all psychopathological research.

The introduction of the method of understanding

Every experienced psychiatrist will be able to recognize how often psychopathological phenomena surpass the possibilities of natural sciences, e.g. by attempting to 'explain' delusion with the energetic theory of psychoanalysis or through measurement of neurotransmitters. Following Dilthey (1955), Jaspers (1912/1968, 1913, 1959/1997, 1963: 301) was early to recognize this particularity of the psychopathological world when he separated precisely what is explainable from what is understandable. With the method of explanation we approach clinical reality in the manner in which physicists study matter, and thus we calculate the size of cerebral ventricles, quantify intellectual capacity, or measure the concentration of catabolites of neurotransmitters in urine, etc. With the method of understanding, by contrast, we have access to phenomena which resist all attempts to quantify them, such as feelings and emotions, the experience of art in general, the world of interpersonal atmospheres, etc., that is, all the world of meaning. How one psychic phenomenon arises from another is something very different from the linear causality of the physical world, and the method of understanding intends to do justice to that difference. To be able to understand the biographical sense of a given illness, or to interpret a delusion within itself and not from supposed extraconscious causalities, are two typical tasks where the psychiatrist has to employ the methods of understanding and hermeneutics in their purest forms. But we have to warn that Jaspers' understanding/explanation distinction is not so valid anymore if one looks at it from the perspective of the new paradigm of natural sciences, also called the paradigm of 'complexity'. The historical evolution of epistemology in the twentieth century has drawn the explanatory methods close to the one of understanding (Hawking and Mlodinow 2010; Kuhn 1970).

To be able to appreciate the value of the introduction by Karl Jaspers of the method of understanding in psychopathology, it is necessary to consider the theoretical postulates of psychiatry of his time. Starting from the nineteenth century and following a period of romantic medicine where passions, faults, and feelings had been crucial in interpreting the genesis of mental diseases, a change of paradigm toward positivism and empiricism took place, which reached its greatest development with Griesinger (1817–1868). This author, when he was only 25 years old, had proclaimed: 'Medical practice has taken leave of empty speculation and finally overcome romantic medicine' (cited by Schifferdecker and Peters 1995) and years later he would formulate his famous principle: 'Mental diseases are brain diseases'. This psychiatry dealt with defining syndromes and then searching for their localization in some brain area. Progressive general paralysis became, consequently, the perfect model, the idea of disease which was completed when its cause, *Treponema pallidum*, was discovered in 1905. Now, in the framework of this organicistic psychiatry arose the figure of Kraepelin, who went beyond the mere register of symptoms, up to the intuition of nosological entities, whose differences he tried to establish on the basis of following the outcome of the disease. And thus he distinguished dementia praecox from manic-depressive illness, because besides the different symptomatology the first evolves toward deterioration and the other towards more or less spontaneous healing. The great nosological problem posed to Kraepelin was that of paranoia, because this illness consisted in a delusion which evolved progressively, such as dementia praecox, but which did not cause deterioration and in that sense resembled manic-depressive illness although with none of its other symptoms.

In reality, Karl Jaspers introduced his concept of understanding and of meaningful psychic connections in 1910, in a work prior to the first edition of *General Psychopathology* (1913), referring specifically to paranoia. It is here for the first time that he distinguishes between static and genetic understanding, on which he would elaborate extensively in his *General Psychopathology*. The first is equivalent to descriptive phenomenology, to which we have already referred and the second would take two forms, the rational and the psychological. Rational understanding allows us to grasp the reasons for which someone acts in one way or another. Psychological understanding, by contrast, captures or intuits how the psychic arises from the psychic: 'When somebody knows that his beloved has been unfaithful with him […], and he falls into a deep desperation and thinks of suicide, we cannot invoke any rational context, there is no purpose to reach for, there are no means to which one appeals with some rationality, and instead, we understand everything by empathy' (Jaspers 1910/1963: 113). To these two forms of understanding Jaspers juxtaposes the 'grasping' (*Begreifen*) of causal relationships, which is analogous to causal relationships prevailing in nature. The maturative processes would be an example of it. Writing prior to the famous work by Gaupp about the Wagner case (1914, 1921) and of the description of the 'Sensitive Delusion of Reference' by Kretschmer (1918/1950), Jaspers states in this foundational article the notion that unlike dementia praecox, which would not be an understandable process, paranoia belongs to the developments category, since delusional ideas, for example, jealousy, would be 'understandable' from the previous personality and also from certain biographical situations. He does acknowledge that there are cases of paranoia that lie between the incomprehensibility of process and the comprehensibility of development. In the next section we will delve deeply into the question of Jaspers' distinction between process and development (see 'The concepts of process and development'). In any case, it is of some interest that in an environment that largely ignored psychology (at least in the field of psychoses) as that prevailing in German psychiatry at the beginning of the twentieth century, Jaspers affirmed the possibility of understanding a psychosis. The only precursor of this more 'psychological' vision of paranoia is the German psychiatrist Heinrich Schüle, who in the first edition of his treatise of 1878 ignores paranoia, but in an 1894 work states, 'the nature and essence of these processes is purely psychological; they are based on thought itself and consequently, they are only psychologically explainable' (cited by Schifferdecker and Peters 1995).

But the problem of understanding, as Jaspers states it, has several weaknesses. In the first place, the fact that it assumes that a community of supposedly healthy persons feel in a similar way in a given sets of circumstances and for that reason they can empathize with what others feel. Second, although the dichotomy comprehensibility/incomprehensibility is based on a 'subjective' incapacity, not being able to understand is transformed into a diagnostic criterion pretending to be 'objective'. Different authors of the psychoanalytical, anthropological, and existential-analytical tradition have questioned this dichotomy (Binswanger 1955: 67–104, 1961: 190–217; Kisker 1963), because psychotherapeutic experiences with schizophrenic patients, for example, have shown that what initially seemed incomprehensible is shown in all its biographical sense in the course of the treatment. But the biggest difficulty with Jaspers' concept of understanding and/or of comprehensibility is that it remains stuck in something like a day-to-day or 'average' understanding. It would be possible, for example, to broaden that horizon and to understand the delusion from the perspective of the psychology of Gestalt psychology, as Conrad did (1958) or from that of existential analysis, in the sense of Binswanger (1957). For this author, the schizophrenic can be shown to us as the specific modification of the a priori structures of Dasein and what in empiricist or even in Jaspers' psychiatry is called symptom, will acquire from the perspective of the Self-world unit the character of the phenomenon containing the world and the Self, since in transcendence not only is the aim of transcending the world constituted, but also the transcended itself, the entity we are in each case. And thus complex and central phenomena of schizophrenia, namely eccentricity (Binswanger 1956) or catatonic postures can be open to understanding. But as transcendence takes root in time, in its evolution from the past to the future, life history acquires great importance in existential analysis. And thus, not only the clinical picture of schizophrenia appears to us as a single meaningful structure, but we can also look into the past for the genesis of these progressive limitations ending in that new image of the world which is psychosis. Existential analysis wonders about lighting, consistency, harmony, temporality, and the spatiality of psychosis and about the characteristics of the world projects which were the condition of possibility of the respective psychotic worlds (see Doerr-Zegers 1997). The authors of the phenomenological-anthropological school have also made fundamental contributions to the knowledge of psychoses insofar as they broke through the limits of Jaspers' comprehensibility, but without the absolute commitment of Binswanger to Heidegger's philosophy. These authors have applied the phenomenological method to the study of psychotic forms in the search for underlying disturbances of fundamental anthropological structures of human being and also of meaningful correlations between life history, previous situation, and psychotic symptoms themselves in a double hermeneutic and psychotherapeutic eagerness. Examples of it are the studies by Zutt (1958) about the paranoid syndrome, by Kulenkampff (1964) about the psychotic crises of adolescence, by Häfner (1959) about hypochondria, by Tellenbach (1961) and Kraus (1977) about melancholy, by Mundt (1984) and Fuchs (2007, 2010) about intentionality in schizophrenia, by Doerr-Zegers (2010) about language disturbances in schizophrenia.

A way to broaden Jaspers' concept of comprehensibility without having to appeal to other paradigms, such as the psychoanalytical or the analytical-existential ones, has been proposed by Blankenburg (1984) in his critical comment to Karl Jaspers' psychopathology. He wonders: 'To what exactly are we referring by speaking of incomprehensibility when faced with a schizophrenic patient?' And he answers himself that this does not mean an impossibility to interpret something, but rather that a person 'does not know how to relate' to the other and consequently is not able to 'make somebody understand'. To be 'mad' or 'insane' (*verrückt*) does not mean that a given behaviour is not intelligible, but only that it is not intersubjectively referred. This being intersubjectively referred as criterion of comprehensibility or incomprehensibility would represent a great advantage, since it restores to these concepts their value in differential diagnosis (between the psychotic and the not psychotic, for example), but without limiting the attempts of psychotherapeutic understanding. And Blankenburg concludes: 'Then, justice could be done to Jaspers' theorem in the sense that it becomes a starting point of a differentiated study of the modifications of intersubjective reference of human experience and/or behaviour' (Blankenburg 1984: 456).

The concepts of process and development

Jaspers introduced the dichotomy process/development in the earlier mentioned article of 1910, in relation to the detailed clinical and biographical study of several cases of jealousy. It is in this article where he also introduces, as we saw, the method of understanding. Strictly, the concept of process comes from somatic medicine. Its application to psychopathology does not pose difficulties when it is a matter of organic-cerebral diseases, such as Alzheimer disease or progressive general paralysis. What occurs here at a psychological level is understood as epiphenomenon of a destructive corporal process. Psychiatry prior to Jaspers also applied this concept to dementia praecox, since this had in common with the organic diseases the beginning in a given moment and the evolution towards some degree of defect or residual state. Moreover, many of the symptoms of what later was called schizophrenia, such as affective flattening or social deterioration, showed certain similarities with what is observed in organic diseases. The fact that the corresponding anatomical-pathological alteration had not yet been proven did not seem a problem, because it was expected to be found later on. Paranoia is what posed a problem, because on the one hand, it gave the impression of 'primary madness', but on the other, it compromised only the content of some ideas (delusions), leaving the remaining functions undamaged.

Kraepelin began to change his definition of paranoia throughout the nine editions of his 'Treatise', but by the fourth (1893) he states the contradiction inherent in this illness of being manifested by 'the chronic development of a persistent delusional system with normal presence of mind'. In the eighth, in 1915, he would specify this contradiction, saying: 'with perfect conservation of clarity and the order of thought, will and action' (cited by Schmidt-Degenhard 1998). Two years later Krüger (1917, cited in Schifferdecker and Peters 1995: 246) would add new elements to this definition, and it has not been surpassed. He also speaks of a delusional system, but:

> Which is constructed and developed logically, which does not occur outside the realm of possibility, which does not generally alter the subject personality apart from a narrowing of his sphere of interest […] which finally does not affect the subject's perception in areas which are not important to the delusional system […] A complete transformation or destruction of the personality does not occur […] even within the delusion, however, the subject's thought remains as comprehensible and logical as the thought of a healthy person and his decisions and actions are logically and clearly derived.

But the great investigator of paranoia was Gaupp, who studied and followed the evolution of a particular case, Ernst Wagner, throughout almost 30 years. At the end of his monograph of 1914 he affirms that Ernst Wagner suffers from 'paranoia', that is, 'a form of mental perturbation gradually developing from the personality and on the basis of degeneration' (Gaupp 1914: 185). As we stated earlier, Gaupp expressly considered paranoia, following Jaspers, as a 'psychologically understandable' development.

In his article, and after an introduction in which he talks about the different forms of jealousy, Jaspers first reports two cases in great detail. In the comment, he states: 'These two clinical histories seem to demonstrate what has frequently been denied, that there are cases which match the definition of paranoia provided by Kraepelin' (1910/1963: 112). Then he proceeds to develop his method of understanding by empathy, previously mentioned, and to establish the differences between a process and a development: 'There where we are not able to grasp the single nature of the development of a personality, there where we find out something new, something heterogeneous with respect to the original disposition, something that does not correspond to the development [of a personality], then it is a process' (Jaspers 1910/1963: 116). And later he adds that 'we call not all pathologic diseases process, but only those leading to a persisting and incurable change' (Jaspers 1910/1963: 117). To provide a distinction from process, he defines development as follows: 'We speak of a development when from an interaction of psychological and rational connections we can understand or explain phenomena which for some reason have been considered pathologic and that in spite of their lack of consistency and harmony are integrated in a uniform psychological context'. And he continues: 'It may be that we have an extreme variation, but the unity of personality in its peculiarity, from growing up to involution, appears conserved' (Jaspers 1910/1963: 116).

Now, the problem Jaspers faced was that when analysing the two mentioned cases of jealousy, he found that delusional jealousy appears accompanied by delusional ideas of persecution and of poisoning and that there is no continuity between life history and psychosis. It is then that he creates his concept of 'psychic process', which forms a boundary concept between the physic-psychotic process inherent in organic-cerebral syndromes and the development of a personality as it is observed in some 'psychopathies' (the generic name given then to personality disorders). In this original work the relationship of nosological entities schizophrenia and paranoia with the concepts of process and development is not clear. In a first approach and as we stated with respect to the introduction of the method of understanding, it seemed that schizophrenia is a process and paranoia more a development. But the symptomatology of the first two cases described by Jaspers greatly exceeds the clinical picture of Kraepelin's paranoia and besides, they do not present that fundamental element of development of a personality, which is the sense of continuity with the life history. On the other hand, they do not present auditory hallucinations or formal alterations of thought, and thus cannot be diagnosed as schizophrenia. Furthermore, cases 3 and 4 present many of the characteristics of paranoia and would fit well into the concept of development, but in a given moment the 'meaningful connections' disappear and 'unconnected delusional ideas' arise (Jaspers 1910/1963: 130–131). Only case number 7, identified as Friedmann's 'light paranoia' by Jaspers himself, seems to match the concept of development of a personality. At the end of the article Jaspers becomes a little sceptical and states: 'And thus, it seems that the criteria for considering delusional jealousy as "development of a personality" or "process" mingle with the predominance of the latter'. And he adds: 'This cannot surprise us, since, as we saw, every life development is a process in which meaningful and rational connections are integrated, but "the process" of normal life can be conceived as a development to the degree that one can grasp in it the unity of the personality' (Jaspers 1910/1963: 140).

In any case, in spite of the fact that these concepts depend on other things, acknowledged, as we saw, by Jaspers himself, they are still used in clinical practice up to the present. And thus, even when they do not appear in the modern systems of classification and diagnosis, such as the fourth revised edition of the *Diagnostic and Statistical Manual of Mental Disorders* (DSM-IV-TR) and the tenth revision of the International Classification of Diseases (ICD-10), many psychiatrists who treat psychotic patients continue speaking of 'process' to refer to schizophrenia and of 'development' to refer to those pictures, now called 'delusional disturbances' that correspond approximately to the different forms of classical paranoia. Notably, five decades ago, German psychiatrist Heinz Häfner proposed a new and interesting way of conceiving of the concepts of process and development, which unfortunately has not gained the publicity it deserves. Häfner starts by pointing out the inadequacy for pathology of the term 'development', given its positive connotation. Next, appreciating its fickleness and ambiguity in the court of somatic medicine, he sets aside Jaspers' concept of a physico-psychotic process. Then, he looks for the broadest possible definition of the concept of process in psychopathology: 'Psychic process is a progressive event necessarily leading to a pathologic defect in the functional capacity of the individual' (Jaspers 1910/1963: 408). Finally, basing himself on Viktor von Gebsattel's important work (1954), Häfner states that addictions, some personality disorders, sexual perversions, and in a certain way obsessive–compulsive neurosis can also represent a form of process, since all these pictures lead to an important, progressive and somehow irrevocable limitation of the ability of an individual to realize his existence. Häfner does distinguish two types of processes, the 'modifying' and the 'restrictive' ones. The former are accompanied by modifications of basic structures of the human, such as interpersonality, spatiality or temporality. This is what occurs in schizophrenias, in schizo-affective psychoses, and in paraphrenias. The second, by contrast, lead to a narrowing of the existence around a theme, such as paranoid delusional jealousy, severe addiction to drugs or to alcohol, etc. The concept of a modifying process is self-explanatory. The manifestations of schizophrenia, for example, cannot be reduced to auditory hallucinations or to delusional ideas. Several authors of the phenomenological-anthropological orientation have been able to demonstrate up to what point the anthropological and constitutive structures of human being are altered in this disease (Binswanger 1957; Blankenburg 1971; Doerr-Zegers 1970, 1997; Gebsattel 1954; Kisker 1963). The restrictive processes, by contrast, require clarification which we will summarize here. Why apply the concept of process to certain forms of addiction or 'philias', as Pelegrina (2006) calls them? What drugs do is to fill an existential emptiness or deficiency. However, drowsiness and the illusory satisfaction of the sensation of void do not last long, and with their end, the same emptiness, which generally occurs upon either the omission of a task or of an actual achievement, is again manifest in an even clearer way. Furthermore, unlike the initial surrender to drugs, feelings of guilt are now added to the emptiness and therefore, the feeling of failure or uneasiness is greater. The compulsion to again consume a drug arises as a consequence. Häfner comments:

> The longer the empirical performance of tasks and possibilities is omitted and emptiness is covered only in an illusory way, the more pronounced will be the distance between real failure (for example, social decline or isolation) and the apparent satisfaction brought by the drug. Herewith this destructive condition, which at the beginning still left some room for a certain freedom, gradually becomes need and compulsion, that is to say, process. (Häfner 1963: 403)

The concept of situation

In Jaspers' time, substantialism was still the dominant thought, which meant that entities, things, were considered realities 'in themselves', whose being is constituted by their inalterable, atemporal 'essence', which in its essence is identical in appearing and metamorphosing. Things would eventually have the capacity of relating to others as external causes of effects on them. This ontology also included, of course, the human being, who was considered as 'in himself' and 'from himself'. Man as substance had been viewed for many centuries as a spiritual being, removed from the materiality of things and who could relate to them, or rather, whose agreement with the world was sustained by God. During the nineteenth century science began to replace God with the absolute universality of scientific laws, and the spiritual essence of man was in turn replaced by an entity, 'consciousness'. The latter confers form to the material given by the senses, thus constructing its 'objects' of consciousness. This consciousness is exposed to the world and is somehow affected by it, provoking in each case a 'reaction'. Strictly, the I-world, subject-object, consciousness-situation relationship was conceived according to the physiological model of stimulus and response. In fact, at that time and until a few decades ago, one talked about 'abnormal experiential reactions', and Jaspers himself used that terminology.

However, in his work *Philosophy* (1932) Jaspers elaborates a new concept of situation, which he later complements with another very important one for his philosophy of liberty, which is that of the 'limit situation'. Even earlier, in his *General Psychopathology* (1913, 1959, 1997) he had dedicated a page to the concept of situation in the chapter about the relationship man-world: 'All life takes place in its own particular surroundings. In abstract physiological terms we say stimulus causes reaction. In real life, the situation releases activity, and gives birth to performance and experience' (Jaspers 1997: 325). Jaspers goes on to explain the manner in which the behaviour of the individual with respect to typical situations becomes an object of the psychology of meaning, and 'the way in which coincidence, opportunity and destiny come to us through the situation itself and how to grasp or lose them' (Jaspers 1997: 325). In this handful of quotes one can appreciate the manner in which

Jaspers' concept of situation moves away from the scheme stimulus-reaction. There is a participation of the subject both in the creation and in the overcoming of it: 'Situations have urgency, their sequence is changeable and unfixed, and the human being can contrive them' (Jaspers 1997: 325). In his *Philosophy*, Jaspers adds new elements to his concept of situation, for example, stating: 'Although, as empirical existence, I am always in situations in which I act or let myself be carried, nonetheless, not for that reason do I know the situations in which in fact I am' (Jaspers 1958: 65). Later he emphasizes this idea, when he writes: 'Empirical existence is a being in situation, I can never get out of a situation without immediately entering into another [...] My action is presented to me with its consequences, in turn as a situation created by me, which is already given' (1958: 66). These considerations are fully in accordance with the deployment of phenomenology starting since the 1940s.

The importance of Jaspers' concept of situation relies on the fact that it is going to represent the model on the basis of which both E. Kretschmer and H. Tellenbach would eventually construct their respective concepts of 'key situation' and 'pre melancholic situation'. In his book *The Sensitive Delusion of Self-reference* (1918/1950), Kretschmer proposes the idea of the existence of an essential relationship between previous personality, psychosis, and triggering situation, which he calls key situation: 'The sensitive delusion of self-reference arises by the accumulative action of typical experiences or life situations, upon typical characterological and constitutional bases, and frequently under the complementary effect of equally typical social constellations' (Kretschmer 1918/1950: 148). Jaspers (1910) and then Gaupp (1914) had already posed the connection or rather the continuity between personality and psychosis in relation to paranoia, but Kretschmer added the concept of a specific triggering situation, which he defines as of 'bashful insufficiency' which was to be crucial in pathogenesis: 'In typical cases the experience or life situation underlying it means everything and without it the illness would be reduced to nothing' (Kretschmer 1918: 148). It was clearly a big step for psychiatry that Kretschmer proposed that a person's key situation has a leading and even causal role in the genesis of a psychosis, since previous authors, such as Kraepelin and Gaupp himself, spoke only of the possibility of understanding the content and not the form, that is, the existence itself of the psychosis. Thus, Kraepelin writes: 'Its content [of paranoia] shows, although in a pathologic way, a notable correspondence with fears, wishes and hopes also arising in healthy persons from the feeling of insecurity and the aspiration to freedom' (1915: 1758).

But undoubtedly we owe thanks to Hubertus Tellenbach (1961, 1980) for his magnificent contribution to the relationship between mental illness, personality, and life situation. Tellenbach's starting point is Jaspers', in the sense that a human situation does not consist only of the action of environmental circumstances over the subject, but also in the action of the subject over the circumstances. According to Jaspers: 'The decision whether a situation is made by a surrounding world or by the individual derives mainly from his knowledge and will: whether he is affected without knowledge by the situation or whether his self-confident will effect it' (Tellenbach 1961, 1980: 132). But Tellenbach goes farther when he states: 'We take the situative as that originality in which the individual and his inner surround are still united [...] Situation is always a cross-section through the existing context of I and world' (Tellenbach 1980: 132). For Tellenbach it is not only that I voluntary can face a situation caused by the environment and alter it (Jaspers' idea), but that I am creating specific typical situations starting from my way of being, from my personality. And thus, the pre depressive personality of unipolar patients, which he called *typus melancholicus,* fundamentally characterized by a fixation to order (orderliness), by a peculiar way of having an order and of being in an order, will tend to go downhill in those situations in which that order is menaced. Tellenbach adds: '[…] always when this order is seriously threatened, this threat will affect the existence itself'. And he continues: 'The specific situation of order is then ready to revert into a situation of disorder, a phase we have occasionally and as yet indeterminately termed "the pre melancholic situation"' (Tellenbach 1980: 135). And this will constitute the starting point of the endogenous-melancholic transformation. This way of framing the situation has allowed us to understand those cases where the pre-depressive situation is presented to a person with an average understanding as something positive, for example, a move to a better house or a promotion at work. The vision of melancholy which Tellenbach poses for us is very comprehensive, from the previous personality and its genesis up to a new understanding of the symptoms of illness, passing through certain characteristic triggering situations that he typifies with the neologisms of *includence* and *remanence.* An excellent interpretation of Tellenbach's ideas can be found in Stanghellini's book *Disembodied Spirits and Deanimated Bodies* (2004: 105). In our opinion, this psychopathological richness of Tellenbach's contributions to pathogenesis of depression would have not been possible without Jaspers' visionary depiction of human situations.

Dialectic thinking in psychopathology

Dialectics dates back to the beginning of philosophical thinking, appearing in different forms in the two great pre-Socratic philosophers: Parmenides from Elea and Heraclitus from Ephesus. For Parmenides, dialectics is a method which allows one to prove the falsehood of appearances that the senses give us and, in this way, to purify the thinking of irrationalities. For Heraclitus, on the contrary, dialectics represents the basic principle which structures and directs all that exists, since reality is ordered in polarities which need one another. Plato uses dialectics as a method to get to the truth through dialogue and by proving the contradictions inherent in nature as well as in thinking. In Hegel the concept of dialectics reaches its greatest universality. Both reality and knowledge would be one and the same process, but the truth of a process is only reached at the end of it, since every cross section will show its internal contradiction: the contradiction between the bud and the blossom that refutes it will be resolved in the fruit; this is the so-called dialectic moment, when the synthesis overcomes the contradiction between the thesis and its denial, the antithesis. Today, dialectic interpretation of reality is present in all of the natural sciences, which deal with the dialectics of contrary elements constituting a unity and not the dialectics of contradictory elements nullifying themselves (see Jasinowski 1957). In the same sense, the Nobel Prize winner in chemistry Ilya Prigogine (1997: 55) asserts that 'the no balance is the fundament of all stability'.

Karl Jaspers was the first to apply dialectic thinking to psychiatry. For Jaspers 'psychic life and its contents are polarized in opposites. It is through the opposites, however, that everything is once more reconnected. Image calls forth counter image, tendencies call forth counter-tendencies and feelings other feelings in contrast' (Jaspers 1997: 340). Jaspers distinguishes categorial, biological, psychological, and intellectual opposites. These opposites manifest themselves in different ways: (1) they reverse through time without consciousness taking part, as inspiration changes into expiration, grief into cheerfulness, etc.; (2) the opposites fight with each other, the one hurling itself against the other; (3) the self decides between the opposites, excluding one in favour of the other. 'The two latter modes lead to radically different dialectical movements: in the one, a synthesis of "this as well as that," in the other a choice—"either-or"' (Jaspers 1997: 342). In the first form a synthesis is produced between the opposites and a new movement arises, which opens the way to the whole. In the second, dialectics engages to the limits of the decision. Both forms carry a special risk for the psyche. Aiming at the whole, the psyche can lose its ground and 'be enticed into pleasing generalities' (Jaspers 1997: 242). On the other side, when the psyche endeavours to reach the sure ground of decision, sacrificing one of the opposites, it may become unnaturally and psychically impoverished.

Among the many contributions of Jaspers to dialectic perspectives, the most interesting is perhaps his attempt to apply it to the understanding of opposites in psychopathology. In patients with schizophrenia, for example, the phenomenon of a drastic emancipation of a tendency without its counter-tendency is given: automatism to the command, echolalia, echopraxia. Likewise, there are examples of failures in the union of the opposites, as it is the case of ambivalence. The emancipation of the counter-tendency can also be produced as occurs in negativism. Jaspers also describes how in most studies of the character and personality of humans opposites have been described: introversion/extraversion, narcissism/object-cathexis, schizoid character versus hyperthymic character, etc. He warns, however, about the risks of the absolute generalization of the opposites and remembers that 'the deeper we grasp the understandable meaning, the more we are directed into the non understandable, extra conscious ground of life and the non understandable, historical absolute of Existence itself' (Jaspers 1997: 345).

But it was Wolfgang Blankenburg (1962, 1965, 1974, 1981) who definitely introduced dialectic thinking into psychiatry. Blankenburg's starting point is the hypothesis that certain positivity can be enclosed in what is negative (the abnormality or illness). The question of the positivity of what is negative is found in many forms in daily life and also in the religious world, e.g. in Christianity: 'the last will be the first', 'it is necessary to die in order to resurrect', etc. And thus Blankenburg underlines the positive aspects of schizophrenia, like the depth of the perception these patients have of the world, their nearness to genius, their metaphysical sense, their authenticity, etc. (Blankenburg 1965) and later the positive aspects of hysteria, as, for example, the lack of rigidity, the easy adaptability, the capacity for entertaining, etc. of hysterical patients (Blankenburg 1974). But the relationships between dialectic thinking and schizophrenia do not end in the question of a possible positivity of the negative. And so, Blankenburg states: 'The modifications of the psychic life that we label as "schizophrenic" show themselves something dialectic insofar ones understands it […] as the openness and sensitivity for every "it is and it is not," for every questioning of the principle of contradiction' (Blankenburg 2007: 167). And then he remembers that Bleuler (1911) has defined ambivalence as a fundamental symptom of schizophrenia.

Following the line suggested by Blankenburg, we tried to advance the dialectic perspective of the great psychopathological syndromes. As the initial model we took the manic–depressive diad, where the polar and dialectical character is evident: mania is the reverse of depression and vice versa. But at the same time each emphatically needs one another so that in some way the one is contained in the other and vice versa. How frequently we perceive, behind the joy and hyperactivity of the manic, infinite sorrow and, inversely, behind the sorrow and inactivity of the depressive patient, feelings of envy and aggressiveness which are almost impossible to emanate from his weakened and harmless appearance. Additionally, what draws one's attention is the fact that situations triggering the two illnesses would seem to be inclined to produce the opposite effect; they are marked by an inverse sign: what would result in joy for any normal person (a move to a better house, the happy marriage of a daughter, the birth of a child who is wanted, promotion at work, etc.), may trigger a depression, while those precipitating mania generally represent intolerable setbacks (the death of a beloved person, financial bankruptcy, the diagnosis of a serious or mortal illness, situations of great pressure, etc.). In other words, the manic develops his mania against depression, while the depressive patient develops his depression against the mania. What is manic can be seen as what is positive with respect to depression, as a defence against that inability, that congealed anguish, that stopping of time. And conversely, what is depressive can be conceived as what is positive with respect to mania, as being saved from exhausting hyperactivity, from continuous disrespect for others or from an inability to maintain both thinking and behaviour within rational and socially acceptable limits. We also observe a dialectic structure in the polarity established between the 'not being able' (*das Nicht-Können*) of the depressive phase and a total ability and availability in the manic phase.

But all the formerly called endogenous conditions can also be seen as distributed between the depressive pole and the schizophrenic pole. The extremes would be represented by unipolar depression on the one side and disorganized schizophrenia on the other. The schizo-affective psychoses would be equidistant from both poles. From these in direction towards the schizophrenic pole we observe the deployment of the rest of the forms of this illness: catatonic, paranoid, and hebephrenic schizophrenia. In the other direction we find cycloid psychoses, delusional manias, delusional depressions, bipolar forms, and finally, unipolar depression. Something similar is suggested by Janzarik (1959) in his description of 'dynamic constellations in endogenous psychoses'. This conceptualization allows a greater fidelity to the clinical fact of the multiple transitions among the different psychopathologic syndromes and resolves the old dispute between the theory of 'unique psychosis' and the one postulating the existence of perfectly different nosological entities (Doerr-Zegers 1987, 1990, 1992).

These structures are not simple reifications as is the case for categorial diagnoses, but 'ideal' types, in the sense of Jaspers (Jaspers 1997: 560). For Jaspers 'dialectics is the form in which a basic aspect of meaningful connections becomes accessible to us' (Jaspers 1997: 345) and that is precisely a structure in the style of the ones we are describing. The ideal types are for Jaspers always self-evident, they do not lead to theories, but rather correspond to patterns through which particular events can be measured. An excellent treatment of this subject matter and of the transcendence of ideal types in daily clinical practice we owe to Michael Schwartz and Osborne Wiggins (1987a, 1987b; Schwartz et al. 1995).

But Jaspers brings dialectic thinking beyond psychopathology, up to human existence itself, explaining how difficult it is for man to achieve the synthesis between the many contradictions in which we are inserted. And so, he states:

> It is fundamentally characteristic of our temporal human situation that we cannot accomplish such a synthesis. This means that in life we select and realize our destiny from among the chances and risks of historical events, while all correct resolutions disappear at the frontiers of tragedy and in the presence of our transcending possibilities. (Jaspers 1997: 343)

Conclusions

Jaspers' *General Psychopathology* constituted, at its time, the creation of an authentic psychopathology at the forefront of medical semiology, and additionally the start of an enhanced clinical praxis from the methodological vantage. Together, the volume continues to have significant heuristic value for clinical as well as theoretical investigation in psychiatry and medicine. Jaspers' work was the fruit of his training as a physician and a philosopher and also his genius for engagement with the issues of his times. We have attempted to show some of Jaspers' main contributions and also the way in which he anticipated future developments in psychopathology with regard, for example, to the concept of situation or to the introduction of dialectic thinking into psychiatry.

From a theoretical point of view, Jaspers knew how to grasp the essentials of the great revolution that was being initiated—at the turn of the century—in the scientific and philosophical vision of reality. This consisted in passing from the 'substantialist paradigm', which saw unities 'in themselves', composed of elements, to the grasping of complex systems, whose connective, communicational dynamics makes the local structures 'emerge', in daily life, as entities or things separate and pre-existing to their causal relations. Thus, the substantialist vision requires a method of analytic-reductionist knowledge and the second demands a dialectic synthetic method. In the end, this overcoming of substantialism has constituted, according to Gastón Bachelard (1934), the greatest intellectual effort of the twentieth century.

Jaspers incarnates in his work the intuition of this revolution of knowledge, with the incorporation of phenomenology as an exploratory method implying a synthetic vision of human existence. This is understood as embodied dialectics stemming from a symbolic communication—of meanings and senses—between the situation and the subject, which simultaneously constructs both the structure of the world and of the subject's personality (see Minkowski 1927). Given the earliness of his work, Jaspers did not reach his objective of grasping the essence of nosological unities, but he undoubtedly opened the way through which this goal has been attained.

References

Apel, K.O. (2003). *Semiótica Trascendental y Filosofía Primera*. Madrid: Editorial Síntesis.

Bachelard, G. (1934). *Le Nouvel Esprit Scientifique*. París: Alcan.

Berrios, G.E. (1992). 'Phenomenology, Psychopathology and Jaspers: A Conceptual History', *History of Psychiatry*, **III**: 303–327.

Binswanger, L. (1947). 'Über Phänomenologie', in *Ausgewählte Vorträge und Aufsätze*, Vol. I. Bern: A. Francke AG Verlag.

Binswanger, L. (1955). 'Erfahren, Verstehen, Deuten in der Psychoanalyse', in *Ausgewählte Vorträge und Aufsätze*, Vol. II. Bern: Francke Verlag, 67–104. (Original work published in 1926.)

Binswanger, L. (1956). *Drei Formen missglückten Daseins: Verstiegenheit, Verschrobenheit, Manieriertheit*. Tübingen: Max Niemayer Verlag.

Binswanger, L. (1957). *Schizophrenie*. Pfullingen: Neske Verlag.

Binswanger, L. (1961). 'Über die daseinsanalytische Forschungsrichtung in der Psychiatrie', in *Ausgewählte Vorträge und Aufsätze*, Vol. 1. Bern: Francke Verlag, 190–217.

Blankenburg, W. (1962). 'In dem phänomenologischen Erkrankungsfeld innerhalb der Psychiatrie (unter Berücksichtigung methodologischer Fragen)', *Schweizer Archiv für Neurologie und Psychiatrie*, **90**(2): 412–421.

Blankenburg, W. (1965). 'Zur Differentialphänomenologie der Wahnwahrnehmung', *Der Nervenarzt*, **36**(7): 285–298.

Blankenburg, W. (1971). *Die Verlust der natürlichen Selbstverständlichkeit*. Stuttgart: Ferdinand Enke Verlag.

Blankenburg, W. (1974). 'Hysterie in anthropologischer Sicht', *Praxis der Psychotherapie*, 19: 262–273.

Blankenburg, W. (1978). 'Grundlagenprobleme der Psychopathologie', *Der Nervenarzt*, **49**: 140–146.

Blankenburg, W. (1981). 'Wie weit reicht die dialektische Betrachtungsweise in der Psychiatrie?', *Zeitschrift für klinische Psychologie und Psychotherapie*, 29: 45–66.

Blankenburg, W. (1984). 'Unausgeschöpftes in der Psychopathologie von Karl Jaspers', *Der Nervenarzt*, **55**: 447–460.

Blankenburg, W. (2007). 'Wie weit reicht die dialektische Betrachtungsweise in der Psychiatrie?', in M. Heinze (ed), *Psychopathologie des Unscheinbares*. Berlin: Parodos Verlag, 149–181.

Bleuler, E. (1911). 'Dementia praecox oder die Gruppe der Schizophrenien', in B. Aschaffenburg (ed), *Handbuch der Psychiatrie*, Vol. IV. Leipzig/Wien: Deuticke Verlag, 1–420.

Bunge, M. (1980). *The Mind-Body Problem: A Psychobiological Approach*. Oxford: Pergamon Press, 6–8.

Cole, J., McGuffin, P., Farmer, A.E. (2008). 'The Classification of Depression: Are We Still Confused?' *British Journal of Psychiatry*, 192: 83–85.

Conrad, K. (1958). *Die beginnende Schizophrenie*. Stuttgart: Thieme Verlag.

Delgado, H. (1966). *Psicología (Estudio Metodológico Del Mundo Anímico)* (8th edn, (revised and updated). Barcelona: Ed. Científico-Médica.

Dilthey, W. (1955). 'Einleitung in die Geisteswissenschaften: Versuch einer Grundlegung für das Studium der Gesellschaft und der Geschichte', in *Gesammtle Schriften*, Vol. 1 (4th edn). Stuttgart/Göttingen: B.G. Teubner Verlagsgesellschaft, VandenHoeck and Ruprecht, 355.

Doerr-Zegers, O. (1970). 'La esquizofrenia como necesidad de la historia vital', *Revista Chilena de Neuro-psiquiatría*, **9**(2): 17–39.

Doerr-Zegers, O. (1980). 'Adicción y temporalidad', *Psicología Médica (Argentina)*, **5**(3): 381–397.

Doerr-Zegers, O. (1987). 'Pensamiento dialéctico y estructuras de personalidad', *Psiquiatría y Salud Mental*, 4: 21–30.

Doerr-Zegers, O. (1990). 'Hacia una concepción dialéctica en psicopatología', *Actas Luso-españolas de Neurología y Psiquiatría*, 18(4): 244–257.

Doerr-Zegers, O. (1992). 'Hermenéutica, Dialéctica y Psiquiatría', *Revista Chilena de Neuro-psiquiatría*, 30(3): 178–188.

Doerr-Zegers, O. (1997). *Psiquiatría Antropológica* (2nd edn). Santiago: Editorial Universitaria.

Doerr-Zegers, O. (2000). 'Existential and Phenomenological Approach to Psychiatry', in M.G. Gelder, J.J. López-Ibor Jr., N.C. Andreasen (eds), *New Oxford Textbook of Psychiatry*, Vol. 1. Oxford: Oxford University, 357–362.

Doerr-Zegers, O. (2010). 'Schizophrenia, Language and Evolution', *Actas Espanolas De Psiquiatria*, **38**: 1–7.

Farmer, A., McGuffin, P. (1989). 'The classification of the depressions. Contemporary confusion revisited', *British Journal of Psychiatry*, 155: 437–43.

Fuchs, T. (2007). 'The Temporal Structure of Intentionality and Its Disturbance in Schizophrenia', *Psychopathology*, **40**: 229–235.

Fuchs, T. (2010). 'Subjectivity and Intersubjectivity in Psychiatric Diagnosis', *Psychopathology*, **43**: 268–274.

Gaupp, R. (1914). 'Zur Psychopathologie des Massenmords, Hauptleherer Wagner von Degerloch', in *Kriminal-Psychologische Studie*. Berlin: Springer Verlag.

Gaupp, R. (1921). 'Die dramatische Dichtung eines Paranoikers über den Wahn', in: Weiterer Beitrag zur Lehre von der Paranoia, *Neurologie und Psychiatrie*, **69**: 182–198.

Gebsattel, V.E. von (1954). *Prolegomena einer medizinischen Anthropologie.* Berlin-Göttingen-Heidelberg: Springer Verlag.

Ghaemi, N. (2003). *The Concepts of Psychiatry: A Pluralistic Approach to the Mind and Mental Illness.* Baltimore, MD: Johns Hopkins University Press.

Häfner, H. (1959). 'Hypochondrische Entwicklungen', *Der Nervenarzt*, **30**: 529–539.

Häfner, H. (1963). 'Prozess und Entwicklung als Grundbegriffe der Psychopathologie', *Fortschritte der Neurologie, Psychiatrie und ihrer Grenzgebiete*, **31**(8): 393–438.

Häfner, H., Wieser, St. (1953). 'Faktorenanalytische Studien zur Formalgenese bestimmter Formen von Schizophrenie', *Archiv für Psychiatrie Nervenkrankheiten*, 190: 394–428.

Hawking, S., Mlodinow, L. (2011). *El gran diseño.* Buenos Aires: Editorial Paidós.

Hegel, F. (1952). *Phänomenologie des Geistes.* Hamburg: Felix Meiner Verlag, 10.

Janzarik, W. (1959). *Dynamische Grundkonstellationen in endogenen Psychosen.* Berlin: Springer Verlag.

Jasinowski, B. (1957). *Saber y dialéctica.* Santiago: Ediciones Universidad de Chile.

Jaspers, K. (1933). *Psychopathologie Générale.* Paris: Ed. Alcan.

Jaspers, K. (1958). *Filosofía*, Vol. II. (F. Vela, trans.). Madrid: Revista de Occidente.

Jaspers, K. (1959). *Allgemeine Psychopathologie* (7th edn). Berlin: Springer Verlag.

Jaspers, K. (1963). 'Eifersuchtswahn, in Beitrag zur Frage: Entwicklung einer Persönlichkeit oder Prozess?', in *Gesammelte Schriften zur Psychopathologie.* Berlin: Springer Verlag, 85–141. (Original work published in 1910.)

Jaspers, K. (1964). *Psicopatologia Generale.* Roma: Il Pensiero Scientifico Editore.

Jaspers, K. (1968). 'The Phenomenological Approach in Psychopathology', *British Journal of Psychiatry*, 114: 1313–1323. (Original work published in 1912.)

Jaspers, K. (1997). *General Psychopathology* (7th edn) (J. Hoenig, M.W. Hamilton, trans.). Baltimore, MD: Johns Hopkins University Press.

Jonas, H. (2001). *The Phenomenon of Life: Toward a Philosophical Biology.* Evanston, IL: Northwestern University Press.

Kessler, R.C., Nelson, C.B., McGonagle, K.A., Liu, J., Swartz, M., Blazer, D.G. (1996). 'Comorbidity of DSM-III-R Major Depressive Disorder in the General Population: Results From the US National Comorbidity Survey', *British Journal of Psychiatry* 168(suppl 30): 17–30.

Kisker, K.P. (1960). 'Psychotherapie als Instrument der psychopathologischen Schizophrenie-Forschung', *Confinia Psychiatrica,* **3**: 1–36.

Kisker, K.P. (1963). 'Gedanken zur schizophrenen Wandlung als einer menschlichen Möglichkeit', in E. Wiesenhütter (ed), *Werden und Handeln. Viktor Emil Frhr. von Gebsattel zum 80. Geburtstag.* Stuttgart: Hippokrates-Verlag, 388–407.

Kraepelin, E. (1893). *Lehrbuch der Psychiatrie* (4th edn). Leipzig: Barth.

Kraepelin, E. (1915). *Lehrbuch der Psychiatrie* (8th edn). Leipzig: Barth.

Kraepelin, E. (1927). *Lehrbuch der Psychiatrie* (9th edn). Leipzig: Thieme Verlag.

Kraus, A. (1977). *Solzialverhalten und Psychose Manisch-Depressiver.* Stuttgart: Ferdinand Enke Verlag.

Kretschmer, E. (1950). *Der sensitive Beziehungswahn.* Berlin: Springer-Verlag. (Original work published in 1918.)

Kulenkampff, C. (1964). 'Über psychotische Adoleszenskrisen', *Der Nervenarzt* **35**: 530–536.

Kuhn, Ç.R. (1970). *The Structure of Scientific Revolutions.* Chicago, IL: University of Chicago Press.

López-Ibor, J.J. (1966). *Las neurosis como enfermedades del ánimo*. Madrid: Editorial Gredos.

Lorenz, K. (1978). *Vergleichende Verhaltensforschung. Grundlagen der Ethologie*. Vienna: Springer.

Luisi, P.L. (2006). *The Emergence of Life. From Chemical Origins to Syntetic Biology*. Cambridge: Cambridge University Press.

Mayer-Gross, S., Roth, M. (1954/1974). *Clinical Psychiatry*. London: Baillière, Tindall and Cassell Limited.

McHugh, P.R., Slavney, R. (1983). *The Perspectives of Psychiatry*. Baltimore, MD: Johns Hopkins University Press.

Merleau-Ponty, M. (1945). *Phénomenologie de la perception*. Paris: Gallimard.

Minkowski, E. (1927). *La schizophrenie: Psychopathologie des schizoides et des schizophrenes*. Paris: Payot.

Mundt, C. (1984). 'The concept of intentionality and the deficiency theory of schizophrenias', *Nervenarzt*, **55**(11): 582–588.

Parker, G. (2006). 'Through a Glass Darkly: The Disutility of the DSM Nosology of Depressive Disorders', *Canadian Journal of Psychiatry*, 51(14): 879–886.

Pelegrina, H. (2006). *Fundamentos antropológicos de la psicopatología*. Madrid: Editorial Polifemo.

Prigogine, I. (1997). *¿Tan solo una ilusión? Una exploración del caos al orden*. Barcelona: Tusquets.

Sarró, R. (1987). *Estructura y dinámica del delirio*. Barcelona: Anthropos.

Schifferdecker, M., Peters, U.H. (1995). 'The Origin of the Concept of Paranoia', in M.J. Sedler (ed), *The Psychiatric Clinics of North America. Delusional Disorders*, Vol. 18(2). Philadelphia, PA: Saunders, 231–250.

Schmidt-Degenhard, M. (1998). 'Zur Problemgeschichte und Psychopathologie der Paranoia', *Fortsch Neurol Psychiat*, **66**: 313–325.

Schwartz, M.A., Wiggins, O. (1985). 'Science, Humanism, and the Nature of Medical Practice: A Phenomenological View', *Perspectives in Biology and Medicine*, **28**: 331–361.

Schwartz, M.A., Wiggins, O. (1987a). 'Diagnosis and ideal types: A contribution to psychiatric classification', *Comprehensive Psychiatry*, **28**: 277–291.

Schwartz, M.A., Wiggins, O. (1987b). 'Typifications. The First Step for Clinical Diagnosis in Psychiatry', *The Journal of Nervous and Mental Disease*, **175**(2): 65–77.

Schwartz, M.A., Wiggins, O., Norko, M.A. (1995). 'Prototyes, ideal types and personality disorders: the return to classical phenomenology', in W.J. Livesly (ed), *The DSM-IV Personality Disorders*. New York, NY: The Guilford Press, 417–432.

Slavney, P.R., McHugh, P.R. (1987). *Psychiatric Polarities*. Baltimore, MD: Johns Hopkins University Press.

Stanghellini, G. (2004). *Disembodied Spirits and Deanimated Bodies: The Psychopathology of Common Sense*. Oxford: Oxford University Press.

Straus, E. (1960). *Psychologie der menschlichen Welt*. Berlin: Springer Verlag.

Tellenbach, H. (1961). *Melancholie: Zur Problemgeschichte, Typologie, Pathogenese und Klinik*. Berlin: Springer Verlag.

Tellenbach, H. (1980). *Melancholy* (E. Eng, trans.). Pittsburgh, PA: Duquesne University Press.

Varela, F.J., Thompson, E.T., Rosch, E. (1991). *The Embodied Mind: Cognitive Science and Human Experience*. Cambridge, MA: MIT Press.

Wiggins, O.P., Schwartz, M.A. (1988). 'Karl Jaspers' Psychopathology and the Problem of Meaning', *Journal of Theoretical & Philosophical Psychiatry*, **8**(1): 16–27.

Zutt, J. (1958). *Das paranoide Syndrom*. Berlin: Springer Verlag.

Chapter 6

Form and content in Jaspers' psychopathology

Chris Walker

Introduction

The distinction of form and content in Jaspers' psychopathology comes straight out of Immanuel Kant's theory of knowledge in his *Critique of Pure Reason* (first edition, 1781, second edition, 1787). Kant was absolutely crucial to Jaspers' work—both psychopathological and philosophical.[1]

Jaspers' interest in philosophy began in his teens: 'when I was still in secondary school, Spinoza was the first (philosophical influence). Kant then became the philosopher for me and has remained so'. As an undergraduate, Jaspers' primary interest was in science and he acknowledges that he 'did not yet understand Kant' (Jaspers 1941/1951: 399). But, as a young doctor, alongside his psychiatric work, he took seminars on Kant with the neoKantian, Emil Lask, a pupil of Wilhelm Windelband and Heinrich Rickert who were to be Jaspers' successive professors on his switch to Privatdozent in psychology in 1913 (Lask was killed in 1915 in the First World War, aged 40). Jaspers (1957a: 86) was particularly impressed with Kant's theory of ideas.

Having graduated to the chair in philosophy in Heidelberg, Jaspers opens his *Philosophy*, 1932, with a list of ten thinkers who had influenced his own philosophizing. At the time, it was unusual for such influences to be spelled out. He writes: 'I rarely refer to them explicitly but I will record their illustrious names here' (Jaspers 1932/1969). The list is given in

---

[1] All translations are mine apart from minor references; for these, e.g. Nietzsche's *Der Wille zur Macht* and Jaspers' *Nietzsche*, I have relied on the published translation. In all cases, I give the original publication date followed by the date of the translation, e.g. Nietzsche 1900/1967, for *Der Wille zur Macht*, 1900, translated as *The Will to Power*, 1967. I am strongly aversive to Nietzsche, 1967, suggesting that Nietzsche was still alive many decades after his death. Ditto for Jaspers who left psychopathology behind in 1946. In referring to *General Psychopathology* I give Jaspers, 1946/1963, p.xxx. I give 1946 as the date of *Allgemeine Psychopathologie* because this was the fourth and final edition. 1963 is the date of the Hoenig and Hamilton translation; this is a translation of the seventh 'edition', 1959, which was a reprint of the fourth edition. The page references are to the Hoenig and Hamilton translation. In referring to Jaspers' early papers on hallucinations I quote not from the original papers, 1911 and 1912, but from *Gesammelte Schriften zur Psychopathologie*, 1963. I give the reference as Jaspers, 1911/1963 and 1912/1963, p.xxx. Ditto for 'The Phenomenological Approach in Psychopathology' as Jaspers, 1912/1968, p.xxx—again the page references are to the English translation. As is the custom, I refer to the two editions of Kant's Critique of Pure Reason as A and B.

chronological order apart from Kant who significantly appears first. He writes of Kant in grandiose terms. Kant is 'the ultimate philosopher, incomparable in the sheer nobility of his humanity as revealed in the purity and acuteness of his endlessly shifting thought' (Jaspers 1932/1969: 2). Then, in his monograph, *Kant*, a part of the *Great Philosophers* series, Jaspers concludes that 'Kant is the nodal point in modern philosophy ... Kant is absolutely indispensable. Without him there can be no critical basis for philosophy' (Jaspers 1957b/1962: 380–1). Jaspers saw the task of his own philosophy as developing and extending Kant's theory of knowledge and critique of metaphysics within a twentieth-century context. The primary topics of Kant's critique of metaphysics—cosmology, the soul, and God—become Jaspers' world orientation, *Existenz* and transcendence.

Jaspers was a fundamentally Kantian thinker to the extent that, late in his life, he was described by a University of Basel colleague as 'the first and last Kantian' (quoted in Ehrlich 1975: 211). Jaspers is more Kantian than Kant.

Form and content in Kant's theory of knowledge

In the *Prolegomena* (Kant 1783: 5), a precis of *Critique of Pure Reason* written between the two editions, Kant described David Hume's empiricism as having 'interrupted my dogmatic slumber'. A primary purpose of Kant's work was to counter Hume's scepticism which claimed that there could be no objective basis for our knowledge about the world, including scientific knowledge. For Hume, knowledge is grounded in, and cannot extend beyond, sensory impressions. Such impressions may be constant and coherent, but they are necessarily subjective rather than objective. Opposing Hume's empiricism was the rationalism of Gottfried Leibniz. For Leibniz, knowledge was founded on innate principles known intuitively to be true.

Kant rejected both; he sought a middle course which preserved the truth, and rejected the error, of each. Kant's conclusion is that: 'though all our knowledge begins with experience, it does not follow that it all arises out of experience. For it may well be that even our empirical knowledge is made up of what we receive through impressions and of what our own faculty of knowledge supplies from itself' (Kant A1). For Kant, there are two stems to knowledge: the sensory or intuitive emphasized by the empiricists and the conceptual or categorical emphasized by the rationalists. Both are necessary so that: 'neither concepts without an intuition in some way corresponding to them, nor intuition without concepts, can yield knowledge' (Kant A50, B74). Each comes from a different source: 'concepts are based on the spontaneity of thought, sensible intuitions on the receptivity of impressions' (Kant A68, B93). 'There are two conditions under which alone the knowledge of an object is possible, first intuition, through which it is given, though only as appearance; secondly, concept, through which an object is thought corresponding to this intuition' (Kant A92–3, B125). The upshot is that: 'thoughts without content are empty, intuitions without concepts are blind' (Kant A51, B75, quoted in Jaspers 1957b/1962: 254).

For Kant, the sensory or intuitive is matter; the conceptual or categorical is form. Matter is the content of sensation or intuition given to cognition; form is the ordering, organizing, determining and constitutive functions of cognition:

> That in the appearance which corresponds to sensation I term its *matter* but that which so determines the manifold of appearance that it allows of being ordered in certain relations, I term the *form* of the appearance. (A20, B34: Kant's italics)

Content or matter is 'from without'; form or concept is 'from within':

> Experience contains two very dissimilar elements, namely the *matter* of knowledge [obtained] from the senses, and a certain *form* for the ordering of this matter, [obtained] from the inner source of the pure intuition and thought which, on occasion of the sense impressions, are first brought into action and yield concepts. (Kant A86, B118)

The distinction of form and matter is a restatement of Kant's theory of knowledge. All experience and knowledge requires the presentation of sensations or intuition (the matter or content) plus its ordering and conceptualizing by cognition (the form). Form provides the 'rule' under which content is brought together in one object: 'a concept is always, as regards its form, something universal which serves as a rule' (Kant A106).

In a different, though still Kantian terminology, matter or content is the 'outer' objective pole and form the 'inner' subjective pole. Form and matter are fundamental to Kant's theory of knowledge. Matter is 'the determinable ... the constituent elements' while form is 'the determination ... the mode in which they are combined in one thing' (Kant A261, B317).

> Matter and form—These two concepts underlie all other reflection, so inseparably are they bound up with all employment of the understanding (*Verstandes*[2]). The one (matter) signifies the determinable in general, the other (form) its determination ... In every being, the constituent elements of it are the matter, the mode in which they are combined in one thing the essential form. (Kant A266, B322, his parenthesis)

Form and content in Jaspers' monograph *Kant*

In the monograph, 1957b/1962, Jaspers outlines the twofold Kantian distinction of form and matter, subject and object, category and intuition, spontaneity and receptivity. For Jaspers, 'within Kantian thinking, there is a two-fold dichotomy at the very basis of things'; he goes on:

> The subject (as the spontaneity of thinking) contrasts with the object (as the receptivity of sensibility) and, within the object itself, form contrasts with matter ... The object is built from the matter of intuition and defined by the form of the category. Matter and form correspond to object and subject. Matter is given (*gegeben*), form is added by thought (*gedacht*). (Jaspers 1957b/1962: 254–255)

Jaspers goes on:

> This is what connects the two contrasting distinctions—matter and form, subject and object. Form arises from the spontaneity of the thinking of the subject; matter arises from the receptivity of the sensibility of the subject. They coincide, on the one hand, with subject, form, a priori, pure and, on the other hand, with object, matter, a posteriori, empirical. (Jaspers 1957b/1962: 255)

[2] In the Kant quotations, I have followed Norman Kemp Smith's translation of Verstand as 'understanding'; but, when Jaspers uses Verstand I have translated it as 'intellect' to distinguish it from empathic understanding (Verstehen).

The contrast is:

matter or content ———— concept or form
intuition ———— category
given ———— added by thought
object ———— subject
receptivity of sensibility ———— spontaneity of thinking
determinable ———— determination

Kant's distinction of conceptual form and intuitive matter or content is the philosophical basis for the form–content distinction in Jaspers' psychopathology. In *General Psychopathology*, he notes (Jaspers 1997: 340; my parenthesis): 'it is a question of a universal form of thinking and a form of being as it appears to us because the intellect can conceive of nothing that does not have something beyond itself. All being presenting itself to the intellect is divided (into form and content); otherwise it is unthinkable'. This reference to the necessary split of all knowledge into form and content becomes the subject–object dichotomy in Jaspers' philosophy.

Form and content in Jaspers' phenomenology

Jaspers (1912) first outlines the form–content distinction in phenomenology in his paper, 'Die phänomenological Forschungsrichtung in der Psychopathologie' ('The Phenomenological Approach in Psychopathology'). He (Jaspers 1912/1968: 1315) contrasts 'simple empathic understanding' of the patient, which is 'subjective in a very special sense', with psychology as a science. For such a science: 'we must be clear from the start that its fully conscious ideal is to present our understanding of psychic life in definite forms'. The former is 'vague, purely personal and subjective as described by a gifted individual and does not get close to the scientific ideal'. He goes on: 'from the beginning, psychiatry has been concerned with the task of the definition and naming of individual forms of experience. Not a single step could have been taken without this basis in phenomenology. It was in this way that delusional ideas, sensory deceptions, depressive and expansive affect and other phenomena were described. This remains the basis for further phenomenological inquiry' (Jaspers 1912/1968: 1319). It is the function of phenomenology to describe, define, differentiate, and classify the patient's experience into the different forms of subjective experience: 'the conscious ideal is to present our understanding of psychic life in definite forms' (Jaspers 1912/1968: 1315). He goes on that: 'phenomenology teaches us the forms in which experience appears to us as psychic reality. It tells us nothing about the contents of individual experience and nothing about that extra-conscious base on top of which the psyche floats like a thin surface of foam on the sea … It is only in these phenomenological forms that we can immediately grasp the reality of psychic life'. Just as in histology where we might expect to account for every cell, so in phenomenology: 'we should account for every psychic phenomenon, for every experience that comes to light in the exploration of our patient and in his self-descriptions. Under no circumstances should we be satisfied with an overall impression or with a few details obtained in an ad hoc fashion. Rather we should get to know, grasp and pass a judgement on every detail'—on every form of experience (Jaspers 1912/1968: 1323).

The form–content distinction is present in all editions of *Allgemeine Psychopathologie*. It is not the case, as is often inferred by common interpretations, that the distinction is restricted to phenomenology. For Jaspers, as a good Kantian, all knowledge entails the form–content distinction. He spells this out in all editions. In the first edition, he writes (Jaspers 1913: 18): 'the distinction of form and content applies from the simplest psychic events right up to psychosis as a whole', and in the fourth edition: 'the distinction of form and content is universal in all knowledge' (1946/1963a/1997: 59). He then outlines the most important implications of the form–content distinction in a statement which is identical in the first three editions, with only minor changes in the fourth:

> 1. In all psychic life, a subject stands in opposition to an object; in the broadest sense, a subject is directed to something objective (to the content of a perception, a thought, an aspiration, etc.). In the broadest sense, we call this object the content of psychic life and the way the individual is presented with the object—whether as perception, idea, thought, etc.—we call the form. Thus, hypochondriacal content can be the content of a voice, a compulsive idea, an over-valued idea or a delusion-like idea. In the same way, we can speak of the content of anxiety and other moods.
> 2. We contrast the form of the psychosis with its particular content, e.g. the periodic phases of low mood as the form of the illness with the particular behavior as the content—whether chronic drunkenness, wandering or suicide.
> 3. We interpret some of the most general variations of psychic life that can only be grasped psychologically as form, e.g. the experiences of the schizophrenic or the hysteric. Within these forms, all human propensities and desires, all possible thoughts and fantasies are to be found as content. It is in these forms that the particular modes of schizophrenia and hysteria are realized.
>
> For the most part, the psychopathologist is primarily interested in form; content appears more incidental and wholly individual. However, not infrequently, content will be of importance and of interest for scientific investigation, e.g. delusion-like ideas in melancholia and its suicidal propensities. (Jaspers 1913: 19, 1920: 23–24, 1923: 23, 1946/1963a/1997: 59)

In the fourth edition, Jaspers (1946/1963a/1997: 58–59) adds that: 'perceptions, ideas, judgements, feelings, drives and self-awareness are all forms of psychic phenomena; forms signify the mode of existence (*Daseinsweise*) in which content is presented to us'. Such forms contrast with the content which might be 'a man, a tree, threatening figures or a peaceful landscape'. 'For the patient, only content is important'; the patient will usually fail to note the mode, the form in which content is presented with the result that hallucinations, pseudohallucinations and delusional ideas are confused. Form is fixed and static while content is changeable, but content is not without importance: 'content modifies the way in which phenomena are experienced … content gives weight and direction to the phenomena, to their conception and interpretation'. Depending on whether it is form or content which occupies our interest, the other will often seem irrelevant. 'For the phenomenologist, form is of the greater interest; to him, content seems more peripheral. But, for the psychologist interested in meaning (*verstehende Psychologen*), content will be essential and form of lesser interest'.

The same content can appear in a diverse range of phenomenological forms. Jaspers gives the examples of hypochondriasis and jealousy as contents which present in a wide variety of forms—the modes in which content is given to us. The patient may have had a long standing preoccupation with illness (the form of an over-valued idea); he may have concluded that he must be ill in the setting of the pessimism and despair of a severe depression (the form of a delusion-like idea); he may have the sudden, compelling, intrusive idea of being ill (the form of a primary delusion); he may hear a voice telling him he is ill (the form of an auditory hallucination); he may have the persistent intrusive thought that he is ill even though he resists the intrusion and knows it to be false (the form of a compulsive idea). All have the same content, hypochondriasis, but they are present in consciousness in different forms. Content is the objective pole, given to consciousness; form is the subjective pole, constituted by consciousness.

Jaspers insists that it is a mistake to speak of these as 'transitions' between diverse forms; 'transition' as a general turn of phrase is a cloak for lazy analysis. It may well be that the individual experience is a mixture of phenomena which can be separately described. For example, the presentation of an acute psychosis is likely to be complex and the patient may not be aware of the differences in the form of the experiences. It is the task of the phenomenologist 'to grasp these differences clearly, to deepen, extend and order them; it is this scientific task which alone can aid in the analysis of our cases' (1946/1963a/1997: 59–60).

To illustrate Jaspers' use of Kantian form I have chosen the phenomenology of perceptual phenomena—normal imagery, hallucination and pseudohallucination—with the emphasis on the pseudohallucination.

Kandinsky, Goldstein, and the pseudohallucination

The term 'pseudohallucination' was coined by Hagen in 1868 in his paper *Zur Theorie der Hallucination* (*A Theory of Hallucinations*). Hagen (1868: 4) considered pseudohallucinations to be 'errors of the senses or illusions'. In the twentieth century, 'pseudohallucination' appeared in an Anglo-American and a German tradition. The Anglo-American tradition began with a German: Kurt Goldstein; the German tradition with a Russian: Victor Kandinsky. The American literature has followed Goldstein, but 'pseudohallucination' appears very infrequently; it appears on just a single occasion in the fourth edition of the *Diagnostic and Statistical Manual of Mental Disorders* (DSM-IV; American Psychiatric Association 1994: 457) in relation to conversion disorder where pseudohallucinations 'generally occur with intact insight in the absence of other psychotic symptoms … (in) more than one sensory modality and often have a naïve, fantastic or childish content'. Jaspers and the German literature follow Kandinsky, although, unusually, Eugen Bleuler belongs to the Goldstein/Anglo-American tradition. Some authors have attempted, unsuccessfully, to span both traditions—Frederick Kräupl Taylor (1981) knowingly, Gary Sedman (1966a, 1966b, 1966c) and Ted Hare (1973) probably unknowingly.

Victor Kandinsky was a psychiatrist in the Asylum of St Nicolas, St Petersburg. He wrote in German. He suffered a lingering psychotic illness complicated by chronic opiate abuse. He was diagnosed as suffering from 'Melancholie' but his own diagnosis was 'primäre Verrückheit'—literally 'primary madness', i.e. schizophrenia. Kandinsky (1884) published his thoughts in a paper entitled 'Kritische und klinische Betrachtungen im Gebiete der Sinnestäuschungen' ('Critical and Clinical Observations in the Field of Sense Deception'), and in a book of the same title the following year. He begins by complaining that, despite a large volume of literature, no clear picture of the phenomena of sense deception had emerged and that very disparate phenomena had been conflated. The clinical phenomena he describes were largely drawn from his own psychotic experiences. For Kandinsky, pseudohallucination is not a perception; it is a compelling and vivid image. He committed suicide in a psychotic episode, aged 40, in 1889 by overdosing on opium taken from the hospital pharmacy. His wife edited and published his work after his death, before committing suicide herself a couple of years later. Kandinsky distinguished 'three types of subjective sensory perception in mentally ill patients':

a. normal sensory images or simple images from memory or in fantasy even though they have an intensity (a liveliness and a resolution) which is greatly increased in comparison with what is normal;
b. true pseudohallucinations;
c. real hallucinations.

(Kandinsky 1884: 482)

A real hallucination is a perception:

- it is a subjective sensory perception which has no object;
- its content is always concrete …
- the sensory elements appear in consciousness with the same character of objective reality as those associated with perceptions which are real outer impressions;
- there can be no gradations in the objectivity of true hallucinations. Either a patient has a hallucination or he does not (in the latter case, it could be a pseudohallucination). In relation to the character of objectivity or reality, there can be no transitional states between those subjective sensory perceptions which do not qualify as hallucinations (e.g. images in memory and my own true pseudohallucinations) and real hallucinations;
- hallucinations are facts of consciousness which … either appear as exactly the same as those objective perceptions taking place alongside them and at the same time as them or they replace these perceptions.

(Kandinsky 1884: 482–483; my bullet points)

Kandinsky distinguishes pseudohallucination from hallucination: 'pseudohallucinations possess all the characteristics present in true hallucinations except for the final and absolutely necessary character of objective reality. It is only for this reason that they are not hallucinations'. There is an absolute gulf between hallucination and pseudohallucination so that 'pseudohallucinations cannot change into hallucinations' (Kandinsky 1884: 484).

Pseudohallucinations and simple images differ from hallucinations because they have no 'objective reality'. Pseudohallucinations differ from simple images not because of 'their incomparably strong intensity (which is not an essential feature) … (but) by virtue of some characteristic features, namely: their passive receptivity (in Fechner's sense), their spontaneity, their compelling quality, their clear sensory definition, their detail, their completeness of the image and their constancy' (Kandinsky 1884: 484). In terms of the intensity of the experience there is a continuum between pseudohallucination and simple image, but a gulf between them and hallucination. The pseudohallucination is a vivid and compelling image.

Influenced by Wilhelm Wundt's associationist psychology and Karl Kalbaum's neuropsychiatry, Kandinsky (Kandinsky 1884:483–4) speculates on whether hallucination and pseudohallucination are of cortical origin. He thinks 'hallucinations cannot appear without the involvement of subcortical centres'. In contrast, 'pseudohallucinations have their origin in the sensory centres of the cerebral cortex'; they are based on 'a general state of abnormally increased excitability'. In his book of 1885, Kandinsky offers eight 'flow-charts' or what might now be described as 'connectionist diagrams' detailing the origins of abnormal perception and imagery in cortical and subcortical centres. In his view, the origin of the pseudohallucination is in the 'centre for abstract, unconscious images' (*Centrum des abstracten, unbewußten Vorstellens*) and the 'centre for apperception' (*Centrum der Apperception*) both of which transmit to the 'centre for clear and conscious thinking' (*Centrum des klarbewußten Denkens*). (Two of Kandinsky's diagrams are reprinted in Berrios and Dening 1996: 757–758.) Kandinsky's theory was hypothetical, highly speculative, and wholly lacking in any empirical support.

Kurt Goldstein was a German Jewish neurologist who studied brain injured soldiers in the First World War. He was arrested by the Nazi regime in 1933 and only released after promising to leave the country, never to return. He left for the United States, gaining citizenship in 1940. He wrote extensively on aphasia, agnosia, and schizophrenic thought disorder. He was greatly influenced by Gestalt psychology. Early in his career, he addressed hallucinations in two lengthy papers entitled 'Zur Theorie der Hallucinationen' ('A Theory of Hallucinations') (1908). Goldstein took the view that pseudohallucination is a perception which the patient knows not to be veridical; it is a perception with insight into its unreality. This became the dominant interpretation in Anglo-American psychiatry.

Jaspers on Kandinsky and Goldstein

Jaspers examined pseudohallucination in his papers, 'Zur Analyse der Trugwahrnehmungen' ('The Analysis of False Perceptions'), 1911/1963b, and 'Die Trugwahrnehmungen' ('False Perceptions'), 1912/1963c, and in *General Psychopathology*. Jaspers (1913/1963a/1997: 191) acknowledges his debt to Hagen and Kandinsky, but Hagen's definition of pseudohallucination was vague so that: 'it was Kandinsky who gave the concept its precise definition and positive meaning'. He (Jaspers 1912/1963c: 271) notes that 'Kandinsky had himself suffered from a hallucinatory psychosis' and that many of his examples were drawn from his own psychotic experiences. He begins:

> In the year 1895, Kandinsky distinguished a group of phenomena from true hallucinations. He explained that these phenomena were not themselves hallucinations but rather they were a pathological variant of sense memories and images. He called these pathological images which up to then had not been precisely defined "true pseudohallucinations." Pseudohallucinations distinguish themselves from both normal images and true hallucinations. (Jaspers 1911/1963b:191, *Jaspers means 1885*).

Pseudohallucinations are 'not hallucinations but rather they are a pathological variant of sense memories and images'. The difference with normal images is that 'pseudohallucinations have a compelling sensory definition … The whole picture is projected in full detail and with total clarity on to the "inner eye" (*innere Auge*) … Pseudohallucinations come and go wholly independent of the will … in a state of receptivity and passivity' (Jaspers 1911/1963b: 191). Normal images are also 'seen' with the inner eye, but they tend to be poor in detail, unclear and dependent on the will, needing to be actively recreated. Following Kandinsky, Jaspers writes:

> There is an unbridgeable gulf between the pseudohallucination and the true hallucination. The pseudohallucination can be recognized by its relationship to an image while the true hallucination has the same tangibility or concrete nature (*Leibhaftigkeit*), the same presence (*Gegenwart*), as an object of perception. The true hallucination has the character of objectivity. The pseudohallucination can be very vivid and distinct and very intense but it does not have the tangibility or concrete presence of an object. In contrast, even the most pallid, indistinct and indefinite hallucination possesses this character of objectivity. (Jaspers 1911/1963b: 191–192)

Connected with this lack of objectivity is 'the fact that pseudohallucinations, exactly like images, are not seen in outer space (*im äußeren Raum*), i.e. objective space, but rather in inner imaginal or representational space (*im inneren Vorstellungsraum*), i.e. subjective space' (Jaspers 1912/1963c: 265–266). Jaspers (1911/1963b: 191) concludes that: 'there is an unbridgable gulf between the pseudohallucination and true hallucination; pseudohallucinations are recognizable by their affiliation to images'.

Jaspers (1911/1963b: 214) is dismissive of Kandinsky's ideas on the pathophysiology of perceptual phenomena: 'Kandinsky's view that the stimulation of subcortical ganglia is the cause of the character of objectivity is mere conjecture with no empirical basis'. He goes on: 'the claim that concrete reality or perceptual quality is the result of stimulation of the sensory cortex is so general as to have no meaning. It has no empirical basis; it is merely a conjecture, an irrefutable postulate'.

The substance of Jaspers' critique of Goldstein is twofold. His first criticism (1912/1963c: 300, citing Goldstein 1908: 617) is that Goldstein sees a 'graded distinction' between hallucination and pseudohallucination: 'Goldstein advances the view that there is a continuum within the hallucination, i.e. between the perception and the image: "a hallucination is a subjective event just like an image; the distinction of hallucination and image is based on a continuum".' In contrast, Jaspers and Kandinsky, see an 'unbridgeable gulf' between perception and image, and thus between hallucination and pseudohallucination (Jaspers 1911/1963b: 191).

Jaspers' second criticism of Goldstein is that he conflates the character of objectivity and reality judgement, and that he attributes this confusion to Kandinsky. For Jaspers (Jaspers 1911/1963b: 192): 'there is confusion here or, at least, the suggestion of confusion for which Goldstein is responsible; this is the confusion between the character of objectivity and reality judgement'. Jaspers goes on: 'Goldstein interprets Kandinsky's distinction between pseudohallucination and hallucination as the distinction between hallucinations in which the patient recognizes the true reality and hallucinations in which there is no such recognition'. This, of course, was Goldstein's view, not Kandinsky's.

Jaspers (Jaspers 1911/1963b: 193) does find confusion in Kandinsky's account, but not the confusion seen by Goldstein: 'Kandinsky does not confuse the concept of objective character with the concept of reality judgement. In fact, he scarcely makes the distinction at all, the result being confusion in his interpretation'. The distinction is anticipated but not explicit in Kandinsky's account; he 'stresses the concrete reality or perceptual quality of hallucinations and their similarity with sense perceptions'. Jaspers goes on that hallucinations are 'present for consciousness and not for judgement or the intellect', but Kandinsky makes nothing more of the distinction.

For Goldstein, the form of a pseudohallucination is of a hallucination in which the patient realizes the unreality of his experience whereas a true hallucination is taken to be a veridical perception. In contrast, Jaspers sees the character of objectivity and reality judgement as distinct. For Kandinsky and Jaspers, the hallucination–pseudohallucination distinction relies on the character of objectivity alone, not on any subsequent reality judgement. But, for Kandinsky, the distinction of objectivity and reality judgement is implicit rather than explicit: 'Kandinsky did not confuse the concept of the character of objectivity and the concept of reality judgement; the distinction was scarcely mentioned' (Jaspers 1911/1963b: 193). For Jaspers (Jaspers 1911/1963b: 192), Kandinsky does offer an account of the character of objectivity such that: 'the character of objectivity is something given. It can be understandably derived from no other aspect of consciousness. It is an "X," a given'; it must have 'some extra-conscious cause'. But, Jaspers goes on, it is 'a very dubious and contentious theory that stimulation of subcortical ganglia is the necessary condition for such a character of objectivity'. Jaspers himself makes a radical distinction between objectivity and reality judgement; objectivity is given, reality judgement is reflective.

Jaspers on the pseudohallucination

Jaspers (1911/1963b: 193) sees his task as 'completing Kandinsky's preliminary suggestions'. He returns to a discussion of the forms of perception and imagery in *General Psychopathology*. The table shown (Table 6.1) is identical in all editions.

Perceptions are objective and concrete; images are subjective and figurative. Between these essential features of perception and imagery there is a phenomenological gulf (*Abgrund*) with no transitional forms; but, between the non-essential features there can be transitions (*Übergänge*). Most perceptions are detailed, clear, full, constant and independent of the will, but a few are incomplete, unclear, insufficient, and dependent on the will with a tendency to dissipate. Most images are the reverse.

A hallucination has the essential and non-essential criteria of a perception; thus, hallucination has the form of a perception—albeit, a perception with no external stimulus.

Table 6.1 Forms of perception

Perception (*Wahrnehmung*)	**Image (*Vorstellung*)**
The essential criteria of perception and image	
1. Perceptions are of concrete reality (*leibhaftig*) with the character of objectivity (*Objektivitätscharakter*);	*Images are figurative (bildhaftig) with the character of subjectivity (Subjektivitätscharakter);*
2. Perceptions appear in outer objective space (*im äußeren objektiven Raum*).	*Images appear in inner subjective imaginal or representational space (im inneren subjektiven Vorstellungsraum).*[a]
The non-essential criteria of perception and image	
3. *Perceptions are clearly delineated and stand before us complete and in full detail;*	Images are not clearly delineated and stand before us incomplete and lacking in detail.
4. *In perceptions, the individual sensory elements have a full sensory freshness, e.g. the colours are bright;*	In imagery, although occasionally the sensory elements are adequate, in the majority of cases, the elements are not adequate and most visual images are grey.
5. *Perceptions are constant and easily retained unaltered;*	Images tend to slip away and break up; they have to be constantly renewed.
6. *Perceptions are independent of the will; they cannot be evoked or altered voluntarily; they are present with a feeling of passivity.*	Images are dependent on our will; they can be evoked and altered voluntarily; they are present with a feeling of activity.

[a] Hoenig and Hamilton omit 'representational' (*Vorstellung*) from their translation, thus allowing the possible misinterpretation that pseudohallucination is a perception from inside the patient's head, rather than an image in 'representational space'.

(Jaspers 1913: 36, 1920: 45, 1923: 49, 1946/1963a/1997: 69)

An image has the essential and non-essential criteria of an image. On the pseudohallucination, Jaspers invokes Kandinsky (1946/1963a/1997: 68): 'for a long time we confused one class of phenomena with hallucination, a class which on closer examination are not concrete perceptions (*leibhaftige Wahrnehmungen*), but rather proved to be an unusual kind of image. Kandinsky carefully described these phenomena as pseudohallucinations'. Pseudohallucination has the essential criteria of an image, but the non-essential criteria of a perception; the form of a pseudohallucination is that of an intense, vivid and compelling image. (It has the italicized features of Table 6.1.)

Form in genetic understanding

It is a common misconception that the form and content distinction applies only to phenomenology. As a good Kantian, Jaspers stresses that this is not the case; all knowledge necessarily splits into form and content. As we have seen, in the first edition of *Allgemeine Psychopathologie*, he writes (Jaspers 1913: 18): 'the distinction of form and content applies from the simplest psychic events right up to psychosis as a whole', and in the fourth edition (Jaspers 1946/1963a: 59): 'the distinction of form and content is universal in all knowledge'. He goes on in the fourth edition: 'throughout psychopathology from the simplest psychic events right up to wholes, the distinction of form and content is in constant use'. The form–content distinction applies to genetic understanding just as it does to phenomenology.

Jaspers (1946/1963a/1997: 307) distinguishes phenomenology (or static understanding) and genetic understanding. Phenomenology or static understanding 'grasps individual psychic qualities and states as they are experienced'; genetic understanding 'grasps the emergence of one psychic state out of another'. Just as phenomenology divides into form and content, so too does genetic understanding. The important difference between phenomenology and genetic understanding is that phenomenology is concerned almost exclusively with form while genetic understanding is principally concerned with content. The form–content distinction is explicit in the subjective psychology of phenomenology and genetic understanding, but only implicit in the objective psychology of observable performances and causal connections. In genetic understanding, Jaspers (1946/1963a/1997: 340) identifies the 'basic forms of the understandable' (*Grundformen der Verstehbarkei*[3]).

There are three aspects to our knowledge of understandable connections—understandable content, the forms of the understandable and self-reflection:

1. *Understandable content: drives* are the source of action in the subject; this takes place within the relationship of the *individual to his world*; the individual understands his being (*Sein*) through *symbols* (we speak of the psychology of drive, the psychology of the real and the psychology of symbols);
2. *The basic forms of the understandable*: the form of the action is *opposition* with its tensions, reversals, reconciliations and decisions. Action is *reciprocal* (we speak of the psychology of opposites and the psychology of reciprocity);
3. *Self-reflection*: a basic phenomenon of all the understandable (we speak of the psychology of self-reflection).

(Jaspers 1946/1963a/1997: 316, his italics)

[3] In their translation of *Allgemeine Psychopathologie*, Hoenig and Hamilton translate 'Grundformen der Verstehbarkeit' as 'basic patterns of meaning', not as 'basic forms of the understandable'; thus missing the Kantian reference (Jaspers 1946/1963a, 340).

Jaspers goes on immediately that:

> These three aspects of understanding (content, form and self-reflection) merge into one interconnected and understandable whole. They are not mutually exclusive but rather the whole is illuminated from each point of view in turn. In order to understand, each must be supplemented by the other two.
>
> (Jaspers, 1946/1963a/1997: 316)

Drives (*Triebe*) as content of the understandable

Jaspers' theory of drive is drawn largely from the philosophy of Friedrich Nietzsche about whom Jaspers was to write a major book in 1936. Nietzsche saw all human motivation as beginning with one basic drive or affect, the will to power (*Wille zur Macht*). From Nietzsche's *The Will to Power*, (1900/1967: 688): 'the will to power is the primitive form of affect, all other affects are only developments of it … All driving force is will to power, there is no other physical, dynamic or psychic force except this'. Jaspers (1946/1963a/1997: 317) is not prepared to follow Nietzsche entirely but he does accept that 'all experience has concealed within it an element of being driven'. Much of our lives involve the modification, sublimation, or distortion of such drives.

Jaspers' favourite example which recurs in his work is drawn from Nietzsche. This is Nietzsche's view of the impact of Christianity—his so-called theory of 'resentiment'. In the Sermon on the Mount, Christianity is a religion for the psychically weak, meek, halt, and lame. Jaspers advances this as an understandable connection based on drive, the Nietzschean 'will to power': 'Nietzsche makes the compelling understandable link between an awareness of weakness, wretchedness and suffering, on the one hand, and moral demands and religions of salvation, on the other. Despite its weakness, the psyche can satisfy its will to power in this round-about way' (1946/1963a/1997: 303). In Nietzsche's typically graphic language (Nietzsche 1900/1967: 781): 'Christianity is a romantic hypochondria for those whose legs are shaky'. Christianity assures our romantic hypochondriac that his weakness and meekness will ultimately triumph in what, for Nietzsche, is a pathological inversion of his will to power.

The individual in the world (*der Einzelne in der Welt*) as content of the understandable

Jaspers begins with the concept of 'situation' (*Situation*). My situation is that of an individual in the world: 'life is interaction with the world'. This interaction is one of 'struggle, influence, creativity … adaptation … knowledge' and, ultimately, one of foundering (*Scheitern*) (Jaspers 1946/1963a/1997: 325). Foundering is a key term in Jaspers' philosophy, indicating the fact that we come up against a block in our attempt to grasp being (*Sein*) such that we can have no knowledge of being; our only access to being is through what he describes as the ciphers (*Chiffren*) of transcendence. The Nietzschean influence is again clear: 'the "world" is only a word for the totality of these actions. Reality consists precisely in this particular action and reaction of every individual part toward the whole' (Nietzsche 1900/1967: 567).

Jaspers writes of the 'typical basic relations of the individual to reality' (*typische Grundverhältnisse des Einzelnen zur Wirklichkeit*). He contrasts (Jaspers 1946/1963a/1997: 327) different styles of 'action and reaction', e.g. the 'contemplation' of the introvert with the 'activity' of the extravert and instances Emil Kretschmer's two dimensional schema of sthenic versus asthenic and expansive versus sensitive. In looking for the relations of the individual to reality, Jaspers follows his friend and intellectual mentor, Max Weber. The building blocks of Weber's *verstehende Soziologie* and Jaspers' *verstehende Psychopathologie* are ideal types. Ideal types are models or templates we hold against reality, models by which understandability can be assessed. There is a problem, however. This is the tension between the 'basic attitude to reality' of the investigator and that of the patient. The result of this tension is that there can be no absolutely secure basis from which to build an understanding psychopathology. In Jaspers' words (Jaspers 1946/1963a/1997: 326): 'when we understand, we must distinguish the validity of the understood person's reality from our own knowledge of that reality. All understanding remains in a state of suspension because of the lack of a final and definitive grasp of reality'.

Again, Jaspers invokes Nietzsche. Nietzsche questions our ability to know anything about ourselves or others and he calls claims to the contrary a 'primordial delusion' (*uralter Wahn*): 'one always stands a few steps too close to himself, and a few steps too far from his neighbour'. The result 'causes us to live in constant self-deception' (Jaspers 1936/1965: 132–133). We are constantly deceiving ourselves and we rely on various mechanisms by which we distort our true reality. Jaspers gives the following examples of mechanisms by which we distort our reality:

a. gaining satisfaction from the unreal
b. the release of tensions in inappropriate ways
c. sublimation
d. forgetting

(Jaspers 1936/1965: 135–7)

Such mechanisms within an understanding psychology look very Freudian but Jaspers draws them from Nietzsche. In Jaspers' view (1946/1963a/1997: 773), Nietzsche dealt with similar issues to Freud but 'more profoundly and at a deeper spiritual level'.

Symbols (*Symbole*) as content of the understandable

With the interpretation of symbols, Jaspers is back with Kant. He gives a lengthy quotation from Kant's *Critique of Judgement* (1946/1963a/1997: 331; citing Kant 1790/1952: 59) in which he says that symbol is 'a concept to which no intuition can directly correspond'. For this reason, symbol cannot be an object of knowledge; it is an idea of reason rather than a form or concept of the intellect. Jaspers goes on: 'the object of a symbol can never show itself directly in an intuitive experience. Thus, all our knowledge of God is purely symbolic'.

Jaspers acknowledges the importance of symbols from the Greeks to Carl Jung. He (1946/1963a/1997: 332) distinguishes symbols as 'carrier of personally valid meanings' and symbols as 'carrier of the encompassing meanings of immanent transcendence'. For Jung, the first are drawn from the personal unconscious, the second from the collective unconscious. Jaspers particularly commends the work of Ludwig Klages and Jung; but, while Klages' interpretations of symbols are vivid, Jung's interpretations lack inspiration. Despite their importance to life and to psychopathology, the interpretation of symbols is fraught with often insuperable difficulties:

- Firstly, the interpretation of symbols is endless; it can never be completed, the ramifications of meaning never stop …

- Secondly, the interpretation of symbols is itself an experience which adds to, augments and throws light on the symbolic. The interpretation of symbols is itself a productive process. There is no firm ground to be found in the interpretation of symbols.

(Jaspers 1946/1963a/1997: 336; my bullet points)

The basic forms of the understandable (*Grundformen der Verstehbarkeit*)

The forms of the understandable are concerned with 'opposing tensions in the psyche and the dialectic of their movement'. These tensions are polarised into opposites at various levels—'logical or categorical, biological, psychological, intellectual'. Opposites interact with one another, and 'this movement is called a dialectic' (Jaspers 1946/1963a/1997: 340). Jaspers begins:

> Psychic life and its contents are split into opposites; but, it is as a result of these opposites that everything comes together again. Images call forth counter-images, tendencies counter-tendencies, feelings contrasting feelings. Sadness turns spontaneously or with minimal cause into gaiety. An unacknowledged inclination leads to an exaggerated emphasis on its opposite. Understanding (*Verstehen*) must always be mindful of such opposites (Jaspers 1946/1963a: 340).

At the logical or categorical level, we have 'otherness (colour and tone), polarity (red and green) and contradiction (true and false)'. At the biological level, we have real polarities of 'inspiration and expiration, systole and diastole of the heart, assimilation and metabolism, sleep and wakefullness, male and female'. At the psychological level: 'the polarity of opposites is universal—activity and passivity, consciousness and unconsciousness, pleasure and displeasure, love and hate'. At the intellectual level, we have 'opposing evaluations—true-false, beautiful-ugly, good-bad, positive-negative'. The result is 'an unlimited number of polarities and opposites … The whole of understanding psychology revolves around such opposites … We call this movement dialectical' (Jaspers 1946/1963a/1997: 340–341).

The movement of opposites has three dialectical modes: 'opposites turn into each other over time … opposites battle with one another … I decide between opposites, in favour of one against other; turn-around results in an event, battle an action, and choice a decision. The latter two modes of the dialectic lead to radically different dialectical movements: a synthesis of "this-as-well-as-that" or an "either-or" decision' (Jaspers 1946/1963a/1997: 342).

Jaspers commends Hegel's dialectic of opposites as the necessary progression from thesis to antithesis resulting in synthesis: 'the riches of these dialectical possibilities—extending far beyond, but enclosing, psychology—is to be found in Hegel's philosophy. Hegel's *Phenomenology of Spirit* (*Phänomenologie des Geistes*) is inexhaustible' (Jaspers 1946/1963a/1997: 343). Comparing the Hegelian dialectic with Kant's forms of the intellect which, Jaspers agrees, are the basis of all knowledge, he goes on: 'the dialectic, in its various modifications, is a universal form of thinking which contrasts with the rational forms of the intellect which it uses and extends. It is indispensable to our understanding of the psyche. It gives a particular quality to our comprehension of the human situation, human facts and movements' (Jaspers 1946/1963a/1997: 343).

Jaspers then turns to the dialectic of opposites in psychopathology. In the healthy individual, there is either 'full integration of opposites in a clear choice or a comprehensive synthesis'. In the sick individual, the dialectic breaks down: 'one tendency stands alone, the other tendency having no influence, or there is no integration, or the counter-tendency achieves dominance'. He concludes (Jaspers 1946/1963a/1997: 343): 'we can make use of such criteria in the understanding of psychosis and neurosis'.

He gives the example of schizophrenia. In schizophrenia, we find examples of 'the extreme realization of the independence of one tendency without its counter-tendency ... (or) a failure to unify'. Clinical examples of the first are automatic obedience, negativism, echolalia and echopraxia; of the second, simultaneous but conflicting actions—what Bleuler called ambivalence. In the neuroses, 'we note both a failure of integration and of choice, for example, an inability to decide ... This dialectic of tension and release is particularly evident in psychotherapy'. Jaspers concludes (1946/1963a/1997: 343): 'when we look at the efforts of understanding psychology and at the study of personality, we see the dominating importance of opposites'.

The conception of psychic life as a whole

The distinction of form and content is universal in all knowledge; it is explicit in Jaspers' phenomenology and psychology of understandable connections (*verstehende Psychologie*), but implicit in the psychology of objective performance and causal connections (*erklärende Psychologie*). However, once we step beyond particular knowledge to psychic life as a whole—to nosology, eidology, and biography—the form–content distinction no longer applies and we are in the realm of Kantian regulative ideas. Kant's system is hierarchical: 'just as the understanding unifies the manifold in the object by means of concepts, so reason unifies the manifold of concepts by means of ideas' (Kant, A644, B672).

Jaspers picks up these themes in *Kants Ideenlehre* (*Kant's Theory of Ideas*) and in *General Psychopathology*. First, *Kants Ideenlehre*, then *General Psychopathology*:

> All objectivity consists of form and matter; each is impossible without the other. All our knowledge begins with intuition based on sensibility, becomes a concept because of the intellect and ends with ideas because of reason ... ideas have no intuition of their own; they relate to the intellect and only through the intellect to intuition. (Jaspers 1919: 465–67)

> Kant grasps and demonstrates brilliantly: when I want to grasp the whole, whether this be the world or the individual, the object eludes me, because what I have in mind is not something particular, enclosed and finite but an idea. What I get to know is never the world but only something in the world. The world is not an object but an idea ... It is no different when it comes to man. He is as comprehensive as the world. He may become an object for me, but I can never know him as a whole. (Jaspers 1946/1963a/1997: 560)

If we try to grasp the world or man as a whole as an object within the form–content distinction then, just as did Kant, we find ourselves trapped in insoluble antinomies and paralogisms. We can know individual facts and theories about the world and about man as 'an infinity of inter-related facts piled one on top of the other'; but the world and man as a whole are beyond our knowledge. The best we can hope is to 'arrange systematically within the idea of a whole what up to now have been dispersed facts. The idea of the whole seems to speak of all the facts as if they were one' (Jaspers 1946/1963a/1997: 560).

Jaspers concludes:

> If I cannot know the whole as an idea, I can get closer to it, in Kant's words, through the schema of the idea. Schemata are types I sketch out. They are false if I treat them as reality or as theories of what underlies this reality but they are true as a methodological aid that can be endlessly changed and corrected. (Jaspers 1946/1963a: 30)

Knowledge is necessarily the combination of form and content; forms of the intellect 'unify' experience or sensibility as everyday knowledge; regulative ideas of reason 'unify' the forms of the intellect as scientific knowledge. But, ideas are not themselves knowledge; rather, they direct the search for knowledge. Regulative Ideas are crucial to Jaspers' schema of diagnosis; he interprets them as Weberian ideal types. The form–content distinction and regulative Ideas constitute the essence of the Kantian philosophy of science standing behind Jaspers' psychopathology.

Form and content in Jaspers' later philosophy

For Jaspers, as a good Kantian, form and content are necessarily ubiquitous to all knowledge. In his *Von der Wahrheit* (*On Truth*), Jaspers (1947: 239) asserts 'form is the means by which being becomes knowable for us'. Two pages later he goes on (1947: 241):

> Form is the general, the rational; matter is the individual, the irrational. It is clear that there can be no matter without form and no form without matter. Whenever I think, I must consider both. If, by way of an experiment, I try to think of matter alone, I am immediately obliged to think of the form of the object of my thinking. Form is implicit in matter. Equally, if I try to think of the form alone, I am obliged to think what it is that this is the form of and this precisely is the matter ... Matter and form cannot exist independently of one another. The two exist together and together they build up the objective world'.

In the *Nachlaß*, Jaspers' posthumous notes, he asserts (Jaspers 1991: 5–6):

> Whatever I am conscious of exists as form. Whatever I think of I think of in terms of form. Whenever I think then all my thinking takes place within the dichotomy that we call the relation of form and matter ... Matter must always be matter of some kind, a formed entity and, in the same way, form must always be the form of a something, the form of a definite and particular object.

Jaspers and Simmel

The sociologist, Georg Simmel, was concerned to dissect social life into a myriad of forms of sociation (*Formen der Vergesellschaftung*). Simmel was a significant influence on Jaspers; much of the philosophy standing behind Jaspers' verstehende Psychologie is drawn from Simmel's *The Problems of the Philosophy of History* (*Die Probleme der Geschichtsphilosophie*), 1907. Jaspers (1946/1963a/1997: 302) acknowledges this debt; but, there is no acknowledgement for the theory of form. Nevertheless, the similarity and mutual debt to Kant is clear. Simmel (1910: 290–292) spells out his debt to Kant in his *Main Problems in Philosophy* (*Hauptprobleme der Philosophie*): 'the point of view here presented is possible only on a Kantian foundation ... no content of knowledge of which we can speak at all can escape formation by the forms of the mind ... Kant's thought has its pivot in the notion of form'.

Conclusion

The following schema summarizes the concept of form as it applies to Jaspers' psychopathology; the debt to Kant's theory of knowledge is clear:

- Form is a category, a language, a taxonomy, a conceptual scheme of the world.
- Form defines all that I experience and all that I know.
- The principles of a form are internal to that form; forms are independent and incommensurable.
- Form implies a selectivity from the flowing chaos of reality.
- All forms are incomplete in that no form can provide an exhaustive classification of the world.
- Form and content are independent; one content can appear in different forms and one form can have many contents.
- Forms are hierarchical; form at one level becomes content for a higher form.

The Kantian distinction of form and content underpins both Jaspers' psychopathology and his philosophy. It is explicit in the subjective psychopathology of phenomenology and understandable (*verstehende*) connections and present, though only implicit in the objective psychopathology of observable performance and causal (*erklärende*) connections. Once we reach the Kantian wholes of disease entity, constitution and biography the form–content distinction no longer applies and we must employ regulative ideas of reason. The form–content distinction also underpins Jaspers' philosophy. Both Jaspers' psychopathology and his philosophy owe a massive debt to Kant's critical philosophy.

Table 6.2 summarizes the influence of Kant's distinction of form and content from *Critique of Pure Reason* on Jaspers' *General Psychopathology*.

Table 6.2 The Kantian structure of Jaspers' psychopathology

Form and content in Jaspers' psychopathology	
Critique of Pure Reason	***General Psychopathology***
Transcendental Aesthetic: intuitive forms of space and time	A minor but very Kantian account of space and time
Transcendental Analytic: all knowledge divides into conceptual form and intuitive content	Part 1: *Individual psychic phenomena*: subjective phenomena (phenomenology) and objective phenomena (objective performance, somatic accompaniments, meaningful objective phenomena) divide into form and content; the first explicitly, the second implicitly Part 2: *Subjective, i.e. understandable, connections* divide explicitly into form and content Part 3: *Objective, i.e. explanatory, connections* divide implicitly into form and content Part 5: *The abnormal psyche in society and history*: psychopathology implicitly takes form and content from the cultural milieu

(Continued)

Table 6.2 *(Continued)*

Form and content in Jaspers' psychopathology	
Critique of Pure Reason	***General Psychopathology***
Transcendental Dialectic: legitimate 'regulative' use of ideas of reason to direct the search for knowledge illegitimate 'constitutive' use of ideas of reason in speculative metaphysics results in antinomies and paralogisms	Part 4: *Psychic life as a whole*: employs regulative ideas of reason as Weberian ideal types as the ideas/ideal types of disease entity, constitution and biography Part 6: *Human being as a whole*: Jaspers' philosophy as an extension of Kant's critique of metaphysics: the idea of the encompassing (*Umgreifende*)

References

American Psychiatric Association. (1994). *Diagnostic and Statistical Manual of Mental Disorders, Fourth Edition*. Washington, DC: American Psychiatric Association.

Berrios, G.E., Dening, T.R. (1996). 'Pseudohallucinations: A Conceptual History', *Psychological Medicine*, **26**: 753–763.

Erhlich, L. (1975). *Karl Jaspers: Philosophy as Faith*. Amherst, MA: University of Massachusetts Press.

Goldstein, K. (1908). 'Zur Theorie der Hallucinationen', *Archiv für Psychiatrie*, **44**: 584–655, 1036–1106.

Hagen, F.W. (1868). 'Zur Theorie der Hallucination', *Allgemeine Zeitscrift für Psychiatrie*, **25**: 1–107.

Hare, E.H. (1973). 'A Short Note on Pseudohallucinations', *British Journal of Psychiatry*, **122**: 469–476.

Jaspers, K. (1912). 'Die Phänomenologische Forschungsrichtung in der Psychopathologie', in *Gesammelte Schriften zur Psychopathologie*. Berlin: Springer. Reprinted in Jaspers, K. (1968), 'The Phenomenological Approach in Psychopathology', *British Journal of Psychiatry*, 114: 1313–1323.

Jaspers, K. (1913). *Allgemeine Psychopathologie* (1st edn). Berlin: Springer.

Jaspers, K. (1919). 'Kants Ideenlehre'; appendix to *Psychologie der Weltanschauungen*. Berlin: Springer Verlag.

Jaspers, K. (1920). *Allgemeine Psychopathologie* (2nd edn). Berlin: Springer.

Jaspers, K. (1923). *Allgemeine Psychopathologie* (3rd edn). Berlin: Springer.

Jaspers, K. (1932). *Philosophie*, Vol. 3. Berlin: Springer. Reprinted in Ashton, E.B. (trans.) (1969). *Philosophy*. Chicago, IL: University of Chicago Press.

Jaspers, K. (1936). *Nietzsche: Einführung in das Verständnis seines Philosophierens*. Berlin: De Gruyter. Reprinted in Wallraff, C.F., Schmitt, F.J. (trans.) (1965). *Nietzsche: An Introduction to the Understanding of his Philosophical Activity*. Tucson, AZ: University of Arizona Press.

Jaspers, K. (1946). *Allgemeine Psychopathologie* (4th edn). Berlin: Springer.

Jaspers, K. (1947). *Von der Wahrheit*. München: Piper.

Jaspers, K. (1951). *Über Meine Philosophie, Rechenschaft und Ausblick: Reden und Aufsätze*. München: Piper. (Original work published in 1941.)

Jaspers, K. (1957a). *Philosophische Autobiographie*. München: Piper. Reprinted in Schilpp, P.A., Lefebre, L.B. (eds), *Philosophical Autobiography: The Philosophy of Karl Jaspers*. New York, NY: Tudor.

Jaspers, K. (1957b). *Kant: Leben, Werk, Wirkung*, München: Piper. Reprinted in Manheim, R. (Trans) (1962). *The Great Philosophers*. New York: Harcourt, Brace and World.

Jaspers, K. (1963a). *General Psychopathology* (7th edn) (J. Hoenig, M.W. Hamilton, trans.). Manchester: University of Manchester Press.

Jaspers, K. (1963b). 'Zur Analyse der Trugwahrnehmungen', in *Gesammelte Schriften zur Psychopathologie*. Berlin: Springer, 191–251. (Original work published in 1911.)

Jaspers, K. (1963c). 'Die Trugwahrnehmungen', in *Gesammelte Schriften zur Psychopathologie*. Berlin: Springer, 252–313. (Original work published in 1912.)

Jaspers, K. (1991). *Nachlaß zur Philosophischen Logik* (H. Saner, ed). München: Piper.

Jaspers, K. (1997). *General Psychopathology* (7th edn) (J. Hoenig, M.W. Hamilton, trans.). Baltimore, MD: Johns Hopkins University Press.

Kandinsky, V. (1884). 'Kritische und Klinische Betrachtungen im Gebiete der Sinnestäuschungen', *Centralblatt für Nervenheilkunde, Pyschiatrie und gerichtliche Psychopathologie*, **7**: 481–485.

Kandinsky, V. (1885). *Kritische und klinische Betrachtungen im Gebiete der Sinnestäuschungen*. Berlin: Verlag von Friedländer.

Kant, I. (1783). *Prolegomena zu einer jeden künftigen Metaphysik die als Wissenschaft wird auftreten können*. Reprinted in Ellington, J.W. (trans.) (1977), *Prolegomena to any future metaphysics that will be able to come forward as science*. Indianapolis, IN: Hackett.

Kant, I. (1781/1787). *Kritik der reinen Vernunft* (1st edn/2nd edn). Reprinted in Kemp Smith, N. (trans.). (1933). *Critique of Pure Reason*. Basingstoke: Macmillan.

Kant, I. (1790). *Kritik der Urteilskraft*. Reprinted in Meredith, J.C. (trans.) (1952). *Kant's Critique of Judgement*. Oxford: Oxford University Press.

Kräupl-Taylor, F. (1981). 'On Pseudohallucinations', *Psychological Medicine*, **11**: 265–272.

Nietzsche, F. (1900). *Der Wille zur Macht*. Reprinted in Kaufman, W., Hollingdale, R.J. (trans.) (1967). *The Will to Power*. New York, NY: Vintage.

Sedman, G.A. (1966a). 'Comparative Study of Pseudohallucinations, Imagery and True Hallucinations', *British Journal of Psychiatry*, **112**: 9–17.

Sedman, G. (1966b). '"Inner voices": Phenomenological and Clinical Aspects', *British Journal of Psychiatry*, **112**: 485–490.

Sedman, G. (1966c). 'Phenomenological Study of Pseudohallucinations and Related Experiences', *Acta Psychiatrica Scandinavica*, **42**: 32–70.

Simmel, G. (1910). 'Hauptprobleme der Philosophie', an excerpt 'Von Wesen der Philosophie', Reprinted in Weingartner, R.H. (trans.) (1959). *The Nature of Philosophy* in K.H. Wolff (ed), *Georg Simmel (1858–1918): A Collection of Essays*. Columbus, OH: Ohio State University Press.

Chapter 7

Jaspers, phenomenology, and the 'ontological difference'

Louis A. Sass

Introduction

It might seem that the study of human consciousness, of the nature of subjective life itself, would necessarily lie at the heart of both psychiatry and psychology. What, after all, could be of greater interest, to us, than the question of what it is like to be us? How can one even speak of recognizing another human being as a human being apart from recognizing him as another subjective centre, embodied and embedded in his own way yet glowing with a comparable self-awareness and awareness of the world? And how can one claim to grasp human differences, whether involving culture, personality, or forms of mental disorder, if one has no inkling, imperfect though it may be, of what it must be like to be that kind of person or to see things as she may do?

In this perspective it can only seem surprising that quite a number of psychiatrists, cognitive scientists, and analytic philosophers, at least from the mainstream of Anglophone scholarship and science, have historically shown little or no interest in consciousness and subjectivity or the related topics of selfhood and self-awareness. Indeed, as is well known, many behaviourists and materialists through the past century and more have even been sworn enemies of any such focus, viewing subjectivity either as a nonentity or an inconvenience that can only undermine the scientific project. Such views survive in the genre of various forms of 'eliminativism' popular in some areas of neuroscience and the philosophy of mind. It is true that, when baldly stated, these extreme objectivist positions are often viewed as implausible and even *outré*. They do however resonate with mainstream tendencies in the now-dominant fields of neuroscience, cognitive science, and evolutionary psychology, where a focus on purported underlying neural patterns, cognitive operations, or evolutionary legacies can displace all interest in understanding 'what it is like' to be the creature in question.

In this chapter I focus on a thinker whose work, perhaps more than that of any other figure, has encouraged and preserved a focus on subjectivity in psychiatry and allied mental-health professions: Karl Jaspers, author of the classic book *General Psychopathology*.[1] Here I would like to consider Jaspers' most general and overall position concerning the nature of human

[1] Jaspers himself rejected the idea that his *General Psychopathology* was the *ur*-text of phenomenological psychopathology, noting that phenomenology is but one chapter in the book. Still, that chapter (in the English translation) is 100 pages long, and issues concerning subjectivity and meaning permeate other parts of the volume as well.

experience and the study thereof, as this is presented in his work on psychopathology. In doing so, I will offer some comparisons with more recent and contemporary views on both phenomenology and the philosophy of mind. My focus is not on Jaspers' views alone but more generally on the central issue of subjectivity: how to conceive of it and of the attendant problems inherent in studying it. In particular I want to bring out the worth of some later developments in phenomenology, largely hermeneutic and post-Heideggerian in spirit, that seem to be absent from Jaspers' discussion of these foundational issues in his work on psychopathology.

I will focus in particular on an article that Jaspers published in 1912 in the *Zeitschrift fur die gesamte Neurologie und Psychiatrie* entitled 'The Phenomenological Approach in Psychopathology' (a translation appeared in the *British Journal of Psychiatry* in 1968), together with some passages from *General Psychopathology*, which appeared, in its first edition, in 1913. The 1912 article offers Jaspers' most complete account of the nature of the phenomenological approach. Jaspers also cites this paper in his final revision of *General Psychopathology*, in the 1940s, and there is no attempt there to distance himself from his earlier statement. I will use this as an occasion to discuss the views that have come to prominence in the now-dominant hermeneutic approach to phenomenology, but that, understandably enough, are largely or wholly absent from Jaspers' early article and book. At the end I will discuss the relevance for phenomenology and phenomenological psychopathology of Heidegger's notion of the 'ontological' dimension of human existence, and of the human, all-too-human tendency to ignore or misunderstand this dimension, which Heidegger referred to with the famous phrase, the 'forgetting of the ontological difference'.

In anticipatory summary, we might say that the vision Jaspers offers seems, at the same time, overly modest and overly confident: overly modest in its views concerning the relevance of what phenomenology might have to offer the field of psychopathology, yet at the same time, rather over-confident about the precision and the certitude of the accounts it might provide. But my goal is not to criticize Jaspers, at least not in any pejorative vein; that would be anachronistic in the extreme. Phenomenology, after all, was in its early stages in 1912: Husserl had not yet begun *Ideas II*, let alone his final, posthumously published *Crisis of European Sciences*; publication of Heidegger's *Being and Time* and of Merleau-Ponty's *Phenomenology of Perception* lay 15 and 33 years into the future. It is hardly surprising, then, that Jaspers' article should offer a vision of phenomenology that is not altogether satisfying to the retrospective gaze of contemporary phenomenology. It is of interest, nevertheless, to consider Jaspers' methodological position and some of its limitations in the light of more recent thought in the philosophy of mind and phenomenology.

I should also say that, in his actual practice of phenomenological psychopathology, Jaspers may not actually follow but actually transcend his own methodological prescriptions. In this vein, one could argue, not only that Jaspers' practice of phenomenology contradicts his principles, but also that the success of this practice owes much to the extent of this contradiction or this transcendence.

But there is also another possible line that would avoid even postulating such a contradiction. This would be to say that Jaspers' methodological pronouncements should not be taken too literally, and perhaps not even too seriously—namely, that one should recognize that these pronouncements postulate distinctions that clearly cannot be sustained in any strict or rigorous sense, and that therefore, the distinctions he makes should be understood as but an exaggerated way of pointing out what are really just certain vague tendencies.

I am sympathetic to both these positions, by the way. I think, however, that it is of some interest to consider this statement, by Jaspers, of his methodological principles in a somewhat more serious, but not overly literalist way, and to consider its limitations when seen in the light of more recent thought in phenomenology and more recent developments in phenomenological psychopathology. That is what I hope to do in this chapter.

Jaspers versus objectivism

At the end of his 1912 article, Jaspers states that the point of the phenomenological approach is to 'further enrich our knowledge of what the psychiatric patient really experiences' (Jaspers 1968: 1323). Naturally enough, he rejects any position that would eliminate or marginalize reference to subjectivity or the first-person perspective. Thus he offers passing criticism of the two major strains of objectivism that have been present in the course of the past century or more.

One of these strains is epistemological: it is the notion that one cannot, in fact, gain access to the reality of subjective life, whether one's own or that of other people. The second is the claim that, even if one could and did, the reality one would discover would be of no great importance, for rather than explaining anything, or being the ground of decision or action, it is but a froth thrown up by deeper structures or more decisive processes taking place outside the realm of our conscious awareness. The theorists who are drawn to such positions are highly diverse, including such strange bedfellows as Foucault and Derrida (in some of their moods) as well as some behaviourists and hyper-materialists of contemporary analytic philosophy of mind or cognitive neuroscience. Perhaps the clearest contemporary examples are Daniel Dennett, a neo-behaviourist, and Pat and Paul Churchland, physicalists who advocate an 'eliminativist' approach to consciousness. What these figures share is an antipathy to any serious study of subjective life as such. In their aversion to exaggerated claims to self-awareness and freedom—claims deemed incompatible with a scientific approach—many such theorists have gone to an opposite extreme in which the availability and relevance, even the very reality, of subjective life is denied or dismissed, and in which subjectivity itself simply disappears as a serious subject of investigation.

Jaspers refers to the first strain of objectivism or eliminativism as 'objective psychology'—which, he says, 'claims to concern itself with objective data only' and whose 'natural consequence is psychology without a psyche', a perspective that would not and could not distinguish between a mechanism, a zombie, or a living person. (It 'does not matter', writes Jaspers, 'whether one is dealing here with a machine, alive but mindless organism, or a human being endowed with a mind'.) By 'eliminating everything psychic, [such a perspective simply] transforms itself into physiology' (Jaspers 1968: 1314).

Jaspers also criticizes materialism or reductive physicalism: those who are drawn, in exclusionary fashion, to studying the supposed 'extra-conscious base on which psychic events [may] seem to float like a thin layer of foam on the surface of the sea'. While acknowledging the attraction of this sort of explanatory approach, Jaspers insists that phenomenology is actually a 'prerequisite for any such investigation'. This, he writes, is because it is 'only in the setting of these phenomenologically established forms that actual life ... unfolds itself, and it is, after all, in order to arrive at a better comprehension of this psychic life that we are prompted to investigate its extra-conscious relations' (Jaspers 1968: 1323).

Jaspers, it seems, would whole-heartedly agree with such contemporary philosophers as David Chalmers, Thomas Nagel, and John Searle. With Chalmers and Nagel he would agree that subjectivity or experience is 'an explanandum in its own right' and that 'without some idea ... of what the subjective character of experience is, we cannot know what is required of physicalistic theory' (Chalmers 1995: 209; Nagel 1979: 71). We must, at the very least, articulate the nature of the explanandum, and this means that the study of subjectivity is indispensable even for the project of naturalizing consciousness or the mind. With Searle (1992) Jaspers would agree that human life and human experience are virtually one and the same, and that any rejection of 'consciousness' or 'subjectivity' flies in the face of all common sense, undermining itself as a position to be taken seriously.

'Empathy' and 'systematic study': Jaspers on phenomenological method

If we turn, however, to Jaspers' articulation of the phenomenological viewpoint, that is, to views about the actual nature of human experience and its study, we do encounter a number of positions that can seem rather dubious from a contemporary standpoint. These do not in any way vitiate the crucial importance of Jaspers' work in psychopathology, which remains indispensable and in many ways unparalleled. It should, however, help us to see some of the problems in Jaspers' metatheoretical positions: how, if taken too literally, these could hamper phenomenological investigation, and how they may have been superseded by more recent work in the phenomenological tradition.

Jaspers presents the phenomenological approach as having two key aspects, both essential to the enterprise: on the one hand 'empathy' (*Einfühlung*) and, on the other, certain techniques for achieving what he calls 'the *systematic* study of subjective experience' (Jaspers 1968: 1314, emphasis added). Empathy, for Jaspers, is as basic to phenomenology as sensory perception is for the objective sciences, given that the 'subjective symptoms' of the patient cannot be directly perceived by the psychopathologist. But Jaspers characterizes empathy as what can sound like a rather mystical or even magical process, something achieved, as he puts it, 'by transforming oneself, so to say, into the other individual's psyche ... by participating in the other person's experience, not by any intellectual effort'. In this way, he writes, the doctor 'can share the patient's experiences ... [and thereby] gain an essentially personal, indefinable and direct understanding' (Jaspers 1968: 1315). This seems to be grounded in the *Einfühlung* notion (borrowed largely, in Jaspers' case, from Dilthey (Wiggins and Schwartz 1997)) that will be sharply criticized by later theorists in the phenomenological as well as hermeneutic traditions. Such theorists are inclined to view interpersonal understanding less as a shedding and a transposition (*Sichhineinversetzung*) and more as a matter of mutual participation in a shared world. In an influential article, 'From the native's point of view', the hermeneutic or interpretive anthropologist Clifford Geertz states, for instance, that 'accounts of other peoples' subjectivities can be built up without recourse to pretensions to more than normal capacities for ego effacement and fellow feeling', and suggests that the achievement of such understanding is more like grasping the shared cultural forms of a proverb or a joke 'than it is like achieving communion' (Geertz 1983: 70).

Jaspers does, in fact, tend to describe empathy as a kind of merger or total identification with the other. This may be why he tends to view it as an either/or achievement, and one that reaches an absolute, unsurpassable limit when encountering something radically unfamiliar, like the 'fabricated' thoughts or moods of passivity experiences in schizophrenia (Jaspers 1968: 1318). Jaspers (unlike Heidegger and Merleau-Ponty) does not emphasize any inherent obscurity in human experience: if we fail to understand, it is because the gap is too great, not because we might be mysterious to ourselves. Jaspers does, however, recognize that empathy alone is hardly suitable to a scholarly or scientific project. Though it can be 'enormously satisfying to individual personalities', empathy alone, he writes, 'deserve[s] to be dismissed as "merely subjective" in a derogatory sense' unless it be integrated with 'more far reaching study of [a] regular system of concepts', thereby allowing its products to be 'discussed or verified' (Jaspers 1968: 1315).

Jaspers' vision of the systematization that is required is highly reminiscent of the phenomenological approach of Edmund Husserl, whom Jaspers acknowledges as having 'taken the first decisive step toward a systematic phenomenology' (Jaspers 1968: 1314) and whose early work, especially the *Logical Investigations* (first edition 1900–1901) seems clearly to be the major influence on Jaspers' approach to the study of subjectivity. The Cartesian or neo-Cartesian elements of Husserl's philosophical approach are well known.[2] Inspired by Husserl's account of a 'descriptive psychology' in the *Logical Investigations* (Wiggins and Schwartz 1997), Jaspers describes phenomenology as an eminently *descriptive* enterprise that is constituted by the 'preliminary work of representing, defining, and classifying psychic phenomena, pursued as an independent activity' (Jaspers 1968: 1314). Jaspers views this process as governed by the Cartesian/Husserlian criteria of the 'clear and distinct', the attainment of which is made possible, in turn, by a form of phenomenological reduction or bracketing that enables a direct seeing which Husserl referred to as 'intuition'. Thus Jaspers writes, 'We must begin with a clear representation of what is actually going on in the patient, what he is really experiencing'; we must 'develop … a fully conscious understanding of mental processes, one that can be represented in definite terms and forms' (Jaspers 1968: 1315). He states that phenomenology's goal is to make 'psychic phenomena' 'more lucid, precise and individually recognizable' (Jaspers 1968: 1321). To accomplish this, all theories and assumptions must be put aside, including all outmoded theories, psychological constructs or materialist mythologies in order to attain the 'freedom from preconception which phenomenology demands' (Jaspers 1968: 1316). The 'phenomenological attitude is to be acquired only by ever-repeated effort and by the ever-renewed overcoming of prejudice' (Jaspers 1968: 1316). Jaspers (like Husserl) is equivocal about how literally this latter goal should be understood, sometimes stating that psychology cannot hope to approach the 'scientific ideal' or that the 'ideal solution remains infinitely remote' (Jaspers 1968: 1315). More often, however, he speaks (again like Husserl) of 'acquir[ing] an unprejudiced direct grasp of these events as they really are' (Jaspers 1968: 1316), through what amounts to a process of reduction or bracketing.

Starting with Heidegger's interventions, the very idea of the reduction has come to be seen as problematic in two ways: one regarding the difficulty of attaining it, the other involving

---

[2] Husserl was perfectly explicit about his Cartesianism. In his 1931 book, *Cartesian Meditations*, based on lectures at the Sorbonne from 1929, he writes: 'Accordingly one might almost call transcendental phenomenology a neo-Cartesianism, even though it is obliged—and precisely by its radical development of Cartesian motifs—to reject nearly all the well-known doctrinal content of the Cartesian philosophy' (Husserl 1969: 1).

problems attendant to adopting its point of view. We might say, in fact, that with later developments in phenomenology, the reduction came to be understood in a highly ambivalent, even paradoxical fashion: as something that is, at the same time, unattainable, misleading, and indispensable: Unattainable in that, as Heidegger and the later Merleau-Ponty will argue, the biases of our being-in-the-world or lived body are so constitutive of our very being that we cannot easily separate ourselves from them or put them aside in an act of bracketing or reflection; misleading in that the form of reflection that reduction engenders may lead us to underestimate the dynamism and ambiguity of the world by making it seem more static and fragmentary than it really is; yet also, and at the same time, utterly indispensable, in that there can be no comprehension without some kind of distancing, no understanding for the person who remains fully within the flux.

Hence Merleau-Ponty's famous statement in the *Phenomenology of Perception*: (1962) 'The most important lesson which the reduction teaches us is the impossibility of a complete reduction' (1962: xiv). And hence Merleau-Ponty's (1968) implicit criticism, in *The Visible and the Invisible*, of Husserl's avowedly Cartesian, transcendental reduction as being what Merleau-Ponty calls the 'illusion of illusions': namely, the illusion that 'we have never been certain of anything but our own acts, that from the beginning perception has been an inspection of the mind, and that reflection is only the perception returning to itself' (Merleau-Ponty 1968: 37). Merleau-Ponty does not, however, reject the very idea of phenomenological reflection. As he notes in *Visible and Invisible*: 'The remarks we made concerning reflection were nowise intended to disqualify it for the profit of the unreflected or the immediate (which we knew only through reflection)' (Merleau-Ponty 1968: 35). But he does insist, in addition, on the 'necessity of another operation beside the conversion to reflection … a sort of hyper-reflection (*sur-réflexion*) that would also take itself and the changes it introduces into the spectacle into account' (Merleau-Ponty 1968: 38).

In light of these later concerns, it is apparent that Jaspers does not express much worry about the problematic nature of the phenomenological reduction, but takes its legitimacy pretty much at face value, roughly in the manner of the early Husserl. As a result, Jaspers has little to tell us about just why it should be so difficult to adopt the phenomenological attitude, or about what doubts we should perhaps entertain about the insights it yields. It is clear, in any case, that Jaspers is very far from adopting the more tolerant view associated with Heidegger's notions of the necessity, for understanding, of what he terms 'fore-having', 'fore-sight', and 'fore-conception' (*Being and Time* 1996: 141 (p. 150 in German edition)), or Gadamer's critique of the 'prejudice against prejudices', in which preconceptions are seen not only as obstacles but as inevitable and enabling components of any process of knowing (Gadamer 1984: 240). One consequence of Jaspers' uncritical stance (towards phenomenological reflection) is that he portrays phenomenological description as having an independent validity that rather isolates it from other sources of knowledge: 'Phenomenology', he states, 'can gain nothing from theory: it can only lose. The accuracy of a particular representation cannot be checked by its conformity to general criteria; phenomenology must always find its standards within itself' (Jaspers 1968: 1322). It is difficult to be sure how to understand this latter statement. Taken in one way, it may seem merely to state the indispensability of paying attention to the plane of phenomenological description—which is noncontroversial in the phenomenological tradition. In spirit and tone, however, it does seem to run rather contrary to the openness to dialogue and reciprocal influence that is called for by recent phenomenological writers, such as Francisco Varela (1996) and Shaun

Gallagher (1997) who have pointed out 'mutual constraints' between phenomenology and cognitive neuroscience and called for forms of 'mutual enlightenment', in which distinctions made in either field may suggest refinements or new avenues for the other.

'Phenomenology' versus 'meaningful connections'

In order to grasp Jaspers' approach to subjectivity, and in particular his attitude towards hermeneutics, it is crucial to understand something I have not yet mentioned. This is the fact that, for Jaspers, what he calls 'phenomenology' is but one aspect of the two-faceted approach to the study of subjectivity that he recommends. In addition to 'phenomenology', there is also what he terms the 'psychology of meaningful connections' or 'meaningful relationships' (Jaspers 1997: chapter V, 1968: 1322); it is here that many of the more hermeneutic or interpretative aspects of knowing come into play.

The basis of Jaspers' distinction between 'phenomenology' and the psychology of 'meaningful psychic connections', sometimes called *verstehende Psychologie*, can be difficult to formulate; Jaspers' presentation can at times seem rather informal and vague. It is clear, however, that Jaspers sees the first as more straightforwardly descriptive and the second as more interpretative as well as explanatory—at least in some sense of the latter, rather ambiguous term. Thus in phenomenology we are 'mainly interested in describing the facts as they presented themselves to us', yet it is true we cannot help but ask as well about 'what might be the source of this or that phenomenon and with what else it might be connected' (Jaspers 1997: 301). As Jaspers notes, the latter enterprise has sometimes been described as offering 'psychological explanation' in terms of a kind of 'internal causality' (Jaspers 1997: 301). Jaspers however warns against equating such 'explanation' or such 'causality' with that offered or discovered in the natural sciences of the objective world. The connections at issue are meaningful and subjective; they can only be apprehended by, e.g. 'sink[ing] ourselves into the psychic situation and understand[ing] genetically by empathy' (Jaspers 1997: 301). The relationships discerned are seen as somehow self-evident on principle, as when one immediately grasps how betrayal engenders jealousy or threat fear. However the application of such relationships in any particular instance is highly speculative and subject to doubt. Jaspers was particularly critical of what he saw as unjustified psychoanalytic genetic interpretations; and these may have contributed to his overall scepticism about *verstehende Psychologie*. Together with his acceptance of a Husserlian confidence about the epistemic grounding of phenomenological observation, this may have motivated him to distinguish rather sharply between 'phenomenology' and what he sees as its more dubious counterpart.

Jaspers offers two overlapping ways of distinguishing the objects of these distinct forms of knowing. Phenomenology concerns itself only with phenomena that are both 'static' and 'individual'—static in the sense of being divorced from any 'genetic' considerations concerning 'how one psychic event emerges from another' (Jaspers 1968: 1322); 'individual' in the (rather ill-defined) sense of being isolated from consideration of how experiences involve 'summation as a whole' or imply a 'frame of reference'. Jaspers' formulation of both these criteria runs counter to the holistic tendencies of many subsequent phenomenologists. The very idea of 'static' phenomena is, e.g. hardly consistent with the essentially temporal quality of human experience first analysed by Husserl and then given such centrality by Heidegger. Indeed one may wonder how true of actual experience a description could be, were it to exclude the element of anticipation (Heidegger speaks of *Dasein* being 'essentially ahead of itself'; *Being and Time* 1996: 373 (p. 406 in original German)) or the grounding in past circumstances that would seem to give it the quality it has. Husserl's analysis of the present moment shows that it is in fact always a 'specious present', constituted by its inherent structure of protentions and retentions.

It is difficult to be sure what Jaspers is getting at when he speaks of avoiding 'basic constructs and frames of reference', contrasting this with 'what is really present in the patient's consciousness' (Jaspers 1968: 1316). By 'frame of reference' does he mean to refer to an aspect of the patient's subjectivity or to an idea in the psychologist's head? It is difficult to see, in any case, how this structure could be compatible with an appreciation of the more encompassing or horizonal aspects of human experience, such as the general sense or feeling of reality, the experience of time, or the implicit sense of ipseity or basic selfhood. Heidegger states that 'Things at hand are always already understood in terms of a totality of relevance', yet this totality typically 'recedes ... into an undifferentiated understanding' (1996: 140 (p. 150 in original German)). All these are potentially important features of the patient's existence, part of the 'form' of experience that Jaspers himself sees as the essential focus of phenomenological study. It is unlikely, however, that the patient himself will be able to describe this sort of feature in spontaneous fashion, and unlikely as well that the psychologist or psychiatrist will be able to discern or describe it without the benefit of a certain theoretical sophistication and the use of 'constructs' whose adequacy could be tested out against the patient's reports and expressive behaviour.

To recognize this sort of aspect or feature is to recognize that the domain of 'what really present[s] itself to the subject's consciousness', of what is 'actually experienced ... "from within"' (Jaspers 1968: 1316, 1322) cannot, in fact, be restricted to the realm of 'individual' or 'static' phenomena; and that there must be some misleading prejudice that makes us think it can. It is not entirely clear that 'individual' and 'static' phenomena really exist; but if they do, their essential nature will not be easily separated from the deeper ground on which, or the larger horizons within which, they occur.

This holism of subject matter (of the essential structure of experience itself) demands a holism of method—a holism that is well expressed by Clifford Geertz when he recommends 'a continuous dialectical tacking between the most local of local detail and the most global of global structure in such a way as to bring them into simultaneous view', in a sort of 'restless' oscillation between 'minutiae' and 'sweeping characterizations' (Geertz 1983: 69). On this view one cannot make any sort of sharp differentiation between description and interpretation or between 'phenomenology' and hermeneutics (*verstehende Psychologie*). This is already very clear in *Being and Time* (1996), where Heidegger says, first, that the very expression 'descriptive phenomenology' is tautological or redundant, and then goes on to state that 'the methodological meaning of phenomenological description is *interpretation*' (Heidegger 1996: 30, 33). Another implication is that the widespread idea that phenomenology is or should be merely descriptive is incorrect, since interrelationships between phenomena—both synchronic and diachronic—are simply unavoidable. This implies that phenomenological accounts are, at the same time, less inherently certain but also more potentially explanatory than is sometimes assumed to be the case (Sass and Parnas 2007).

Forgetting the 'ontological difference'

Perhaps the most general statement of the latter view of the true nature of phenomenological accounts, and of how this view is likely to be neglected, is Heidegger's famous notion of what he calls the 'ontological difference', and of the 'forgetting' of this difference. This notion of the ontological difference is perhaps the key, organizing idea running through the entirety of Heidegger's work, from *Being and Time* (1996) and its predecessor lecture courses through to his final writings on the end or ends of philosophy. Heidegger uses it to explain the principal mistakes of that itinerary of error that (in his view) is the Western philosophical tradition, and also the mistakes which any contemporary student of subjectivity is likely to commit. These ideas clearly influenced Merleau-Ponty's final work, *The Visible and the Invisible* (1968), and may well permeate Merleau-Ponty's earlier work as well. The relationship to Husserl is more unclear, for though rooted in some aspects of Husserl, the idea of the 'forgetting' is also directed against various tendencies present in Husserl as well as in his, in this respect, disciple Karl Jaspers.

Heidegger defines the ontological difference as the difference between 'Being', the 'ontological realm', and 'beings', which he defines as the realm of the ontic. To forget this difference is to ignore the encompassing 'fact' of awareness or what might be called the very presencing of the world itself, and the modalities in which this can occur, in favour of a focus on the 'what', on the particular entities or objects that seem to occur 'within' the horizon, or 'against' the background of this awareness or this presencing. But what, we may ask, are the 'sources' of this forgetting, and why is it so difficult to overcome?

One answer focuses on the all-encompassing nature of the ontological. That which is everywhere is also nowhere, or at least nowhere in particular, which is to say, nowhere to be discerned. So just as the proverbial fish is unaware of the water in which it swims, so the human being will be unaware of the very condition of *Dasein*, or presencing itself, which could be aptly described (in Jean-Paul Sartre's words) as the very 'light of his eye and the atmosphere of his thoughts' (Sartre 1950: 81). According to Heidegger, this unawareness is an 'existential', which is to say, a constant or universal of the human condition in general. The same may hold, in a less universal level, of the individual human being, on what Heidegger called the 'existentiell' level, as when a person with paranoia or depression cannot attain the degree of self-distance that might relativize their suspicion or their despair, and therefore holds these visions to be unquestionably true, simply a reflection of the way things are.

A second answer centres on the question of reflexivity or self-awareness. Here the proverbial expression concerns the eye that cannot see itself seeing or, in more complex form, the foveal blind-spot that makes seeing possible (it is the portal of the optic nerve) yet is itself invisible to our gaze. Here the idea is not, as with the fish, that the everywhere is necessarily nowhere, but that the here cannot be there, namely, that the foundation, origin, or essence of my knowing or experiencing can be itself an 'object of' this knowing. These two answers may, in fact, turn out to be variants of the same, given that what is everywhere, for the human being, is *Dasein* or presencing itself, which is to say: a form of consciousness that is inseparable from some form of *self*-consciousness (for as Heidegger puts it, *Dasein* 'understands itself in such a way that this understanding'—which is a form of self-consciousness—actually 'constitutes' its being (Heidegger 1996: 298; p. 325 in original German)).[3]

It is crucial to understand that the obscurity in question is inseparable from, indeed coextensive with, the illumination that is consciousness or manifestation itself. The mystery of the world is in this sense unavoidable, never to be fully plumbed; yet it lies right here before us, in the visible or in the manifest. This fact implies an unavoidable element of mystery even within the experience that is most familiar to oneself, an element that seems at odds with Husserl's belief in the possibility of direct, certain, and precise observation of one's own mental life. Subjectivity is therefore described by Heidegger and Merleau-Ponty in terms of a complex, often paradoxical-sounding set of metaphors that include the intertwining or interdependence of light and dark, visibility and invisibility, surface and depth, and nearness and distance.

Heidegger (1996) himself explained the pervasive forgetting in several ways. Partly it results from our practical involvement, what he called our 'entanglement' with tools, obstacles, and concrete goals, all of which orient us towards these items themselves rather than towards anything so nebulous and trivial (from the practical point of view) as the fact *that* there is a world, a form of presencing, or a subjectivity capable of witnessing. More detached or contemplative modes can also be conducive to such a forgetting—in this case because of a focus on isolated, present-at-hand objects that are contemplated at a remove. This is central to Heidegger's critique of Descartes, who has often been viewed as serving Heidegger as a proxy for Husserl. According to Heidegger, Descartes fixates on a 'deficient' or derivative mode of being, namely, the kind of contemplative detachment that can occur when our practical activity breaks down—as when one contemplates the broken hammer that had been transparent in one's grip so long as it functioned properly. Such a mode of perception has an isolating or fragmenting effect on its field of awareness while also imposing, on this field, the criteria of clarity and distinctness as markers of the real (as in Descartes' famous demand for 'clear and distinct ideas' and Husserl's criteria of clarity and precision).

Engaged activity and detached reflection are antithetical in many ways, as Heidegger repeatedly emphasizes. Still, they both encourage us, though for different reasons, towards modes of understanding that are ontic rather than ontological. Either we live in the flux of practical activity or we stop and stare; but in either case we are likely to be oriented towards beings rather than Being as the underlying truth of things.

The coup de grâce of this forgetting is delivered by a third factor that reinforces and preserves the previous two. This is what Heidegger (1996: 118–122 (pp. 126–130 in original German)) calls our 'falling-prey' to the 'inauthenticity' of the 'idle talk' of 'the They'—which is a way of referring to the profoundly social/conventional nature of all discourse and understanding, which is always rooted in and dependent on what is generally believed in one's particular linguistic community, grounded in the authority of what Heidegger calls 'the They'. Any attempt to call the ontic mode of self-understanding into question, or to replace it with a conceptualizing of Being, is liable to strike common-sense as weird or self-indulgent, and may even be subject to ridicule.

---

3 The idea that, by its very nature, consciousness includes a kind of implicit self-awareness, can be traced back to Aristotle. See Caston (2002).

It is interesting to consider a shift in the way Heidegger conceived the origin of this error. As we have seen, in *Being and Time* (1996) the forgetting is a most natural event: a product of the most basic features of the human condition itself. But in later years Heidegger adopted a different view, now seeing the 'forgetting' more as an aberration—a kind of mistake, avoidable on principle, that results from the advent, in human culture, of a kind of self-centeredness, of the 'subjectivism' and 'enframing' inherent in refusing to recognize the reality of anything that does not fit into *our* categories, which are the ontic ones that serve *our* practical or technological needs but that tend to block out the appreciation of Being or presencing itself.[4]

Conclusion: Jaspers and the 'forgetting'

As already noted, Jaspers follows a Husserlian line in his methodological pronouncements, and it is the relatively early, avowedly Cartesian Husserl who is in question. It is hardly surprising, therefore, that many aspects of Jaspers' approach should illustrate the 'forgetting' that Heidegger surely attributed to his mentor and phenomenological predecessor. The very idea of viewing phenomenology as concerned with purely 'static' and 'individual' phenomena suggests a vision of human experience that is more ontic than ontological—as if subjectivity could be understood as, in essence, a matter of objectified quasi-entities that, if properly recognized in a presupposition-less way, would emerge in clear and distinct fashion before the distancing contemplative gaze.

Jaspers' famous attitude towards schizophrenic incomprehensibility can perhaps be understood in a similar light. The focus, for Jaspers, seems to be on certain individual symptoms, such as thought broadcasting or the experience of 'made' emotions—experiences that, taken in their individuality, do seem to be radically unfamiliar and perhaps beyond the pale of any imaginable form of empathic comprehension. Jaspers' version of phenomenology emphasizes, on the one hand, a form of empathy that is immediate or spontaneous and essentially non-intellectual ('participating in the other person's experience, not by any intellectual effort' (Jaspers 1997/1963: 1315)), and, on the other hand, an isolating of individual experiences in a controlled, focused, and purified reflection. What this does not allow, or at least does not encourage, is the appreciation of overall ontological or horizonal changes—of, say, fundamental mutations of pre-reflective self-experience or of the implicit temporality that constitutes the flow of our experience (see, e.g. Fuchs, 2013; Sass and Parnas 2007). Aberrations such as these would seem to require some more general theoretical speculation to be understood. And, once grasped in a partially intellectual fashion, they might not be fully recalcitrant to all forms of empathy, at least if these forms allow for the incorporation of certain theoretical speculations and insights—thereby, however, giving up on the ideals both of immediate empathy and of the presupposition-less gaze. Such a mode of understanding might be described as a form of 'radical empathy' (Ratcliffe, 2012). It is the kind that is probably required if one is to gain any real grasp of the most severe forms of psychopathological experience, such as schizophrenia but also, perhaps, forms of melancholia that take the patient beyond any recognizable emotional

[4] See, for example, the following essays by Heidegger: 'The question concerning technology' (1953), 'Building dwelling thinking' (1951), and 'The end of philosophy and the task of thinking' (1966), all in Heidegger (1993: 311–341, 347–363, 431–449).

state, no matter how exaggerated. In the case of such conditions as these, any 'forgetting of the ontological difference' will be particularly problematic, for it is likely to create a sense of difference and of distance that will seem absolute and unbridgeable.

References

Chalmers, D. (1995). 'Facing up to the Problem of Consciousness', *Journal of Consciousness Studies*, **2**: 200–219.

Caston, V. (2002). 'Aristotle on Consciousness?', *Mind*, **11**: 751–815.

Fuchs, T. (2013). 'Temporality and Psychopathology', *Phenomenology and the Cognitive Sciences*, 12(1): 75–104.

Gadamer, H.G. (1984). *Truth and Method*. New York, NY: Crossroad. (Original work published in German in 1960.)

Gallagher, S. (1997). 'Mutual Enlightenment: Recent Phenomenology in Cognitive Science', *Journal of Consciousness Studies*, **4**: 195–214.

Geertz, C. (1983). 'From the native's point of view': On the nature of Anthropological understanding', in C. Geertz (ed), *Local Knowledge: Further Essays in Interpretive Anthropology*. New York, NY: Basic Books, 55–70.

Heidegger, M. (1993). *Basic Writings* (D. Farrell Krell, ed and trans.). New York, NY: Harper Collins.

Heidegger, M. (1996). *Being and Time* (J. Stambaugh, trans.). Albany, NY: SUNY Press. (Original work published in German in 1927.)

Husserl, E. (1969). *Cartesian Meditations: An Introduction to Phenomenology* (D. Cairns, trans.). The Hague: Martinus Nijhoff. (Original work published in French in 1931.)

Jaspers, K. (1963). *General Psychopathology* (7th edn) (J. Hoenig and M.W. Hamilton, trans.). Chicago, IL: University of Chicago Press.

Jaspers, K. (1968). 'The phenomenological approach in psychopathology', *British Journal of Psychiatry*, 114: 1313–1323. (Original work published in *Zeitschrift fur die gesamte Neurologie und Psychiatrie*, 1912; 9: 391–408.)

Jaspers, K. (1997). *General Psychopathology* (7th edn) (J. Hoenig, M.W. Hamilton, trans.). Baltimore, MD: Johns Hopkins University Press.

Merleau-Ponty, M. (1962). *The Phenomenology of Perception* (C. Smith, trans.). New York, NY: Routledge & Kegan Paul. (Original work published in French in 1945.)

Merleau-Ponty, M. (1968). *The Visible and the Invisible* (A. Lingis, trans.). Evanston, IL: Northwestern University Press. (Original work published in French in 1964.)

Nagel, T. (1979). *Mortal Questions*. Cambridge: Cambridge University Press.

Ratcliffe, M. (2012). 'Phenomenology as a form of empathy', *Inquiry*, 55(5): 473–495.

Sartre, J.P. (1950). *Baudelaire* (M. Turnell, trans.). New York, NY: New Directions. (Original work published in French in 1946.)

Sass, L., Parnas, J. (2007). 'Explaining Schizophrenia: The Relevance of Phenomenology', in M.C. Chung, K.W.M. Fulford, G. Graham (eds), *Reconceiving Schizophrenia*, Oxford: Oxford University Press, 63–95.

Searle, J. (1992). *The Rediscovery of the Mind*. Cambridge, MA: MIT Press.

Varela, F. (1996). 'Neurophenomenology', *Journal of Consciousness Studies*, **3**: 330–349.

Wiggins, O.P., Schwartz, M.A. (1997). 'Edmund Husserl's influence on Karl Jaspers' phenomenology', *Philosophy, Psychiatry, & Psychology*, **4**(1): 15–36.

Chapter 8

Jaspers on explaining and understanding in psychiatry

Christoph Hoerl

In one of the later editions of *General Psychopathology*, Karl Jaspers writes that, when the book was first published, his discussion of the distinction between explaining and understanding was 'greeted as something radically new, although all I had done was to link psychiatric reality with the traditional humanities' (Jaspers 1997: 302). There is not a little tension between the apparent modesty of this remark and the somewhat grandiose picture of the psychiatrist that emerges from some of the other pages of the book, where we learn, for instance, that only 'a lifelong study of poets such as Shakespeare, Goethe, the ancient dramatists and such moderns as Dostoevsky, Balzac, etc.' (Jaspers 1997: 314) can furnish a person with the kinds of understanding abilities called upon in psychiatry.

Related to this tension within the book, there is an optimistic, but also a rather more cynical, take one might have on why the distinction between explaining and understanding, as articulated by Jaspers, came to enjoy a great deal of influence on work in psychiatry. According to the optimistic take, that influence is due to the fact that Jaspers correctly identified a key element of psychiatric practice, and for the first time provided the conceptual resources required to give it a precise theoretical articulation. According to the cynical take, the influence is rather to be seen as a result of the flattering picture Jaspers paints of the psychiatrist as a Renaissance man, whose insights are as much to do with a scientific understanding of brain physiology as with 'a close association with poetry and human reality at its greatest' (Jaspers 1997: 314).

In what follows, I will largely set aside Jaspers' claims about how the understanding abilities needed in psychiatry are acquired—which is where the cynical view takes its departure from—and focus instead on looking at how the optimistic view might be fleshed out. That is to say, my aim is to get clearer about what exactly Jaspers has to say about the nature of understanding abilities, and their role within psychiatry. What I want to argue is that there is some more recent philosophical work, in particular work on causation, that might be used to shed light on how exactly Jaspers thought of the distinction, but that also brings out where some of the challenges to Jaspers' position might lie.

Understanding versus explaining: the epistemic dimension

In a key passage, Jaspers characterizes the basic distinction between understanding and explaining as follows.

> 1. We sink ourselves into the psychic situation and *understand genetically by empathy* how one psychic event emerges from another. 2. We find by repeated experience that a number

of phenomena are regularly linked together, and on this basis *we explain causally*. (Jaspers 1997: 301)

As this passage indicates, at least part of the thought is that the understanding/explaining dichotomy marks a difference in epistemic method. Explaining, Jaspers thinks, requires repeated experience—it is achieved by 'observation of events, by experiment and the collection of numerous examples' (Jaspers 1997: 302), which allow us to formulate general rules and theories. Understanding, by contrast, is achieved (if it is achieved) directly upon confrontation with a particular case. As Jaspers also puts it, '[p]sychological understanding cannot be used mechanically as a sort of generalized knowledge but a fresh, personal intuition is needed on every occasion' (Jaspers 1997: 313). We might thus say that Jaspers subscribes to a form of *epistemic particularism* regarding understanding. Understanding is not achieved by bringing certain facts under general laws established through repeated observation. Rather, the grasp it delivers of how one psychic event emerges from another in a particular case strikes us 'as something self-evident which cannot be broken down any further' (Jaspers 1997: 303).

Jaspers is careful, though, to distinguish between this self-evidence of understanding and epistemic certainty. The immediacy with which it strikes us as intelligible that certain psychic connections obtain in a particular case should not be mistaken for a proof that they do in fact obtain. He illustrates this with the example of Nietzsche's *Genealogy of Morality* (Nietzsche 1994). Genealogy too, as used by Nietzsche, engages the faculty of understanding. As Jaspers writes, '[w]hen Nietzsche shows how an awareness of one's weakness, wretchedness and suffering gives rise to moral demands and religions of redemption, […] we experience the force of his argument and are convinced' (Jaspers 1997: 303). Yet, this is compatible with the possibility that the account Nietzsche provides of the 'particular event of the origin of Christianity' (Jaspers 1997: 303) is in fact false. Jaspers marks this point with a terminological distinction that can be seen to mirror the distinction between knowledge and belief: Just as there can be mere belief, falling short of knowledge, we can also fall short of genuine understanding, even though we may not realize that we are doing so.[1] In such cases, as Jaspers puts it, all we have is an *interpretation* of the circumstances.

The distinction between genuine understanding and mere interpretation, as Jaspers conceives of it, plays a key role in the way in which he positions himself with respect to Freud. On Jaspers' reading of Freud, the latter uses theoretical constructs modelled on understandable relationships to postulate unconscious mental states that are supposedly responsible for the patient's conscious beliefs, desires, and feelings. For Jaspers, there are at least two things wrong with this methodology. First, it blurs the epistemic distinction between understanding and explaining. Understanding is treated as though it yielded knowledge of general causal laws—in particular, laws that can also operate outside consciousness. Second, and as a consequence, this methodology can at best be said to yield '"as if" or pseudo-understanding' (Jaspers 1997: 307, compare also 539). By Jaspers' lights, Freud can at best be seen to be offering mere interpretations, rather than genuine understanding. We might also put the point here by saying that, from Jaspers' perspective, Freud's approach

1 See also Wiggins and Schwartz (Chapter 2, this volume).

ultimately involves a form of fictionalism.[2] Rather than making genuine assertions about his patients' mental life, Freud in fact engages in a form of pretence. Doing so may not be completely without purpose: imagining that the patient has the kinds of propositional attitudes Freud postulates may provide a useful tool in organizing observations and deriving predictions of their behaviour. However, this is insufficient reason for thinking that it is actually true that the patient in fact has those propositional attitudes, or that we are being provided with a genuine insight into what it actually is about the patient him- or herself in virtue of which they behave the way they do.

Conversely, a crucial aspect of Jaspers' construal of understanding is that understanding, when it is achieved, is factive: it does not just amount to a useful tool; it captures an objective fact of the matter about the patient's mental life. As Jaspers puts it, its role is to 'make[] something visible to our experience' (Jaspers 1997: 312). Moreover, understanding, as Jaspers conceives of it, is capable of playing that role because it deals specifically with connections between elements of a person's *conscious* life. What makes it possible to 'sink ourselves into the psychic situation' of the other is that, to put it in more recent terminology, there is *something it is like* to be in that situation. Grasping what it is like for the other, however, can also make intelligible how the psychic situation they find themselves in may give rise to certain other psychological phenomena.[3] Or so the thought goes.

'Meaningful connections': the ontological dimension

Jaspers also casts his disagreement with Freud in terms of the idea that '[t]he falseness of the Freudian claim lies in the mistaking of meaningful connections for causal connections' (Jaspers 1997: 539). This points to a second dimension the distinction between understanding and explaining has for Jaspers. We have already seen that this distinction, as Jaspers conceives of it, is in part a distinction on the epistemic level. However, there is also, for him, an ontological dimension to the distinction. In other words, it is not just that understanding and explaining involve two different ways of gaining knowledge; what they provide us with knowledge of is also different. *Meaningful psychic connections* is the term Jaspers uses to describe that which understanding provides us with knowledge of. Explaining, by contrast, establishes *rules of causality* (Jaspers 1997: 304).

What exactly are meaningful connections, for Jaspers? As can be seen from the passage quoted at the beginning of this section, he sometimes writes as if they must, in some sense, be non-causal ones (see also, Jaspers 1997: 28). Yet this claim is quite difficult to make sense of. One problem here is that, if meaningful connections were really non-causal, it would make it quite obscure what genuine epistemic gain understanding could deliver. Adolf Grünbaum makes this point by distinguishing between causal connections and mere 'thematic affinities' between psychic events. Thematic affinities between two psychic events

[2] See Yablo (2001) for a discussion of various forms of fictionalism.

[3] Jaspers acknowledges that there may be factors of the patient's psychic situation that are unnoticed by the patient himself, and that understanding may require realizing how such factors can be present in consciousness albeit being unnoticed. But he insists that being unnoticed, in this sense, needs to be clearly distinguished from being extra-conscious (Jaspers 1997: 306).

may make it possible for us to draw, in our *own* minds, a connection between them. Yet, this does little to establish the existence of an objective connection between them also within the mental life in which they occur. As Grünbaum puts it:

> [N]arratives replete with mere hermeneutic elucidations of thematic affinities are explanatorily sterile or bankrupt; at best, they have literary and reportorial value; at worst they are mere cock-and-bull stories. (Grünbaum 1990: 575)[4]

Thus, it seems that, if understanding is to yield any genuine epistemic gain, it must be concerned with more than just thematic affinities. It must be concerned with what is actually causally responsible for the specific psychic state that the patient is in.[5]

There is also a second, exegetical, problem with the idea that meaningful connections, as Jaspers conceives of them, are non-causal ones. On the face of it, much of what Jaspers himself writes about them, and about understanding, seems incompatible with this idea. Consider, for instance, the following passage:

> Psychic events 'emerge' out of each other in a way which we understand. Attacked people become angry and spring to the defence, cheated persons grow suspicious. (Jaspers 1997: 302)

What Jaspers describes as 'emergence' here clearly goes beyond the mere idea of a thematic affinity, as articulated by Grünbaum. And, arguably, it does so precisely because the relevant notion of 'emergence' at issue here is a causal one. There are also other terms Jaspers uses when describing examples of meaningful connections—such as 'reacting', or 'growing out of'—which are difficult to understand as anything other than causal terms.

It therefore makes sense to see whether there is a way of construing what Jaspers is trying to get at that is compatible with the thought that understanding, like explaining, deals with connections that are ultimately to be thought of in causal terms, even though the two don't deal with exactly the same (type of) connections. I think we can see how this might be done if we look at a concrete example he uses to illustrate the idea of an understandable connection. He writes:

> [T]he frequency of the understandable connection between autumn and suicide is not confirmed by the suicide-curve, which shows a peak in the spring. This does not show that the understandable connection is wrong since one actual case can furnish us with the occasion to establish such a connection. (Jaspers 1997: 304)

The specific point Jaspers seems to be making here is that there can be an understandable connection, in a particular case, between one factor, A, and a certain event E, even if, in general, that type of event is less likely to occur in the context of A than it is in the context of another factor, B. Straight off, it should be obvious that this point does nothing to

---

[4] Grünbaum takes himself to be criticizing Jaspers and his followers here, but I think it is arguable that Jaspers was in fact very much aware of the difference between a mere thematic affinity and a genuine connection between aspects of a person's psychic life. See, e.g. Jaspers (1913: 178), and also the discussion later in this chapter.

[5] Compare also Jaspers' distinction between understanding and mere interpretation, as discussed earlier.

undermine the idea that the relation between A and E is a causal one.[6] However, a point of this kind is sometimes made in the context of arguing for a distinction between two different types of causal claims, viz. what are sometimes called *singular causal claims* (e.g. 'David's taking paracetamol caused him to have a headache') and *general causal claims* (e.g. 'Taking paracetamol causes headaches'), respectively.[7] How exactly this distinction is to be construed is vigorously debated in the philosophical literature on causation, but there is one particular construal of it that in fact displays striking affinities with some of the remarks Jaspers makes about the distinction between understanding and explaining. On this construal, singular causal claims are in some sense more fundamental in capturing the real nature of the relation between causes and their effects, and general causal claims are mere generalizations over singular ones. This kind of view, sometimes referred to as singularism about causation, has been defended by Elizabeth Anscombe, who writes:

> [C]ausality consists in the derivativeness of an effect from its causes. This is the core, the common feature, of causality in its various kinds. Effects derive from, arise out of, come of, their causes. [A]nalysis in terms of necessity or universality does not tell us of this derivedness of the effect; rather, it forgets about that. (Anscombe 1981: 136)

Against the background of a view such as Anscombe's, we might understand Jaspers' view as follows. When he talks about (mere) causal explanation, what he has in mind are general causal claims linking types of events. Understanding, by contrast, is concerned with singular causation in the psychological domain—i.e. with the particular way in which one psychic event emerges from or arises out of another on a particular occasion. Furthermore, only understanding makes manifest what causation between one element of a person's mental life and another ultimately consists in. Insofar as there are true generalizations or laws in psychology at all, these obtain in virtue of the kinds of singular causal connections that understanding makes manifest. The obtaining of such generalizations or laws is not what makes it the case that one psychic event causes another on any particular occasion.

Interpreting Jaspers in this way does make it possible to preserve his idea that there is a difference in kind between what understanding provides us with knowledge of and what explaining provides us with knowledge of, whilst allowing that there is nevertheless a sense in which they are both dealing with causal relationships. It also has the added virtue of helping to bring into focus a particular challenge Jaspers faces. For there is considerable opposition in contemporary philosophical work on causation to the kind of approach advocated by Anscombe. I will discuss one expression of such opposition in the next section, and then consider the bearing it might have on how exactly we should understand Jaspers' view.

The 'level' of understanding

That mental phenomena be amenable to understanding is important to Jaspers for a specific reason. For he thinks that it is in fact constitutive of mental phenomena that

6 For some material on the relationships between causation and probability that is relevant here see, e.g. Cartwright (1979), Hitchcock (1995).

7 See, e.g. Sober (1985).

they do stand in meaningful connections to each other, and it is understanding that uncovers such meaningful connections. Any attempt to approach the mental merely by bringing it under causal laws, by contrast, ends up 'losing the object of the enquiry'[8] (Jaspers 1997: 302).

The basic intuition here is familiar from other writers. It shows up, for instance, in the following passage, in which Christopher Frith (1992) argues that delusions such as thought insertion have to be accounted for 'at the right level':

> [C]onsider statements of the type 'alien thoughts are caused by inappropriate firing of dopamine neurones.' Let us assume that it is true that there is an association between alien thoughts and abnormal dopamine neurones. Nevertheless, the explanation is clearly inadequate. It says nothing about the nature of the [delusion] and the processes that underlie [it]. (Frith 1992: 26)

The general idea in the background here is of a hierarchy of different possible levels of description, such as the physical, biological, and psychological, each featuring a specific set of variables. And the more specific claim is that accounting, e.g. for psychological phenomena and their specific nature requires linking them to other variables on the same level, i.e. the psychological level.

A particularly influential version of this latter claim can be found to be at work in authors such as Davidson and Dennett, who claim that ascribing propositional attitudes such as beliefs, desires and intentions to a person is a matter of rationalization, i.e. of making rational sense of particular beliefs, desires or intentions in light of the person's other propositional attitudes and the situation they find themselves in.[9] Fleshed out in this way, though, the idea that psychological phenomena must be accounted for 'on the psychological level' might in fact be seen to have paradoxical consequences when it comes to psychopathology. For it seems to force upon us a choice between two ways of treating phenomena such as delusions, neither of which seems plausible. Either they would have to be seen as responses that, despite appearances, can in fact be made good rational sense of, say, given certain unusual experiences. Or we would have to say that, despite appearances, the patient does not in fact hold the bizarre beliefs they seem to report.

Already from the point of view of common sense, this seems a false choice.[10] The possibility of an illness that befalls our rational endowment, whilst leaving intact the basic capacity to have beliefs and desires, seems all too real. Especially from the standpoint of the psychiatrist, though, it appears obvious that such cases actually exist. Led by considerations such as this, John Campbell (2008) has argued against both the general idea of a 'psychological level' on which psychological phenomena have to be accounted for, and the more specific idea that ascription of propositional attitudes is necessarily a matter of rationalization. For Campbell, both ideas in fact rest on the same mistake, which lies

---

8 See Eilan (2000) for further discussion of this ingredient of Jaspers' view, and also Sass (Chapter 7, this volume) for a connected critique of Jaspers' characterization of 'phenomenology'.

9 Cf. e.g. Davidson (1980) and Dennett (1987).

10 Which is not to say that there haven't been attempts to argue that one of those two choices mentioned earlier is in fact correct. Thus, Maher (1988) adopts what is in effect a version of the former view, whereas Berrios (1991) opts for the latter. Compare also Evnine (1989).

in the thought that causal connections must possess a certain form of intelligibility. He writes:

> We naturally seek a certain kind of intelligibility in nature; we naturally try to find explanations that will show the world to conform to reason, to behave as it ought. Hume's point is that there are no such intelligible connections to be found. This point has generally been accepted by philosophers thinking about causation. […] Hume's comments nonetheless do leave us in an uncomfortable position, because we do tend to look for explanations that make the phenomena intelligible to reason. We are prone to relapse, to think that after all we must be able to find intelligibility in the world. This tendency survives, I suspect, in the idea of 'levels of explanation.' The idea is that within certain levels of explanation, we will find a particular kind of intelligibility. [T]he lesson from Hume is that there is no more to causation than arbitrary connections between independent variables of cause and effect. We have to resist the demand for intelligibility. (Campbell 2008: 201)

The specific approach to causation Campbell himself subscribes to is often referred to as interventionism. One key idea behind interventionism is that causal relationships are relationships that are exploitable for the purposes of manipulation and control. Put very crudely, what it is for A to be a cause of E, according to the interventionist, is for there to be a way of manipulating E through manipulating A (see Woodward 2003, for a considerably more refined articulation of this basic idea).

What causes what, on this type of view, clearly has nothing to do with intelligibility. It is simply a matter of whether certain truths hold as to what would happen if we performed certain interventions. Campbell illustrates this point with the example of research carried out by Kendler and colleagues on depression following catastrophic life events (Kendler et al. 2003). This research suggests that the best predictors amongst catastrophic life events for a subsequent occurrence of major depression are episodes of humiliation, especially humiliation with some significant social dimension. As Campbell points out, alongside this type of research also stands other research that assigns serotonin transporters a causal role in depression. Thus, the question arises how we are to think of the relationship between these two factors, that both seem to play a role in the genesis of major depression. Campbell's suggestion is that we should simply see humiliation and serotonin function as two different variables that can be 'put together in a single causal account of the disorder' (Campbell 2008: 205). He goes on to say:

> Is there any reason why we should rule out such explanations a priori and say that they somehow involve a confounding of variables of different types? On the interventionist approach, it is difficult to see why there should be any such prohibitions. […] Intervene on the humiliation, and there will, in some cases at any rate, be a difference in the risk of depression. Intervene on serotonin function, and there will, in some cases at any rate, be a difference in the risk for depression. Do we need any more than this to establish the legitimacy of the many-sorted causal explanation? Isn't it perfectly obvious that the many-sorted causal account is legitimate? (Campbell 2008: 205)

Just to make absolutely explicit what the issues at stake here are, note two implications of the view Campbell sketches here. First, whilst in the example Campbell uses there is both a psychological cause (the humiliation) and a biological one (the serotonin), there is in fact nothing in his view that guarantees that there must be at least some factors 'on the psychological level' amongst the causes for any given psychological phenomenon. In interventionist terms, there may simply be no other psychological variable interventions on which would make any difference to a given aspect of a subject's psychic life. Second, there is, on this view, also no reason to think that causal links *within* the psychological domain need to be intelligible. As long as the right kind of interventionist counterfactuals hold between two mental states, the first one can causally explain the second one, irrespective of whether there are any intelligible connections between them. This is in fact what, according to Campbell, happens in psychosis. As an example, he uses the case of delusions of reference. He says:

> [On my] analysis, for one belief to be the cause of another is for intervening on the first belief to be a way of changing the second. Suppose you believe:
>
> (1) that this man is stroking his chin, and
> (2) that this man believes you need a shave.
>
> [...] What is it for the first belief to be a cause of the second? On the interventionist analysis, it is for intervention on the first belief to be a way of changing whether you have the second belief. So if some external force changed your belief that this man is stroking his chin, you would no longer believe that he believes you need to shave. (Campbell 2009: 143)

What we have here, then, is a view of causation, and of causal explanation in psychology, that is radically at odds with the thought that, in order to spell out what it is for two psychic events to be causally connected in the first place, we have to appeal to the idea that such events '"emerge" out of each other in a way which we understand' (Jaspers 1997: 302). As such, it is also at odds with the reading of Jaspers' distinction between explaining and understanding that I have offered in the preceding section, which turned on this thought. On Campbell's view, the idea of a 'meaningful connection' plays no essential role in accounting for causation between psychic events. Moreover, Campbell thinks that we have to abandon the thought that it does so precisely in order to do justice to the very idea of psychopathology—of a mental life marked by an impairment to one's rational endowment.

A third position?

How might Jaspers respond to the kind of argument Campbell puts forward? Perhaps we can make a start on this issue by looking again at the two examples Campbell actually mentions. Arguably, in each of the two cases, there is in fact still a sense in which understanding can get some kind of grip. What they might not involve is a transition between mental states that can be fully explained in terms of rules of rationality. But it is also not true that we have no idea how humiliation might give rise to some of the patterns of thought and feeling characteristic of depression, or how one might read a message about one's needing a shave into seeing someone else stroke his chin. What this shows is that our common sense notion of understanding encompasses more than the idea of rationalization. Common sense, in other words, finds a form of intelligibility in connections between mental phenomena that is not just a matter of rational intelligibility. Indeed, for Jaspers, psychology, properly speaking, only starts when we engage in a type of understanding that goes beyond a mere grasp of rational connections. He writes:

> Rational understanding always leads to a statement that the psychic content was simply a rational connection, understandable without the help of any psychology. Empathic understanding, on the other hand, always leads directly into the psychic connection itself. Rational understanding is merely an aid to psychology, empathic understanding brings us to psychology itself. (Jaspers 1997: 304)

We can think of Jaspers' position here as one that tries to establish an alternative to both the kind of view exemplified by Davidson and Dennett, on the one hand, and Campbell's view, on the other. Jaspers does subscribe to a 'levels of explanation' approach of the kind Campbell wants to abandon, insofar as he thinks that it is constitutive of psychic phenomena that they stand in meaningful connections with each other, which can (at least to a certain extent) be uncovered through understanding. Giving up the idea that there is thus a specific way in which psychic phenomena can be made intelligible would mean 'losing the actual object of the enquiry' (Jaspers 1997: 302). Yet, contrary to Davidson and Dennett, the relevant type of intelligibility here has to be distinguished from mere rational intelligibility.

This, however, gives us only an extremely schematic picture of Jaspers' position, and it has to be said that some interpretative effort is required to extract from *General Psychopathology* materials that might help to flesh it out in more concrete terms. In the book, Jaspers' initial theoretical characterization of the distinction between explaining and understanding is followed by a number of examples of what Jaspers takes to be types of meaningful connections. In this context, he makes use, for instance, of a Nietzsche-inspired notion of drives, or the idea of opposing tendencies that psychic life is always subject to. But, even setting aside the question as to whether these constitute psychological categories in good standing, it is very difficult to distil a systematic picture out of Jaspers' discussion that would help make clearer, e.g. how exactly he might respond to the type of argument put forward by Campbell.

Perhaps a better source for material that might help us flesh out Jaspers' position is an article, also published in 1913, which starts with close variants of the more programmatic remarks on the distinction between understanding and explaining that can be found in *General Psychopathology*. In contrast to the book, however, the article follows up these remarks with two extremely detailed case studies, each including an 'analysis' containing subsections that are explicitly identified as dealing with causal and meaningful connections, respectively.

What emerges from Jaspers' discussion of the two cases as issues to be addressed as a matter of (mere) 'causal explanation' is whether (and to what extent) the psychosis was, for instance, caused by imprisonment or homesickness, or by an innate 'hysterical constitution', or whether it reflects a pathological process of the type that is characteristic of schizophrenia (Jaspers 1913: 203). Much of what Jaspers writes here in fact fits in quite well with an interventionist approach to causation, insofar as it involves identifying particular non-psychic variables in play in each case. Specifically, Jaspers seems to think that we can identify which particular kind of such variable is in play because they make a difference to the particular form the psychosis takes. Thus, for instance, hysterical psychoses are characterized by a clouding of consciousness and often have a theatrical aspect, whereas schizophrenic psychoses don't have these features. Yet, there is also a respect in which, even here, Jaspers' interest can be seen to go beyond merely identifying particular causally relevant variables. What he also seems to be interested in is what we might refer to as the ontology of the non-psychic factors that made a particular psychotic episode possible: are they themselves episodic, do they exist in the form of something like a standing disposition, or in the form of an unfolding process?

Jaspers provides the most detailed discussion of what, by contrast, he regards as *meaningful connections* in connection with the case of 'Joseph Mendel'. In particular, one central claim he puts forward is that Mendel's psychosis can be understood, in part, against the background of a general sceptical disposition, understood as a lack of an ability to form firm opinions. This, Jaspers believes, leads to a preoccupation with philosophy—a 'metaphysical need' (Jaspers 1913: 253) or 'need for a system' (Jaspers 1913: 253). Yet, once Mendel actually starts to study philosophy, prompted by this need, the study of philosophers such as Kant, Brentano, and Husserl just reinforces the feeling that nothing can be asserted with any confidence.

Can an example such as this help to clarify how exactly understanding, according to Jaspers, can lend intelligibility to psychoses, and what kind of intelligibility might be at issue? Jaspers does stress in connection with both of the case studies that understanding of meaningful connections in psychosis can only ever be achieved to a degree (Jaspers 1913: 257). To the extent that it can be achieved, though, the kind of understanding Jaspers has in mind seems to be especially connected to notions such as 'psychic upheaval' or 'psychic disintegration', where these have mainly to do with aspects of the mental such as fears, wishes and motivation. Thus, for instance, Jaspers says of Mendel that he didn't suffer from intellectual defects, but that his psychoses rather have to be understood against the background of changes to the 'life of the will' (*Willensleben*) and his values (Jaspers 1913: 258).

On one possible reading, what Jaspers might be seen to be drawing attention to in these passages are features of human psychology that are simply left out by the idea of the mind as governed purely by principles of rationality, but that, in turn, have some bearing on the extent to which the subject can be rational. For instance, as Jon Elster (1985) has pointed out, whilst a given set of evidence may make it rational to form a certain belief, the question as to when he or she should stop collecting further evidence is not ultimately one a subject can answer purely by relying on principles of rationality. Whilst the subject 'knows, from first principles, that information is costly and that there is a trade-off between collecting information and using it, […] he does not know what that trade-off is' (Elster 1985: 69). As a consequence, even within the context of rational deliberation, the subject has to rely on 'shadow decisions' (Elster 1985: 69) as to when to stop collecting evidence, which cannot themselves be accounted for purely rationally.

So we might conjecture that understanding, for Jaspers, insofar as it is to be contrasted with or go beyond mere rationalizing, is in fact concerned with features of psychology of the latter type, that are in some sense preconditions for, and constraints on, rational thought. In this category we might further include, for instance, the conditions under which certain thoughts occur to us in the first place, or come to occupy us, or indeed become difficult to shake off despite some evidence to the contrary. Intuitively, it does seem that we have at least some idea, from our own case, how other psychic factors can have an impact on these features so that we become, for instance, more prone to jumping to conclusions or more prone to prevaricating. And if this is what Jaspers means by psychological understanding, we can see how it is indeed different from purely rational understanding, and perhaps also how it might be thought to have a special role to play in psychiatry. The thought, in short, would be that it is an understanding of this type that must be brought into play if we are to get at least some grip on what psychic illness actually consists in.

At the beginning of *General Psychopathology*, Jaspers characterizes the concept of psychic illness as being concerned with cases in which human beings' distinctive 'freedom and infinite possibilities are themselves a cause of illness' (Jaspers 1997: 8). If what I have been saying is along the right lines, we might see Jaspers as signalling here that, as long as we focus only on the idea of rationality, or of an absence of rationality, we will not get a proper grasp of what it is for someone to have a psychic illness. Rationality is impaired in psychic illness, but not every case of impaired rationality is a case of psychic illness. Rather, to get right the specific nature of psychic illness, we have to bring in the idea of a specific way in which rationality is affected in psychic illness. And what makes that idea available is the thought that rational thought is itself dependent on, and constrained by, other cognitive and volitional preconditions that are not themselves a matter of rational decision. In psychic illness, particular features of the patient's psychic situation affect these preconditions to such an extent that the very capacity for rational thought is impacted upon. However, even outside the context of psychic illness, the particular shape and content of a person's psychic life is never dictated by purely rational considerations alone. And we can therefore have at least some insight, from our own case, into the general kind of 'emergence' of constraints on one's mental life from features of one's psychic situation that, in psychosis, leads to a pathology.

The un-understandable in schizophrenia

Having sketched one possible interpretation of Jaspers' views on understanding and its role in psychiatry, I want to finish with a few remarks about a particular type of limit to understanding Jaspers talks about specifically in connection with schizophrenia.

Psychology will always come up against limits where understanding, as Jaspers conceives of it, is no longer possible. In most of *General Psychopathology*, the understandable is set off against the un-understandable primarily in the guise of that which falls outside the contents of consciousness. As Jaspers says, 'the act of understanding presupposes and implies something that cannot be understood' (Jaspers 1997: 308). This is true, he thinks, in two quite different senses. First, our mental life is shaped by the particular nature of our embodied existence and our interactions with our environment. These condition the contents of our consciousness causally from outside. Secondly, the very existence of a conscious life itself is also something that falls outside the scope of possible understanding.[11] Understanding can only encompass meaningful connections within consciousness; it cannot illuminate the conditions of the possibility of its own existence.

In a small number of passages in the book, though, the un-understandable also appears in a further, somewhat different guise—in the context of the idea that, in schizophrenia, some

[11] This, at any rate, is one way of understanding some of the more enigmatic remarks of Jaspers (1997: 308).

aspects of the patient's conscious mental life itself become in principle un-understandable. Jaspers writes:

> The most profound distinction in psychic life seems to be that between what is meaningful and *allows empathy* and what in its particular way is *ununderstandable*, 'mad' in the literal sense, schizophrenic psychic life. (Jaspers 1997: 577)

The idea of the un-understandable, in the specific sense at issue here, is meant to capture a sense in which certain schizophrenic symptoms are particularly puzzling. For it is to be distinguished from the idea that, in any concrete situation, there will be limits to understanding beyond which only interpretation is possible. The latter idea has to do with how much detailed information we possess about the patient. By contrast, Jaspers seems to think that there is something in principle un-understandable about schizophrenic psychic life. Yet, at the same time, schizophrenic un-understandability also has to be contrasted with cases in which, as we might say, there is really nothing left that calls for understanding. Jaspers makes this point by using the example of general paralysis and contrasting it with that of schizophrenia:

> In the one case, it is as if an axe had demolished a piece of clockwork—and crude destructions are of relatively little interest. In the other it is as if the clockwork keeps going wrong, stops and then runs again. In such a case we can look for specific, selective disturbances. But there is more than that; the schizophrenic life is peculiarly productive. (Jaspers 1997: 576)

What Jaspers seems to have in mind here is that there is a sense in which the schizophrenic un-understandable calls for understanding at the same time as precluding it. Schizophrenia, by contrast with general paralysis, is productive of genuine mental phenomena and—in line with Jaspers' position as sketched in earlier sections—it is in fact constitutive of such mental phenomena that they stand in meaningful psychological connections to other aspects of the patient's mental life. But there is a particular feature of the mental phenomena produced in schizophrenia that, at the same time, stands in the way of us being able to uncover the relevant meaningful connections through understanding.

Is there a way of fleshing out this line of thought in more concrete terms? I think the kind of interpretation of Jaspers I have offered might help us see a way to do so, especially once we note that there is one specific 'productive' aspect of schizophrenic life, in particular, that Jaspers seems to have in mind when he talks about the schizophrenic un-understandable. These are what he refers to as 'made phenomena', such as thought insertion. Against the background of the reading of Jaspers' position I have offered, we can perhaps see why he would find such phenomena particularly puzzling. For what is remarkable about them is that the patients in fact think of their own mental lives in the interventionist way suggested by Campbell: as being potentially manipulable by any variable whatsoever (even without any involvement of the rest of their own psyche). And this may be seen to make any attempt at understanding them a particularly paradoxical endeavour. On the one hand, to attempt to understand them, in the way envisaged by Jaspers, means that we must suppose that the patient's attitude towards their own thoughts somehow emerges from other, prior, aspects of their psychic life. Yet, actually 'sinking ourselves into the psychic situation' of the patient in fact means giving up, within the project of trying to understand the patient, on this very conception of psychic states as emerging from in each in a meaningful way. Thus, in schizophrenia, the content of the delusion that we are trying to understand—the idea of a 'made' mental life—conflicts with the very conception of the mental that governs the project of emphatic understanding.

Acknowledgements

Thanks to the members of the Wednesday philosophy of mind discussion group at Warwick for a number of very helpful comments. I am also grateful for additional written comments I received from Eileen John and Giovanni Stanghellini.

References

Anscombe, G.E.M. (1981). 'Causality and Determination', in *Metaphysics and Philosophy of Mind: Collected Philosophical Papers II*. Oxford: Basil Blackwell, 133–147.

Berrios, G.E. (1991). 'Delusions as "Wrong Beliefs": A Conceptual History', *British Journal of Psychiatry*, **159**: 6–13.

Campbell, J. (2008). 'Causation in Psychiatry', in K.S Kendler, J. Parnas (eds), *Philosophical Issues in Psychiatry*. Baltimore, MD: Johns Hopkins University Press, 196–215.

Campbell, J. (2009). 'What Does Rationality Have to do with Psychological Causation?: Propositional Attitudes as Mechanisms and as Control Variables', in L. Bortolotti, M. Broome (eds), *Psychiatry as Cognitive Neuroscience*. Oxford: Oxford University Press, 137–149.

Cartwright, N. (1979). 'Causal Laws and Effective Strategies', *Noûs*, **13**: 419–437.

Davidson, D. (1980). 'Mental Events', in *Essays on Actions and Events*. Oxford: Clarendon Press, 207–227.

Dennett, D. (1987). 'True Believers. The Intentional Strategy and Why it Works', in *The Intentional Stance*. Cambridge MA: MIT Press, 13–35.

Eilan, N. (2000). 'On Understanding Schizophrenia', in D. Zahavi (ed), *Exploring the Self: Philosophical and Psychopathological Perspectives on Self-Experience*. Amsterdam: John Benjamins, 97–113.

Elster, J. (1985). 'The Nature and Scope of Rational-Choice Explanations', in E. LePore, B.P. McLaughlin (eds), *Actions and Events: Perspectives on the Philosophy of Donald Davidson*. Oxford: Blackwell, 60–72.

Evnine, S.J. (1989). 'Understanding Madness?', *Ratio*, **2**: 1–18

Frith, C.D. (1992). *The Cognitive Neuropsychology of Schizophrenia*. Hove: Lawrence Erlbaum Associates.

Grünbaum, A. (1990). '"Meaning" Connections and Causal Connections in the Human sciences', *Journal of the American Psychoanalytic Association*, **38**: 559–577.

Hitchcock, C. (1995). 'The Mishap at Reichenbach Fall: Singular vs. General Causation', *Philosophical Studies*, **78**: 257–291.

Jaspers, K. (1913). 'Kausale und Verständliche Zusammenhänge zwischen Schicksal und Psychose bei der Dementia Praecox (Schizophrenie)', *Zeitschrift für die gesamte Neurologie und Psychiatrie*, **14**: 158–263.

Jaspers, K. (1997). *General Psychopathology* (7th edn) (J. Hoenig, M.W. Hamilton, trans.). Baltimore, MD: Johns Hopkins University Press.

Kendler, K.S., Hettema, J.M., Butera, F., Gardner, C.O., Prescott, C.A. (2003). 'Life Event Dimensions of Loss, Humiliation, Entrapment, and Danger in the Prediction of Onsets of Major Depression and Generalized Anxiety', *Archives of General Psychiatry*, **60**: 789–796.

Maher, B.A. (1988). 'Anomalous Experience and Delusional Thinking: The Logic of Explanations', in T.F. Oltmanns, B.A. Maher (eds), *Delusional Beliefs*. Chichester: John Wiley and Sons, 15–33.

Nietzsche, F. (1994). *On the Genealogy of Morality* (C. Diethe, trans.). Cambridge: Cambridge University Press.

Sober, E. (1985). 'Two Concepts of Cause', in P. Asquith, P. Kitcher (eds) *PSA*, Vol. II. East Lansing, MI: Philosophy of Science Association, 405–424.

Woodward, J. (2003). *Making Things Happen: A Theory of Causal Explanation*. Oxford: Oxford University Press.

Yablo, S. (2001). 'Go figure: A Path Through Fictionalism', *Midwest Studies in Philosophy*, **25**: 72–102.

Chapter 9

Jaspers and neuroscience

Matthew R. Broome

Introduction

One of the recent surprises in the history of ideas is that the rebirth of interest in the philosophy of psychiatry followed closely on the heels of 'the decade of the brain' and advances in neurosciences. As has been pointed out (Fulford 2003), perhaps this shouldn't in fact come as such as a surprise: with empirical scientific advances comes the pressure to think deeply about their significance, their place within existing knowledge, and how prior discourse and practice stands in relation to the new findings. Given this volume marks the centenary of Jaspers' publication of the first edition of *General Psychopathology*, as Fulford and colleagues point out, the historical moment now, one hundred years after this publication and after the 'decade of the brain', is similar to the conceptual terrain that Jaspers found himself in the early twentieth century and the 'first biological psychiatry' (Shorter 1997). As such, psychiatry is intensely interested in the nature of the experiences our patients relate to us (Broome et al. 2013; Ratcliffe and Broome 2012), their relationship to the classificatory systems we employ, and how in turn such experiences can be investigated scientifically (Broome and Bortolotti 2009; Broome et al. 2012).

In this contribution, Jaspers' views on neuroscience and its relationship to psychopathology will be described. Firstly, there will be a brief historical discussion of neuroscience and its place in the 'first biological psychiatry' of the late nineteenth century, secondly, this will be followed by a detailed exegesis of Jaspers' views on the psyche and neuroscience in the translated 1959 edition of *General Psychopathology*. Thirdly, a brief survey of Jaspers' later general views on science and pluralism will be presented.

The historical background

Engstrom's rich book, *Clinical Psychiatry in Imperial Germany* (2003), charts Wilhelm Griesinger's reforms to psychiatry and in particular the shift from asylum and alienist-led psychiatry to one based in university clinics, with a concurrent emphasis on laboratory science and the investigation of the brain. As part of this shift, the subject matter of psychiatry also changed. On Engstrom's account, academic psychiatrists drew less on the clinical experience of admitted patients, but, in the 1870s and 1880s, on more basic scientific techniques, with a resultant shift in the object under investigation.

> Their observations were directed not so much at institutionalized patients, as at histological specimens, and vivisected animals. They drew less upon skills derived from years of asylum experience and more upon practices and techniques learned as students and honed in rudimentary laboratory facilities. Their ideal was not the practicing alienist, but rather the diligent

> researcher who spent long hours in front of the microscope and at the autopsy table. The psychiatric knowledge that they extracted from their objects of study was the product of disciplined laboratory conduct in handling microscopes and specimens, in opening the cranium, in applying electrodes. For them, psychiatry was a natural science with its own rigorous techniques and modes of observation. (Engstrom 2003: 89)

This vivid picture of Engstrom's is helpful to bear in mind: these are the academic psychiatrists of the generation just before Jaspers, those who trained in the last decades of the nineteenth century prior to Jaspers' writing of the *General Psychopathology* and undoubtedly, this mindset would have influenced Jaspers. Engstrom goes on to note that Griesinger referred to alienists as 'fossils from a distant past' (Engstrom 2003: 90) and indeed, the younger psychiatrists chose not the title of alienist (*Irrenheilkünstler*) but rather that of 'cerebral pathologist' (Engstrom 2003: 90). With this paradigm and ideological shift, the bright young psychiatrists saw their object of study not the person or the patient but rather the brain or nervous system, and further a nervous system that was viewed through complex microscopic, staining, and histopathological techniques.

Engstrom cites the Jena Professor of Psychiatry, and Nietzsche's psychiatrist, Otto Binswanger, writing in 1892 of the scientific optimism of the prior two decades:

> A degree of disdain for imponderable psychic influences became the norm. This [scientific] progress literally intoxicated the heads [*Gemüter*] of many; in heated efforts to derive the cause and manifestations of all normal and pathological life processes from the fundamental precepts of biological research, from chemical, physical, and mechanical processes, the old facts derived from observing nature [*Naturbeobachtung*] were jettisoned as irrelevant and unproven, and hence inexplicable ballast as they could no longer be fitted into the framework of so called exact research. (Engstrom 2003: 98)

What here Binswanger is already picking up on is that the zenith of biological psychiatry was short lived: the spectacular advances of the 1860s and 1870s were not continued into the 1880s and psychiatrists like Meynert and Flechsig (psychiatrist to Schreber) were accused of over extending neuroscientific theories into mental illness and charged with a term that Jaspers uses, 'brain mythology'. Hence, Jaspers' concerns regarding the somatic dominance of psychiatry were very much of their time and part of a wider concern as to the ideological excesses of the 1860s to 1880s.

In his own philosophical autobiography, Jaspers (1981) echoes some of the historical trends Engstrom details and recounts working under the supervision of Nissl. Jaspers describes him thus: 'He was an excellent research man, a brain histologist' (Jaspers 1981: 13) and notes that although Nissl had started working to the Griesinger maxim of mental illnesses as diseases of the brain, his own research undermined this proposition and his interest in clinical psychiatry developed and grew. Jaspers too notes the disappointment in the promise of biological psychiatry that he and his colleagues keenly felt:

> The realization that scientific investigation and therapy were in a state of stagnation was widespread in German psychiatric clinics at that time. The large institutions for the mentally ill were built constantly more hygienic and more magnificent. The lives of the unfortunate inmates, which could not be changed essentially, were controlled […]. In view of the exceedingly small amount of knowledge and technical knowhow, intelligent, yet unproductive psychiatrists, such as Hoche, took recourse to a sceptical attitude and to elegant sounding phrases of gentlemanly superiority.

> In Nissl's hospital too, therapeutic resignation was dominant. In therapeutics we were basically without hope, but we were humane and kind and prevented, as far as possible, any calamity which might unnecessarily result from the condition of the mentally ill. (Jaspers 1981: 16)

Jaspers describes much of the psychiatric literature, in terms reminiscent of positivist philosophy, as 'unfounded chatter' (Jaspers 1981: 16) and criticizes the obscurity, jargon, and lack of common theoretical language in discourse. Jaspers makes a diagnosis of this difficulty of psychiatric thinking: psychiatry had forgotten that its subject was man, rather than his body. As such, Jaspers describes how he turned to philosophy, philology, social and cultural science, and psychology and utilized the thought of Husserl, Dilthey, and Weber (Broome et al. 2013; Jaspers 1981), emphasizing the importance of methodological reflection and pluralism regarding theories. Hence from a more widespread theoretical disaffection, Jaspers launched his attempts to diagnose the crisis in psychiatry and to reground its practice.

General Psychopathology

Jaspers views on biology, and on the nervous system, are scattered throughout the two volumes of the 1959 edition of *General Psychopathology*, but with some important, key concepts detailed in the introduction. From the opening of the book, Jaspers (1959) is clear that:

> The psychiatrist as a practitioner deals with individuals, with the human being as a whole. (Jaspers 1959/1997: 1)

and that:

> Psychopathology is limited in that there can be no final analysis of human beings as such, since the more we reduce them to what is typical and normative the more we realise there is something hidden in every individual that defies recognition. We have to be content with partial knowledge of an infinity which we cannot exhaust. (Jaspers 1959/1997: 1)

Here are two themes, announced in the introduction, around the scope of psychiatry and psychopathology and go against the model of psychiatry as 'cerebral pathology', as described earlier. Firstly, psychiatry is about the human as a whole and as an individual, a theme linked to his neo-Kantian heritage (Broome 2008), and secondly, it is limited, partial and incomplete. He goes on to describe psychopathology's subject matter as 'actual conscious psychic events' (Jaspers 1959/1997: 2) but stresses the importance of somatic events as causes of mental states, and the relationship between mind and body.

> In every individual event soma and psyche form an inseparable unity. The two stand in mutual reciprocity which shows itself more directly in psychopathology than it does in normal psychology […]. [I]nsight into the aetiology of psychic events cannot be achieved without some knowledge of somatic function, more particularly the physiology of the nervous system. Thus psychopathology finds in neurology, internal medicine and physiology its most valuable auxiliary sciences.
>
> Investigation of somatic function, including the most complex cortical activity, is bound up with investigation of psychic function, and the unity of soma and psyche seems indisputable. Yet we must remember that neither line of enquiry encounters the other so directly that we can speak of some specific psychic event as directly associated with some specific somatic event or of an actual parallelism. The situation is analogous with the exploration of an unknown continent

> from opposite directions, where the explorers never meet because of the impenetrable country that intervenes. We only know the end links in the chain of causation from soma to psyche and vice versa and from both these terminal points we endeavour to advance. Neurology has discovered that the cortex with the brain stem provides the organ most closely associated with psychic function and its researchers have reached their highest peak so far in the theory of aphasia, agnosia, and apraxia. It seems, however, as if the further neurology advances, the further the psyche recedes; psychopathology on the other hand explores the psyche to the limits of consciousness but finds at these limits no somatic processes directly associated with such phenomena as delusional ideas, spontaneous affects and hallucinations. In many cases, which increase in number as we gain in knowledge, the primary source of psychic change is found to lie in some cerebral disorder. Yet we always find that no one specific psychic change is characteristic for any one of these disorders. The facts seem to be that cerebral disorders may be responsible for almost all possible psychic changes though the frequency with which they may appear may vary in different disorders (for example, in *General Paralysis of the Insane*). (Jaspers 1959/1997: 3–4)

This is a dense section and, metaphysically, offers a detailed conception of the relation between psyche and soma. His first point is that psyche and soma are an 'inseparable unity' and stand in a reciprocal relationship to one another. This seems to suggest that both can affect one another and are in turn constrained by one another. Further, this reciprocity is perhaps clearer in psychopathology than in normal mental function, the thought being perhaps that these mutual constraints and interdependence are clearer, or stronger, in mental illness. Moving on from this statement of unity, Jaspers makes a trenchant approval of what may be called neuroscientific method. He stresses the importance of studying the nervous system including, in a phrase resonant with the work of contemporary functional neuroimagers, of 'the most complex cortical activity'. However, despite stressing the unity of psyche and soma, Jaspers then introduces the idea of an epistemological void or abyss, 'an impenetrable country', which separates our knowledge of how precisely to link up our comprehension of psychic events with somatic events. Despite being convinced of general unity between these events, Jaspers claims that we cannot speak of connections between specific psychic and somatic events. What is not clear, at this point, is what stops us knowing the precise causal connections linking these two classes of events: whether, for Jaspers, it is a conceptual '*Mysterianism*', as in the work of Colin McGinn (1991) on consciousness where the human intellect is posited as simply not capable of solving the problem of consciousness, or is an empirical problem that may be resolved with scientific advances. Jaspers again reiterates the claim that the primary source for many psychic changes lie in the brain, yet there is not a clear tight connection between a given cerebral change and a resultant psychic change. Hence, we have both some positive views of Jaspers regarding the unity of psyche and soma, and the importance of neuroscience, but some pessimistic views as to how precise physical changes are mapped onto discrete mental states. Further, there is a seeming worry: that with the progress of neurology, the psyche recedes, and as such the soma and somatic models of illness have explanatory and ontological dominance. This worry is brought out more explicitly by Jaspers (1959/1997) later in the introduction in his discussion of the 'somatic prejudice'. He defines this 'prejudice' thus:

> Tacit assumptions are made that, like everything else biological, the actual reality of human existence is a somatic event. Man is only comprehensible when he is understood in somatic terms; should the psyche be mentioned, this is in the nature of a theoretical stop-gap of no real scientific value. A tendency arises to discuss all psychic events as if their essence were something

> somatic, already in one's grasp, or as if such a concept merely pointed the way to discoveries of a somatic nature. (Jaspers 1959/1997: 18)

For Jaspers, having stressed the unity and equal importance of psyche and soma, he addresses the prejudice that the soma and its study is the locus of true scientific endeavour and that this in turn leads to 'resignation' when considering matters psychologically. Indeed, the psyche is a 'theoretical stop-gap': so much like the contemporary eliminative materialism of Paul and Patricia Churchland (1986, 1988), Jaspers' worry is that for those enthralled by the somatic prejudice they may view the psyche much like folk psychology is viewed for the Churchlands (who in turn cite the example of phlogiston as a scientific construct and theoretical concept now abandoned by natural science), and that the psyche will vanish and be eliminated through the endeavours of the somatic researchers. As a warning of this view, again resonant with contemporary scientific psychopathology, Jaspers gives an example of the 'somatic prejudice' as 'all psychological interest in schizophrenia will vanish when the morbid somatic process that underlies it is discovered' (Jaspers 1959/1997). Jaspers discusses his predecessors in late nineteenth- and early twentieth-century psychiatry who felt that for the psyche to be discussed scientifically it had to be in the guise of physiology or anatomy and as a somatic function. As such, early theoretical biological constructs and mechanisms were more preferred, and viewed as more 'scientific', than any psychological account. Jaspers endorses the term 'Brain Mythologies' to denote the target of the criticism of this use of non-empirical, fantastic, theoretical, 'pseudo scientific' explanatory accounts and entities. Jaspers here remains not anti-science, or anti-neuroscience specifically, but coherently with his later views on science more generally, ecumenical and pluralistic. His reason for emphasizing the 'somatic prejudice' is not to limit biological research or critique it but rather to challenge its hegemony and dominance. As such, Jaspers maintains his view of the unity and inter-dependence of the psyche and soma, a unity where emphasizing one element of investigation ('neurology') over another ('psychopathology') is not warranted.

Later in the introduction there is a clue as to why for Jaspers the relationship between psyche and soma is more apparent in psychopathological states. Essentially, the idea here is that in some morbid states, the classic example for Jaspers being the primary delusions of schizophrenia, folk psychology 'runs out' as an explanatory tool: we cannot follow the person's thought processes we are interviewing and it is here, in this failure to follow the psychic processes of the other that, rather than holding up our hands and saying we can go no further, we turn to causal processes. As Jaspers puts it:

> In psychopathology our genetic understanding (or perception of meaningful connection) soon reaches its limits. […] In psychopathology psychic phenomena appear suddenly as something entirely new, in a way we cannot understand at all. One psychic event follows another quite incomprehensibly; it seems to follow arbitrarily rather than emerge. Stages of psychic development in normal people, psychic phases and episodes in abnormal people are all incomprehensible events and appear as purely temporal sequences. It is equally difficult to understand the whole range of the person's psychic development and its full meaning in genetic terms. We can only resort to causal explanation, as with phenomena in the natural sciences, which, as distinct from psychological phenomena, are never seen 'from within' but 'from the outside' only. (Jaspers 1959/1997: 28)

So, for both psychopathology and in the full understanding of a person's whole psychic development, understanding fails: our narrative resources are not sufficient, on Jaspers' account, to follow through the meaningful connections and instead of accepting ignorance, objective, external, causal explanation is turned to. Jaspers uses the term 'genetic' in the passage quoted not in the same way as Brentano—namely, to refer to an explanation that is causal and draws upon physics, physiology, and anatomy (Broome et al. 2013)—but rather to refer to an empathic understanding of how one psychic event arises from another. The distinction between understanding and causal explanation in this excerpt then launches Jaspers' influential discussion of 'understanding' (*Verstehen*) and 'explanation' (*Eklären*), where he suggests these are different, but both are legitimate sources of knowledge (see Hoerl, Chapter 8, this volume, for an extended discussion).

Moving deeper into the *General Psychopathology* (Jaspers 1959/1997), part III 'The Causal Connections of Psychic Life' pursues some of the themes from the introduction in greater depth. Specifically, the relationship between cause and effect in psychic life. Jaspers makes a few points that are as timely now as then:

- Between cause and effect there may lie 'an infinite number of intermediary events' (Jaspers 1959/1997: 451).
- A given phenomena may have a number of causes, either at the same time or on different occasions.
- More direct causes (i.e. those that are more proximal to the effect on the causal pathway) have 'more uniform and regular sequences' (Jaspers 1959/1997: 452).

Jaspers suggests that in psychopathology 'nowhere do we know any real direct cause' (Jaspers 1959/1997: 452) and 'the more causes, the less knowledge' (Jaspers 1959/1997: 453). This suggests that the only causes we have at present are distal from the psychic events we are interested in, and as noted earlier, at this distance such causes are various and at a given alternate time point or in a different individual the same psychic phenomenon can be caused by different factors. Hence, as we spread our net wider for the causes we invoke, Jaspers seems to imply that as we may pull in causes that are less tightly linked to effects, and hence we can make less of claim to having knowledge. For Jaspers, the direct, proximal causes that map neatly and tightly onto effects are where knowledge lies—but for Jaspers we do not have these in psychopathology, and thus lack knowledge. Or more generously, we lack the precise kind of knowledge that Jaspers views as worthy of the name: that is to say, a knowledge where we can link a precise cause to a definite and specific psychopathological effect.

When talking further about causes and meaning, Jaspers offers another means of demarcating these two methods for studying psychic life. Perhaps in an aside to Freudian theory, Jaspers tells us that the psychology of meaning 'remains by definition within consciousness' (Jaspers 1959/1997: 457), whereas causal investigations penetrates into the 'extraconscious foundations of psychic life' (Jaspers 1959/1997: 457). So, here Jaspers can be read as implying that we are transparent to ourselves and there is nothing hidden when one attempts to understand oneself or another through meaning: there is no non-conscious locus of meaning. If this in turn fails, then causal explanation is outside of consciousness and has its foundation in 'somatic events' (Jaspers 1959/1997: 457). What doesn't seem to be an option, on Jaspers' account, is to look for meaning anywhere other than in consciousness. We see here what has been referred to as Jaspers' scientific pluralism (Ghaemi 2007)—the idea that multiple methodologies and approaches are required and options are not closed off. Hence, despite Jaspers' block to thinking about non conscious meaning, one can investigate psychic life through the use of the traditional disciplines of the humanities and social sciences, including literature, philology, sociology, and history, and in turn, can use causal science to investigate non-conscious foundations of the psyche. As noted earlier, this links in with wider understanding of the *Geisteswissenschaft* that was a dominant for philosophers and social scientists in Germany at the turn of the century, such as Nietzsche, Dilthey, Weber, and the Southwest NeoKantians (Broome 2006, 2008; Broome et al., 2013) and an attempt to bring methodological rigor to the social, historical and 'human' sciences, much as Kant had brought to the natural sciences.

Jaspers then moves to discuss findings in neuropathology and psychiatric illness. As mentioned earlier, here he reiterates that the specificity and lack of tight relationships imply that we cannot presume that brain changes are direct causes of psychic events. This is not, to repeat, to argue that Jaspers believes that brain changes do not cause mental illness, but rather, based upon his understanding of direct cause, they are not close enough on the causal pathway to the event and hence a given brain change that is not specifically linked to a given psychic change cannot serve as a direct cause. For Jaspers, 'we postulate that all psychic events, normal and abnormal, do have a somatic base, this has never been demonstrated' (Jaspers 1959/1997: 458). Jaspers then comments on the clarion call of Griesinger's psychiatry 'mental illness is cerebral illness':

> This declaration is as dogmatic as its negation would be. Let us clarify the situation once more. In some cases we find connections between physical and psychic changes taking place in such a way that the psychic events can be regarded with certainty as consequences. Further, we know that in general no psychic event exists without the precondition of some physical basis. There are no 'ghosts.' But we do not know a single physical event in the brain which could be considered the identical counterpart of any morbid psychic event. We only know conditioning factors for the psychic life; we never know the cause of the psychic event, only a cause. So this famous statement, if measured against the actual possibilities of research and the actual findings, may perhaps be a possible, though infinitely remote, goal for research, but it can never provide a real object for investigation. To discuss statements of this sort and to try and solve this problem in principle indicates a lack of critical methodology. Such statements will vanish from psychiatry all the more quickly in proportion as philosophic speculations vanish from psychopathology and give place to a philosophical maturity in the psychopathologist. (Jaspers 1959/1997: 459)

Jaspers then more positively mentions that this doctrine has at least spurred on contemporary research into the brain but has led to psychiatrists abandoning psychopathology as unscientific. Causes remain important for Jaspers, not only to understand aetiology, but as a way to see opportunities for treatment. In discussing therapy, Jaspers suggests two poles: at one extreme, a biological intervention with no role for meaning ('Injections may perhaps bring about effective therapy without any personal engagement of doctor and patient' (Jaspers 1959/1997: 461)) and at the other extreme 'the therapy in which the doctor becomes personally engaged and through the patient's activity affects both his environment and attitude and makes possible those inward reversals and decisions which become the source of cure' (Jaspers 1959/1997: 461). For Jaspers, there are many grey areas between these poles where these are intermingled: he offers examples of drilling versus education, mere doing versus stimulation and encouragement.

Later in part III, when discussing the effect of the environment and of the body on psychic life, there is an extended discussion of cerebral localization (Jaspers 1959/1997: 480–495). After reviewing briefly the history of the theory of localization, Jaspers tells us that since the late nineteenth century 'localisation has become a fact' (Jaspers 1959/1997: 481). However, he says a question remains as to what it is that is localized. He offers a précis of the work of Meynert as an example of how brain and psychic events are connected:

> Meynert designed a comprehensive chart of brain psyche activity. The unthought-out postulate- the principles of which were hardly conscious—ran as follows: the objects of observation in psychopathology (psychic phenomena, experience, character properties, meaningful connections, etc.) must be conceived in terms of corresponding to the spatial events in the brain or, to put it differently, the structure of the psyche, as we variously conceive it in our psychological thinking, must be embodied in the structure of the brain; or put differently again, the structure of the psyche and the structure of the brain must coincide. This postulate has never been proved. It cannot be proved, because it is meaningless. What is heterogeneous cannot coincide, but at best one can be used as a metaphorical expression of the other. (Jaspers 1959/1997: 481–482)

Again, Jaspers praises this approach as being a spur to neuroscientific knowledge, with some valid gains being made. However, Jaspers says that simply expressing psychic events in the jargon of neuroanatomy is an empty move and accuses Meynert's imagination of masquerading 'quite unscientifically in a scientific disguise' (Jaspers 1959/1997: 482). Unarguably, the work on aphasia, apraxia, and agnosia has served as the model and inspiration for the localization paradigm. Jaspers rightly points out we observe, on one hand, the 'crude, focal cerebral lesions; and on the other we observe disturbances of function that are partly psychic (speech and action), which usually but not always appear together with these focal lesions' (Jaspers 1959/1997: 489). However, the rub comes for Jaspers in what we might call today 'the explanatory gap': 'between the two aspects of these more detailed analyses no relationship can be found, nor can we define any one elementary function through our analysis which can be localised as such' (Jaspers 1959/1997: 489). Here Jaspers seems to say that despite even a very tight correlation between a change in anatomy and a change in psychic function, we cannot localize or find the relationship that in turn mediates the connection from anatomical to psychic change. Based on these concerns and others Jaspers claims that we do not know 'what or where to localise' (Jaspers 1959/1997: 493). Echoing contemporary discussions in philosophy around connectionism and in cognitive neuroscience around functional connectivity, Jaspers suggests that function may be dependent not on discrete areas, but on relationships between many different parts of the brain.

> The interplay of anatomical parts and physiological functions forms a whole, within which, when there are particular lesions, they replace and compensate for each other; a whole within which, when they stimulate each other, facilitate and inhibit each other in an infinitely complex structure, which so far has only been recognised in part as regards the neurological connections and as far as psychic connections are concerned remains mere metaphor. (Jaspers 1959/1997: 489)

His related concern of 'what' to localize is based upon both the idea of how we cut up parts of mental life and whether it is possible (in functional imaging jargon: fractionating mental states)—can we study this part of mental life in isolation from another? But also by focusing on specific functions Jaspers says we miss the psyche as a whole and instead only see 'psychic tools', speech, recognition, etc., and features that are distal from that of the personality.

He ends this discussion on localization with two cautions:

> The idea that different psychic disturbances could be caused by a different localisation of the same disease process is purely theoretical and has no basis in fact. (Jaspers 1959/1997: 495)
>
> Further, we have to remember that in principle cerebral changes may also be the result of primary psychic phenomena, though such an effect has not been empirically demonstrated. (Jaspers 1959/1997: 496)

But he returns to some of the themes when discussing Wernicke and his work on attempting to reduce psychic life to reflex arcs and the creation of false association or the breaking of associations (sejunction) in a section on 'Examples of Theory Formation in Psychopathology' (Jaspers 1959/1997: 534–537), specifically with Wernicke's thought that the 'elements and connections of psychic life are seen as identical with the elements and structures of the brain. The psyche becomes spatially represented' (Jaspers 1959/1997: 534).

Towards the close of *General Psychopathology*, when discussing nosology, Jaspers reiterates the ongoing theme that summarizes his relationship to biological psychiatry. That is to say, one that values it, but one that is cautious of such an approach being hegemonic and instead advocates both an independence, to some extent, of psychopathology ('it can be said that psychopathology still has the task of studying abnormal psychic processes in *General Paralysis*, even after the discovery of cerebral processes' (Jaspers 1959/1997: 576)) from neuroscience but also a pluralism of method to understand mental illness:

> We must guard against any one viewpoint becoming an absolute even if such a viewpoint proves fruitful for research and might now and then even be decisive for radical therapy. The fact that a classification of disease entities into generic groups—a diagnostics proper—is not applicable to the psychoses but only to cerebral processes has probably led to our seeing in brain research not only one task among many but the task of psychiatry. On the other hand the poverty of the so far recognised relationships between abnormal events in the brain and abnormal psychic events, the restricted outlook for further results in psychopathology and the self evident assumption that psychopathology has to deal with psychic life may all heave lead psychopathology to reject, sometimes perhaps a little too abruptly, this over estimation of anatomy and of the somatic for psychiatry. As brain research is nowadays still more firmly anchored as a science than psychopathology this is perhaps an understandable rejection on the part of psychopathologists who are still too much on the defensive. (Jaspers 1959/1997: 577)

To conclude this survey of Jaspers' views on neuroscience, as expressed in *General Psychopathology*, we can say a few things in summary. In no sense is Jaspers anti-science or opposed to biological psychiatry. Indeed, reading him on cerebral localization and on extra-conscious causal factors he is likely to have been impressed by the advances that have been made to understand psychopathology through neuroscience. However, what he is clear on is that such work can never be the sole means to understand the psyche and mental illness. Jaspers constantly warns throughout *General Psychopathology* of one mode of study being dominant and blocking out others, and this theme, of scientific pluralism, is one that Jaspers continues in his later philosophy.

Philosophical writings on science

In *Way to Wisdom* Jaspers (1951/2003) argues for an interdependence of science, as *Wissenschaft*, and philosophy and with that the call that philosophers should have a scientific training. Jaspers urges for philosophy to turn against both those who are superstitiously fervent in their beliefs of science as well as those who are of contemptuous of science, and instead argues that 'philosophy grants its unconditional recognition to modern science' (Jaspers 1951/2003: 160). His thoughts on the nature of science remain constant throughout his philosophical writings and are coherent with the views expressed in *General Psychopathology*. For Jaspers (1986) in *The Origin and Goal of History* science has the following characteristics: it is methodical, compellingly certain, and universally valid (Wallraff 1970). Methodical means, on this account, that the scientist is consciously aware and reflective on the methods he or she uses in their research and how such methods themselves have limitations. Scientific results are still reliant upon presumptions, interpretation, etc. yet still he suggests that there is some greater degree of 'factuality and reliability of scientific results' (Jaspers 1986: 43) than in the conclusions drawn by philosophical thought. Validity is the implication that scientific truths are true for all people at all times: it is true objectively for all men. Together with these key attributes, Jaspers suggests that science is also progressive, ever moving forward, and is all inclusive. It aspires to totality and coherence and all facts are to be taken into account. Finally, he suggests there is a distinctive scientific style or personality that Wallraff (1970) translates as 'scientificalness': a style characterized by the ability to relentlessly question and criticize, and scrutinize every finding as to the method utilized in the research. It aspires to a clarity and precision of expression and avoids dogmatism. Philosophy, strictly, is not scientific for Jaspers: it has some awareness and reflection on its methods, but lacks a specific object of enquiry (Jaspers 1951/2003). It lacks the universally validity that Jaspers claims is a central feature of science. Further, philosophers rely on science to bring its findings into real world outcomes and changes.

Further on in *The Origin and Goal of History*, Jaspers breaks *Wissenschaft* into *Geisteswissenschaft* (human or mind sciences) and *Naturwissenschaft* (natural science). As in *General Psychopathology*, he views the natural and human sciences as a polarity, yet suggests that the limits demarcation between a psychology and a biology of the mind 'remains hidden' (Jaspers 1986: 361) with perhaps this view on their methodological differences of these sciences paralleling the views expressed in *General Psychopathology* on the 'impenetrable country' separating psyche and soma. However, at these extremes he reiterates his belief in the validity of science, greater in the natural sciences, such that these scientists can understand one another clearly and unequivocally, yet the understanding between mind scientists is constrained by historical limits (Jaspers 1986: 360). However 'between the two groups there usually yawns an abyss, and very few will even glance across it at the other side' (Jaspers 1986: 360). On this account, psychology straddles both *Geisteswissenschaft* and *Naturwissenschaft*—drawing on physical and biological sciences as well as the sciences of meaning making up *Geisteswissenschaft*. Hence, more generally, Jaspers argues, as for psychiatry and psychopathology, psychology needs to draw on both somatic and psychic/hermeneutic studies.

The former, biological, approach to psychology Jaspers defines as 'non-*Verstehen* research' (Jaspers 1986: 361) and 'comes from interest in knowing things in their externality, in the transparency of this externality as an event proceeding necessarily under cognizable laws as well as the capacity to control what is transparent within limits due to cognition'. However, this approach fails to capture the Alien, the Other, and *Existenz*. 'Nature does not respond; it does not speak to me as *Existenz*; it is not mind' (Jaspers 1986: 361). *Existenz* is a key term for Jaspers in his philosophy and one that is difficult to grasp.

It refers to the 'innermost core' of the self, of the soul, that is irreducibly free and can never be any object for science (Wallraff 1970). The crucial point here then in the biological study of the mind is around the idea that natural science is limited to the study of the objective world and the development of universal laws and doesn't see, what is for Jaspers, the transcending nature of man, due to man's inherent freedom and participation in ideas. However, the mind sciences are not a unity and, as with *General Psychopathology*, rely on *Verstehen* that now finds itself as a method limited by two boundaries. Firstly, existent objects as the actuality of nature (as with the study of the psyche), and secondly the other is *Existenz*. The one boundary is dealt with natural science and the other by communication. Mind is embedded and part of nature, and hence to some extent world oriented, yet incomprehensible to scientific laws. 'Mind, taken by itself, keeps its flanks open toward two sides, towards the incomprehensibility external of actuality and the universally inwardness of *Existenz*' (Jaspers 1986: 363).

Concluding remarks

As I hope this chapter demonstrates, by no means does Jaspers espouse an anti-science position nor is he against neuroscientific research. Indeed, in several passages in *General Psychopathology*, Jaspers praises the work and advances generated by biological psychiatry. What he constantly reiterates is the problems in a psychiatry that is purely based upon the study of the brain and the problems for this approach, problems he brings out with great lucidity in his discussion of German psychiatry in the second half of the nineteenth century. As in his later philosophy, Jaspers argues for psychiatry and psychopathology, as with other human sciences, to draw on and utilize all methods. As such, his work resonates with the approach of his contemporaries in sociology, history, and philosophy but also with contemporary philosophical work on psychiatry as a science (Broome 2008; Cooper 2007). Jaspers' understanding of biological research is sophisticated, as his discussions of Meynert and Wernicke attest, and he grasps the fundamental conceptual issues at stake, as well as the institutional and professional pressures impacting on researchers, issues that remain as timely and as relevant now as then.

Acknowledgements

Many thanks to Professor Giovanni Stanghellini for his helpful comments on an earlier draft of this paper, and to Drs Ken Ma, Marek Marzanski, Moli Paul, Adrian Vann, the King's College London Philosophy of Medicine Group, and the Edinburgh University Philosophy, Psychology, and Informatics Reading Group for useful feedback and questions when this paper has been presented.

References

Bortolotti, L., Broome, M. (2009). 'The Future of Scientific Psychiatry', in M. Broome, L. Bortolotti (eds), *Psychiatry as Cognitive Neuroscience: Philosophical Perspectives*. Oxford: Oxford University Press, 365–375.

Broome, M.R. (2006). 'Taxonomy and Ontology in Psychiatry: A Survey of Recent Literature', *Philosophy, Psychiatry, & Psychology*, 13(4): 303–319.

Broome, M.R. (2008). 'Philosophy as the Science of Values: South West NeoKantianism and Psychiatric Interviewing', *Philosophy, Psychiatry, & Psychology*, 15(2): 107–116.

Broome, M.R., Bortolotti L. (2009). 'Psychiatry as Cognitive Neuroscience: An Overview', in M. Broome, L. Bortolotti (eds), *Psychiatry as Cognitive Neuroscience: Philosophical Perspectives*. Oxford: Oxford University Press, 1–9.

Broome, M., Dale, J., Marriott, C., Merino, C., Bortolotti, L. (2012). 'Neuroscience, Continua and the Prodromal Phase of Psychosis', in P. Fusar-Poli, S. Borgwardt, P.K. McGuire (eds), *Vulnerability to Psychosis: From Psychopathology to Neurosciences*. London: Routledge, 1–22.

Broome, M.R., Harland, R., Owen, G., Stringaris, A. (eds) (2013). *The Maudsley Reader in Phenomenological Psychiatry*. Cambridge: Cambridge University Press.

Churchland, P.M. (1988). *Matter and Consciousness* (Revised edn). Cambridge, MA: MIT Press.

Churchland, P.S. (1986). *Neurophilosophy*. Cambridge, MA: MIT Press.

Cooper, R. (2007). *Psychiatry and Philosophy of Science*. Stocksfield: Acumen.

Engstrom, E. J. (2003). *Clinical Psychiatry in Imperial Germany*. Ithaca, NY: Cornell University Press.

Fulford, K.W.M., Morris, K.J., Sadler, J.Z., Stanghellini, G. (2003). 'Past Improbable, Future Possible: The Renaissance in Philosophy and Psychiatry', in B. Fulford, K. Morris, J. Sadler, and G. Stanghellini (eds), *Nature and Narrative: An Introduction to the New Philosophy of Psychiatry*. Oxford: Oxford University Press, 1–41.

Ghaemi, S.N. (2007). 'Pluralism in Psychiatry: Karl Jaspers on Science', *Philosophy, Psychiatry, & Psychology*, **14**(1): 57–66.

Jaspers, K. (2003). *Way to Wisdom: An Introduction to Philosophy*. New Haven, CT: Yale University Press. (Original work published in 1951.)

Jaspers, K. (1959). *Allgemeine Psychopathologie* (7th edn). Berlin: Springer Verlag.

Jaspers, K. (1997). *General Psychopathology* (7th edn) (J. Hoenig, M.W. Hamilton, trans.). Baltimore, MD: Johns Hopkins University Press.

Jaspers, K. (1981). 'Karl Jaspers "Philosophical Autobiography"', in P.A. Schlipp (ed), *The Philosophy of Karl Jaspers*, La Salle, IL: Open Court, 3–75.

Jaspers, K. (1986). *Karl Jaspers: Basic Philosophical Writings*. Atlantic Highlands, NJ: Humanities Press.

McGinn, C. (1991). *The Problem of Consciousness*. Oxford: Wiley-Blackwell.

Ratcliffe, M. Broome, M. (2012). 'Existential Phenomenology, Psychiatric Illness and the Death of Possibilities', in S. Crowell (ed), *Cambridge Companion to Existentialism*. Cambridge: Cambridge University Press, 361–382.

Shorter, E. (1997). *A History of Psychiatry*. New York, NY: Wiley.

Wallraff, C.F. (1970). *Karl Jaspers: An Introduction to His Philosophy*. Princeton, NJ: Princeton University Press.

Chapter 10

Karl Jaspers the pathographer

Matthias Bormuth

Introduction

Karl Jaspers is one of the classic representatives of modern pathography (Bormuth 2007; Hilken 1993). His study *Strindberg und van Gogh. Versuch einer pathographischen Analyse unter vergleichender Heranziehung von Swedenborg und Hölderlin* (*Strindberg and van Gogh: An attempt of a pathographic analysis in comparative relation to Swedenborg and Hölderlin*) was published twice in his early years as a philosopher (Jaspers 1922/1926). The guiding question concerning the influence which mental disorders exert on the creative process was motivated by Jaspers' interest in psychiatry at that time. And yet the investigation simultaneously shows indications of the existence-philosophical dimension first sketched out in his 1919 book *Psychologie der Weltanschauungen* (*Psychology of World Views*) (Jaspers 1919). Jaspers develops this way of thinking psychiatrically *and* philosophically even more clearly in the extensive case history incorporated into his 1936 monograph *Nietzsche: Einführung in das Verständnis seines Philosophierens* (*Nietzsche: An Introduction to the Understanding of His Philosophical Activity*) (Jaspers 1936). Here he determined a biological process as the cause of mental breakdown whose psychopathological impact, he claimed, had influenced Nietzsche's work even before his last year of creative productivity. Jaspers addressed the issue of pathography a third time in 1947 when he formulated a clinical casuistry of the prophet Ezekiel for a *Festschrift* dedicated to his student of psychiatry Kurt Schneider (Jaspers 1951). Here he ascribed a schizophrenic psychosis to the Old Testament figure on the basis of passages from the Bible.

The article at hand explores the three pathographical studies conducted by Jaspers in the context of a history of ideas. It will focus initially on three exemplary representatives of modern pathography, a discipline whose emergence in the late nineteenth century was closely connected to the triumphal march of the natural sciences and the introduction of psychiatric doctrines of understanding. Then Jaspers' approach will be introduced, starting with methodological considerations concerning his *General Psychopathology* followed by three sections devoted to detailed analyses of his pathographical studies. Lastly, Jaspers' philosophical premises will be explored in greater detail. These express themselves most saliently in the polemical way in which Jaspers distinguishes van Gogh's art from that of modern Expressionism and from works of the mentally ill included in Heidelberg's 'Prinzhorn Collection'. In this sense the pathographic studies conducted by Jaspers can also be read as philosophical texts which give an impression of existence philosophy *in statu nascendi* during the Weimar Republic.

Methodologically speaking they are instances of scientific casuistry which transcend disciplinary boundaries from the very start through the chosen subject of investigation.

They also show how closely psychiatric and philosophical understanding are connected in Jaspers' work and that he sometimes failed to meet his own demand to distinguish subject value judgements clearly from scientific propositions.

Pathography before Jaspers

The history of modern pathography is closely associated with Friedrich Nietzsche. Little notice was taken of his works, which were strikingly unusual in philosophical as well as stylistic terms, during his lifetime. His radical way of calling into question traditional values deeply unsettled bourgeois society. His complete mental breakdown posed a challenge for psychiatry long before academic philosophy even recognized his importance. Due to his provocative theses, Nietzsche was usually pathologized, however. For those with no desire to engage with his thoughts, it was easy and seemed only too natural to discredit his radical destruction of bourgeois and Christian conventions in the wake of the debate on genius and madness as a more or less clearly pronounced expression of pathological influences. A year before his breakdown in Turin, Nietzsche himself anticipated this tendency, giving it a name: 'One constantly expiates such a peculiar status—through ever increasing, ever icier, ever sharper isolation [...]. Words like "eccentric," "pathological," "psychiatric" are resorted to now' (Nietzsche 1986: 212).

The tendency towards discrediting his thoughts in clinical terms recognized so clairvoyantly by Nietzsche evidences itself to a high degree in the casuistry of the psychiatrist Paul Julius Möbius from Leipzig, who coined the term pathography (Schneider 1922: 4). Before we examine his Nietzsche study as an exemplary work of this border-crossing genre more closely, it should be placed in the context of a history of ideas.

At the time pathography was rooted—whether affirmatively or disaffirmatively— in the tradition of Cesare Lombroso, whose work *Genio e Follia* appeared in Germany in 1887 under the title *Genie und Irrsinn* (*Genius and Madness*) (Lombroso 1887), being received with storms of enthusiasms. In 1926 Karl Jaspers speaks in a letter to his pupil Kurt Kolle of the 'Lombroso wave' which, as a fantasy of sorts, had dispersed again (German Archive of Literature, Jaspers Papers). What he identifies as particularly problematic is the fact that during the Kraepelin era, criminal psychologists had only a very imprecise set of concepts at their disposal and these evidenced one-sided social-Darwinistic and antimodernist tendencies. The doctrine of degeneration, which incorporated the prejudices against individualistic artists and their lack of societal conformity held by bourgeois society, was a decisive force here.

Thus the concept of 'decadence' as it emerged around 1900 adopted the pejorative meaning of liberation from traditional conventions. It became relevant most importantly for the artistic avant-garde whose cultural ambitions aimed at effecting political, social, and economic change. According to Max Nordau, who developed the doctrine of degeneration in Germany systematically, Lombroso was one of the 'proudest appearances of the century' by virtue of his animosity towards the avant-garde (Nordau 1892: viii).

In stylizing Lombroso as a saviour of culture in his 1892 standard work entitled *Entartung* (*Degeneration*), Nordau promoted the psychiatrization of large segments of society such as modernistic artists and their supporters, who did not conform to the values of the dominant civil society. Thus he insinuatingly portrays the metropolitan population as inmates of a 'hospital', claiming that in 'infirm times' one could also find 'degeneration and hysteria' in art, literature, and philosophy (Nordau 1892: 496): 'The degenerates are not always criminals, prostitutes, anarchists and declared madmen. Sometimes they are writers and artists', Nordau writes (Nordau 1892: vii). For him the physician takes on the task of the lonely preacher in the desert during these times of societal crisis. Nordau's pointed remarks on the allegedly pathological genesis of intellectual works constitute an effort to prevent them from influencing the public through proof of their morbid nature. The unfettered emotionality of the modern man is interpreted by Nordau as a result of social fragmentation as well as of biological determination which, he claims, manifests itself in individual physiognomic and anatomical stigmata. So the artist became around 1900 an ambivalent legend (Gockel 2010).

Since Möbius founded his knowledge of pathography on the doctrine of degeneration as formulated by Lombroso and advanced further by Nordau, it comes as no surprise that his 1902 study entitled *On the Pathological in Nietzsche* is clearly informed by resentment against this thinker. According to his argument, Nietzsche developed an 'irreligious individualism' which opposed itself full of hatred and derision to civil society in the name of 'aristocratic anarchism' (Möbius 2000: 67). In diagnostic terms, Möbius founds his derogative psychiatric judgement on the assumption that a slow, progressive form of paralysis had set in which influenced Nietzsche's work from the very start, leading to a dramatic escalation of psychopathological symptoms in the last year of creative productivity. To be sure, he also makes the consequences of an abnormal personality responsible for what he views as questionable elements in Nietzsche's philosophy. Möbius speaks of the 'stigma of immoderateness' and a 'lack of *sophronsyne*'. His judgement is nurtured by the idea of Aristotelian moderation guaranteed by the individual capacity for balancing extremes. Formally speaking, Möbius deems to detect an absence of this capacity in the stylistic peculiarity which weds Nietzsche with Pascal and the French moralists: 'With his exorbitance, the tendency towards aphorism, which is to say, a breaking off of thoughts, grows as well' (Mobius 2000: 61). He speaks of a 'mild form of degeneration' evidenced, moreover, by renouncement of marriage and an excessive enthusiasm for new ideas.

On the basis of the gradually increasing 'insanity' ascertained by him, the pathographer advises his readers to take extreme care in engaging with all of Nietzsche's works. The study of Nietzsche is claimed to be dangerous for one's mental health because, as Möbius purports, only one out of every one hundred readers is capable of judging for himself, not allowing himself to be deluded by the glow of individual passages and managing to recognize the fragmentary aspect of Nietzsche's work. As he writes, 'if you find pearls do not think that the whole is a string of pearls. Be wary, for this man is mentally ill' (Möbius 2000: 178).

More than two decades later, Wilhelm Lange-Eichbaum took upon himself the task, in his 1928 study entitled *Genie, Irrsinn und Ruhm* (*Genius, Madness and Fame*) of founding pathology as a systematic science and compiling a bibliography of previous research (Lange-Eichbaum 1967). His approach was rooted in a social-Darwinist critique of modernity and decadence as well, which viewed the loner qua genius as the expression of a degenerate type of personality. In keeping with this approach, Lange-Eichbaum views Nietzsche in particular as a curious artist with an uncontested capacity for formulating admirable ideas but who, as a psychopath, had become the exponent of the degenerated masses. Only too often, he argued, this psychopathic genius adopted the role of a negative model for the masses (Lange-Eichbaum 1967: 434).

During the time when pathography as it was pursued in the German-speaking world invoked the doctrine of degeneration, William James was already criticizing 'medical materialism' in North America. In his work *The Variety of Religious Experiences. A Study in Human Nature*, this psychiatrist, psychologist, and philosopher who taught in Harvard contended that unusual works in religion, art, and philosophy should not be generally discredited by indicating pathological influences. The clinically retrospective debasement of the legendary calling of Paul the Apostle by modern scientists served as a monitory example of the now classic discipline of pathography. James writes: 'Medical materialism finishes up Saint Paul by calling his vision on the road to Damascus a discharging lesion of the occipital cortex, he being an epileptic'. James attributed such hasty tendencies towards general pathologizing to the human need for invalidation of rather than argumentative engagement with disagreeable intellectual attitudes: 'We are surely all familiar in a general way with this method of discrediting states of mind for which we have an antipathy. We all use it to some degree in criticizing persons whose states of mind we regard as overstrained', James writes (James 1929: 13). He dismisses this tendency by querying rhetorically: 'But now, I ask you, how can such an existential account of facts of mental history decide in one way or another upon their spiritual significance?' (James 1929: 14) According to this view, the attempt to ascertain biological facts cannot liberate oneself from confrontation with cultural value judgements.

Thus James vehemently opposed the doctrine of degeneration as it was developed as an ostensibly objective argument of pathographic thought by Max Nordau following mainly Lombroso. James writes: 'One disciple of the school, indeed, has striven to impugn the value of works of genius in a wholesale way (such works of contemporary art, maybe, as he himself is unable to enjoy, and they are many) my using medical arguments' (James 1929: 18).

He also spoke out against the 'newest fashion', i.e. psychodynamically oriented pathography, which—at least from a psychoanalytic perspective—viewed religious phenomena as a questionable expression of repressed sexuality. For James this constituted a 'fashion, quite common nowadays among certain writers, of criticizing the religious emotions by showing a connection between them and the sexual life' (James 1929: 11).

In the context of a history of ideas, Nietzsche is associated with the propagation of the biological topos of degeneration as well as with the new focus on the power of unconscious emotions. James might have suspected this when he spoke out against the theory of resentment created by Nietzsche. With ironic reluctance he responded to the provoking ideas of Nietzsche to the effect that in Christian ethics in particular, the envy and resentment of the weak had led to the announcement of the ideal of justice and love as a means of preventing the strong from living out their nature. James writes: 'For Nietzsche the saint represents little but sneakingness and slavishness. He is the sophisticated invalid, the degenerate par exellence, the man of insufficient vitality. His prevalence would put the human type in danger' (James 1929: 364). Although James is not completely free of this tendency in his remarks on such pathologizing critique of Christianity, the decisive aspect of his evaluation lies in the observation that one cannot clarify the question as to which norm should be valid by pointing out any unconscious dynamic. As he argues, 'Poor Nietzsche's antipathy is itself sickly enough, but we all know what he means, and he expresses well the clash between two ideals. […] Shall the seen world or the unseen world be our chief sphere of adaption?' (James 1929: 365)

In formulating this question James articulated precisely what Max Weber, who was quite taken with the *Gifford Lectures*, as he confessed in a letter to Jaspers 1912 (Weber 1998: 729), had said about cultural-scientific understanding in principle. Any rational clarification or ascertainment of a fact, be it biological or historico-psychological in nature, comes up against limits when it comes to value judgements. These can never be comprehended and explained completely by the factors on whose basis they are formed. An irrational moment of human freedom always remains which Weber, following Kant, referred to as the 'transcendental prerequisite' of cultural scientific thought. In other words: in order to grasp the human being as capable of judgement, one cannot get around conducting one's own examination, quasi congenially, on the basis of value assumptions whose sense cannot be fully testified logically or empirically (Bormuth 2006, 2010: 64–70).

In this vein Jaspers, who viewed himself as a student of Max Weber in methodological terms, pointed out the tendency which pathographies—like that of Nietzsche—had of harbouring a philosophical prejudice, often under the 'objective veneer of a devastating psycho-pathological ascertainment of fact' (Jaspers 1936: 102). Already in the first edition of his *General Psychopathology* one finds indirect indication of his ambivalence towards pathographic attempts—especially the one made by Möbius—when Jaspers ascertained: 'Pathography is a touchy issue' (Jaspers 1913: 309). That his own pathographic analyses were informed by personal value judgements to a greater degree than he himself liked to believe is yet to be elucidated.

His pupil Kurt Schneider distanced himself during the Weimar years from the overconfidence in pathography expressed by some psychiatrists in no uncertain terms. His lecture *Psychopathology and the Poet* invokes the danger of attempts to medically domesticize or marginalize artistic idiosyncrasy: 'Only too often—particularly during our time—physicians have tried to dismiss everything new, everything extraordinary, everything unusual, everything which exceeds their own horizon as "pathological" and "degenerated"' (Schneider 1922: 5).

Methodological considerations

The concept 'boundary situation' plays a central role in pathographic studies (see Schlimme, Chapter 11, this volume). Jaspers had used it for the first time in his 1919 *Psychology of World Views* to describe the boundary situations comprising 'struggle, death, chance and guilt' which, as he says, force us to engage in philosophical contemplation (Jaspers 1919: 202–204). For him, serious mental illnesses without any hope of healing also counted as boundary situations of this kind. When commenting on the price which an individual had to pay for the deepened perspective of psychosis if he possessed talent, Jaspers writes in the conditional: 'It is possible that the greatest depth of metaphysical experience, the consciousness of the absolute, of horror and blessedness in the conscious perception of the supernatural is to be found where the soul is loosened up to such an extent that it is destroyed and left behind' (Jaspers 1926: 98); a boundary situation of this kind, determined by psychic pathology, can provoke the intellectual substance of a human being in dangerous ways. For his doctrine of understanding this means that the personal 'connoisseurship and art' which should enable the psychiatrist working in the borderland of art and illness to gather clear 'evidence' of psychopathological connections must always possess a philosophical horizon as well (Jaspers 1913: 71). In a late retrospective of his *Psychology of World Views*

Jaspers acknowledged the existential element of his objectifying thought: 'My philosophical impulse strove for wholeness in the cloak of psychology' (Jaspers 1960: xii).

As his essay 'The Phenomenological Approach in Psychopathology', written in 1912, shows, Jaspers had originally operated on the assumption that it was possible to perform a neutral evaluation of individual psychic phenomena through empirical procedures (Jaspers 1968). Here the limit of the comprehensible for the psychopathologist constituted the objectifiable criterion of whether a process or phase-like psychosis could be ascertained or not. Thus the pathograph looks to the works and biographical reports of those artists who show indications of a serious process psychosis and attempts to grasp 'the incomprehensible though understanding'. Jaspers speaks of the 'abyss' which opens up between patients with a psychosis and those with a neurosis during the attempt of understanding. As he observes, a schizophrenic process always constitutes something 'inaccessible' and 'foreign' to the psychologist engaged in such an attempt (Jaspers 1926: 7).

This foreign psychic aspect and the foreign existential aspect are thus the two dimensions which limit the understanding of the pathograph, as it were, in regard to the boundary situations experienced by the ill artist. In the last edition of *General Psychopathology* Jaspers observes that not only the process pathology but also the level of the existential is barred from psychological understanding. In consequence, he places the artist above his time, putting him on the pathographical pedestal of the incomprehensible, as it were. Illness and existential experience are somehow corresponding in his life and work provoking the others to understand although there will always be limits. Psychopathological and metaphysical understanding are both necessary ways to approach not only great artists but also average people whose psychic deep disorder may open up the eyes for border perspectives of life of which we are normally not aware:

> He [man] is not only an empirical reality to us but under the scrutiny of our metaphysical understanding, he, like everything else that is real, becomes a meaning we cannot verify. He is not only meaningful like a tree or a tiger but meaningful in his own unique way as a human being. This metaphysical experience of him is not a matter for the science of psychopathology but the latter can help in clarifying facts that will refine the experience for instance, the fact that extreme psychotic states offer us a human parable, containing inverted and distorted attempts to realise and elaborate marginal situations, which are common to us all. There is also the fact that patients see into depths which do not so much belong to their illness as to themselves as individuals with their own historical truth. Finally there is the fact that in psychotic reality we find an abundance of content representing fundamental problems of philosophy: nothingness, total destruction, formlessness, death. Here the most extreme of human possibilities actually breaks through the ordinary boundaries of our sheltered, calm ordered and smooth existence. The philosopher in us cannot but be fascinated by this extraordinary reality and feel its challenge. (Jaspers 1997: 309)

Although this perspective of limits of understanding is very fascinating there emerges out of it a constant problem for the pathographic viewpoint. Jaspers can only demarcate the realm of the foreign in diseased artists from the outside with a large degree of imprecision. For this reason his pathographies remain substantially vague when they speak of the 'other atmosphere', the 'qualitatively other' or the 'singular plus' which he sees as distinct marks of schizophrenia in the artist (Jaspers 1926: 32). How he gets the feeling of the otherness is often not clear and due to his personal impressions of the works of art and other documents which give testimony of the life and ideas of the artist.

Just how touchy this 'subjectivist turn' proved to be in scientific terms for the psychopathological approach in general is discussed by Häfner in his retrospect of the discussion on 'Process and Development' (Häfner 1963); later Janzarik, a critical follower of Jaspers' tradition of psychopathology in Heidelberg, pointed to the problematic aspect of using the notion of 'inaccessible' madness as a fundamental criterion (Janzarik 1974).

Strindberg and van Gogh—Jaspers' first pathography

Jaspers designated his study entitled *Strindberg and van Gogh* as 'the attempt of a pathographic analysis'. His project restricted itself to revealing the irrational core of artistic creativity without striving to uncover its mysteriousness in rational terms, however. Beyond the limit of the objectifiable he discovered the world of multivocal subjectivity whose philosophical contours Jaspers had sketched out for the first time in his *Psychology of World Views.* Jaspers admitted indirectly that his pathographic analysis was shaped by his own personal values, for the second edition of *Strindberg and van Gogh*, which appeared in 1926, was no longer published in the series called 'Studies on applied psychiatry' (Jaspers 1922); instead the monograph came out under the rubric 'Philosophical Investigations' (Jaspers 1926). The existence-philosophical self-understanding which informed his pathographic studies was not developed by Jaspers for another ten years, however, when his cultural-critical *Die Geistige Situation der Zeit* (*Man in the Modern Age*) and the three-volume *Philosophie* (*Philosophy*) made him known to a larger public (Jaspers 1931, 1932).

If one reads his pathographies, their existence-philosophical contours do not announce themselves immediately, for Jaspers seems to inquire from an exclusively psychiatric perspective whether a schizophrenic process was involved in the case histories of the artists or not and if so, how this had influenced the lives and works of these creative individuals. His considerations are premised on the assumption that in all three cases, serious psychoses had merely intensified these artists' 'original talent' to the extreme without having changed the original direction of their work substantially: 'What matters is, what soil schizophrenia loosens up, which previously given possibilities it turns into unconditional experiences which stop nowhere'. Thus as Jaspers contends, the 'mind' of the artist cannot become ill and the 'process' merely offers an 'opportunity and condition' for the artistic breakthrough into mental boundary regions of human existence, with this occurring almost in the sense of 'godly madness' (Engelhardt 1991). In the image used by Jaspers 'just like a diseased mussel allows pearls to form, schizophrenic processes could allow unique works of the mind to emerge' (Jaspers 1926: 100).

In his pathography Jaspers devotes himself primarily to 'Classic Modernism', the movement which August Strindberg and Vincent van Gogh—two of the most controversial figures in bourgeois society of the time—contributed to. Jaspers also gives some attention to the poet Friedrich Hölderlin, who had lived in the Tower in Tübingen for almost 40 years from the early nineteenth century on during the final stage of a schizophrenic psychosis; Jaspers' interest in him stemmed in no small part from the fact that Hölderlin's work had shaped the style of the literary avant-garde around 1900. Jaspers had a great appreciation of the Swabian poet and van Gogh alike, having seen over 100 paintings of the latter in the large Cologne exhibition of 1912, which had done much to create a public awareness of Expressionism as an art movement. Jaspers looked upon the Dutch painter as a modern brother of Friedrich Hölderlin. For Jaspers, both artists were characterized by the fact that they had liberated themselves from the deceptive conventions of the times—Hölderlin by freeing himself from metric form, van Gogh by dynamizing stroke and palette. As Jaspers contended, their new poetic and painterly language had given them the capacity to diagnose the crisis of a heralded and eventuated disintegration. As Jaspers argued, the price both had had to pay for an artistically stimulating process was terminal schizophrenia and suicide respectively. As he writes: 'In Hölderlin's case it was as if the string, violently plucked, snapped the very moment the tone was produced' (Jaspers 1926: 131).

In his pathography Jaspers does all he can to underscore the aesthetic and ethical unity behind the 'formative and disciplining power' of van Gogh's and Hölderlin's works. What evidenced, in his eye, Hölderlin's 'formidable spirit' was the fact that despite his previously unstable psyche, the poet had worked and lived 'with a conscious will, an active understanding, an instinctively formative power and a capacity for figurational expression' (Jaspers 1926: 110). Of van Gogh Jaspers writes: 'In his case personality, actions, ethos, existence and artistic work are to be grasped as a whole to an unusual degree' (Jaspers 1926: 128). Jaspers actually had a high appreciation of the ill painter who, like Hölderlin the poet, had no longer been capable of producing the 'perfect work of art'. The pathograph sees van Gogh's 'tense search' as a 'fragment of that sought-after perfection' which already constituted its 'fulfilment' since all that counted in modernism was perpetual striving on the way. Both artists impressed the existence philosopher with their ability to sketch the metaphysical horizon of the age of decline in their resistance against psychosis and the ultimate failure which resulted from it. As Jaspers said, because they had done this as artists under the conditions of illness but also as representatives of us all, the beholders of these artists' works could participate in their experiences of substantial failure without needing to abandon the protective space of their normal bourgeois existence. Jaspers elevated his view that only a few, usually ill artists saw themselves confronted with this difficult task into a metaphysical dimension: 'The gods are cautious with their touch' (Jaspers 1926: 112).

In contrast to the enthusiastic portraits of van Gogh and Hölderlin, Jaspers viewed August Strindberg as the negative type of modern man. As he contended, Strindberg did not possess the 'metaphysical or religious' depth which the psychopathograph ascribed to Hölderlin and van Gogh. Instead, Jaspers interpreted Strindberg's autobiographical novels as indications of a form of artistic creativity which was eccentric in the first place, for, as he observed, it had not been invested with any extraordinary formal quality as a result of the schizophrenic process, only with experiential material laid out by the author as the critical expression of a modern loss of standard. In keeping with this judgement, Jaspers commented in a critical vein to the effect that Strindberg's work evidenced his superficially restless, sceptical-playful, self-exposing and sexually debaucherous life conduct (Jaspers 1926: 82–85). As he saw it, the psychosis had intensified his genuine tendency to lack 'any strong awareness of the need for a connection, a goal-oriented development in thought as well as in life'. As Jaspers claimed, the life of the poet had shattered into a questionable pluralism which the pathograph dismissed as a 'conglomerate of various vehemently advocated viewpoints' (Jaspers 1926: 14).

When Jaspers raises the issue of delusional jealousy in connection with Strindberg—a topic he had been quite familiar with since 1910—the degree to which Jaspers' own values informed his pathographic perspective becomes only too apparent. As he writes: 'In the passionate merging there is never any mutual understanding, any loving communication, any struggle for clarity'. With a moralizing gesture Jaspers attributes the failure of Strindberg's first marriage in particular to his having perpetually resisted 'the desire to become transparent in a boundless way' despite his many literary self-exposures. Consequently, Jaspers assumes that Strindberg's schizophrenia had only intensified, to the extreme, this original 'dislike of real, complete communication'—an ideal consciously held up by Jaspers from 1915 on (Jaspers 1926: 78).

Fundamentally speaking, Strindberg represents, for Jaspers, the 'world view of current times'. His psychosis had merely aggravated an attitude typical of the times. Thus in Jaspers' eye, the Expressionist poet who, ethically speaking, had shattered 'truth into many isolated fragments' and proved himself incapable of any disciplined way of life, reflected a negative variation of modernity in aesthetic terms (Jaspers 1926: 84). Strindberg stands as an exponent of the Expressionist generation in general, whose eccentric and fragmentary life conduct manifested itself in his work. As Jaspers contended, the mentally ill poet no longer understood how to draw his personal life out of an inner, metaphysical centre which would justify all real failure in regard to an unfulfillable aspiration of totality. Jaspers has no use for the poet whose world view differed so decidedly from his own. As Jaspers writes, 'I confess that my relationship to Strindberg is indifferent, that my interest in him is almost solely of a psychiatric and psychological nature' (Jaspers 1926: 149). Thus Strindberg does not fulfil the norm established by Jaspers: 'The contrast between a moving life and disciplining, rationalizing and formative order is common to all human spirit' (Jaspers 1926: 110).

It has been shown that psychopathological judgements made in the case of Strindberg in particular did not gain clarity until the word 'schizophrenic' appeared, albeit without the reader ever discovering how Jaspers had reached such 'certainty' of a psychically foreign element. The fact that the pathograph coupled his imprecise diagnostics of Strindberg's 'purported' schizophrenia with derogatory descriptions of his moral behaviour is taken as an implicit indication—and justifiably so—of Jaspers' own 'value system' and 'image of humankind' (Glatzel 1986: 175).

Nietzsche's illness

The ideal-typical contrast between the daunting figure August Strindberg and the admirable artists van Gogh and Hölderlin is brought together in Jaspers' pathographic analysis of Nietzsche in 1936. Having only made marginal note of what he presumed to be a paralytically diseased philosopher in 1922 (Jaspers 1926: 141), Jaspers now devoted an entire chapter to Nietzsche's medical history in his philosophical monograph (Jaspers 1936: 91–117). According to Jaspers, the deeply disturbed philosopher Nietzsche had been afflicted by the modern 'experience of a world crisis' earlier and more intensively than anyone else (Jaspers 1936: 109). According to Jaspers, his work, as determined by this pathology, ascends into previously unfathomed heights and plunges into absurd abysses simultaneously. The esteem held by the pathograph for the one author and the condemnation held for the other now converged as a pair of opposites attributed to one and the same figure, Friedrich Nietzsche.

In doing so, Jaspers presupposes a biologically determined psychosis which had exacerbated the original heterogeneous tendencies in this individual. This lead Nietzsche into 'philosophical boundary experiences' and to articulate these 'consuming truths' in a good as well as a bad sense almost a decade before the paralytic collapse of 1889 (Jaspers 1936: 104). Jaspers writes: 'Nietzsche's work is not such that we could derive pure satisfaction from it. The emotional turmoil of quintessential drives, the enhancement of seriousness and the illumination of the gaze do not prevent Nietzsche from seeming to fail when he quasi thrusts into emptiness or from appearing oppressive due to narrowness and exorbitances and absurdities' (Jaspers 1936: 105). It is not surprising that Lange-Eichbaum criticized Jaspers severely in his late works. Apparently his Nietzsche pathology failed to take the development of the abnormal personality into consideration; instead, it seems to have narrowed his view, in particular through the assumption of a purely biological process (Lange-Eichbaum 1946: 22).

In this pathographical study on Nietzsche, due to the assumption of biological process underlying it, one gains only a vague idea of how to grasp the connection between artistic-philosophical and psychopathological aspects: 'It is in fact one of the unsolvabilities of the entering into existence, namely the specific assumption […] that Nietzsche does not reach his actual culmination until the leap of 1880. The factors of "disease" […] had not been disturbing yet; maybe they even made things possible which would not otherwise have evolved', Jaspers writes (Jaspers 1936: 108). To be sure, he recommends exploring the hypothesis that Nietzsche's pathography involved a gradual, progressive paralysis by comparing clinical observations with those of other artists' *vitae*. He does not take this path himself, however, for fear of getting lost in pathographic speculations beyond the realm of psychopathological description. As he writes: 'Since no certain knowledge can be gained today, the simple task which remains is to gain a descriptive knowledge of the course of the diseases and psychologically ascertainable conditions Nietzsche suffered from, these not even being graspable as diseases, without discovering what comes together to form a disease' (Jaspers 1936: 93). The foundation of his diagnostic judgement, the 'overall impression' of the work gained through 'precise chronological reading', is not spelled out either; instead, the reader is challenged to discover the pathographic relations for himself through 'his own study of Nietzsche', particularly, as is stated, since 'no proof' for such relations exists.

It is only in regard to the corpus of letters that Jaspers elucidates in detail what 'leaps' it was possible to ascertain in this case history. Independent of a vague 'overall impression', he speaks of three phases during which pathological influence is exerted on Nietzsche's work, the first of which he identifies as beginning with a general sickliness in the year 1873. The second caesura, in 1880, is of psychiatric significance, it being the result of—biologically based—manic and depressive conditions. For this period, from which *Zarathustra*, written in 1883/1884, issued, Jaspers speaks in exemplary ambivalence of an 'oeuvre-generating inspiration' as well as a 'terrifying inscrutability' (Jaspers 1936: 95). The pathologist concedes that in these years 'parallels between the intellectual development of the oeuvre and biographically ascertainable or presumed psychophysical changes' evidence themselves without drawing any close connection between the increasingly polemic critique of Christianity and the development of the metaphysics of the will to power on the one hand and the incidence of disease on the other (Jaspers 1936: 103). Not until he turns his attention to the beginning of the year 1888, which constitutes, for him, the decisive caesura, does Jaspers become more pointed. He describes the 'new tone of self-assurance' on the part of Nietzsche, which, as he claims, issued from the belief in being able, as a thinker, of deciding 'world history as a whole' (Jaspers 1936: 108). Now a clear connection is drawn between the loss of a continuous sense of tact, the 'uninhibitedness' and the fact of Nietzsche's mental breakdown on the one hand and the occurrence of an organically psychotic process on the other (Jaspers 1936: 109).

While Jaspers postulates that narrow limitations are placed on understanding in pathography, he also expresses his belief that any philosophical approach to Nietzsche encounters a hermetically sealed core of existential thought which cannot be objectified. Instead, he argues, every individual should utilize Nietzsche's inner flexibility and incomprehensibility in order to encounter him or herself: 'Through this, each and every individual can only become what he or she is', Jaspers writes (Jaspers 1947: 30). And he places a group of privileged philosophers to whom he ascribes the 'gift of differentiation' on eye level with psychopathologists of special rank to whom he attests the capacity to clearly determine the limits of understanding. These groups, he says, could penetrate to the 'essence of truth' in their engagement with Nietzsche despite the extreme ambiguity of his work. Only such initiates are capable, he contends, of ascending to the 'possible rank of existences in themselves' through such an approach, whereas the broad masses succumb to the 'seduction' which lies in drawing from Nietzsche's writings 'doctrines and laws in their seeming unambiguity as something generally valid' (Jaspers 1936: 31).

In other words: the postulate of the limits of understanding in philosophical as well as psychiatric terms makes it possible to remain aloof from the ideologized debate on Nietzsche conducted during the years of National Socialism. And yet this rigid drawing of boundaries also meant that possible connections between disease and oeuvre were hardly vocalized by Jaspers.

The prophet Ezekiel—a pathographic sketch

The last pathography written by Jaspers originally in 1947, his study of the Jewish prophet Ezekiel, demonstrates once again with urgency the problem which lies in vague ascriptions of symptoms and diagnostic statements influenced in no small degree by the author's own value perspectives. In writing this work Jaspers emphasized, as William James had decades earlier, the 'self-evident truth that psychopathological analysis revealed nothing about the factual and historical value of intellectual substance' (Jaspers 1951: 105). And yet the pathographic sketch of the prophet which ends with Jaspers' diagnosis of a schizophrenic process is not the expression of any unbiased examination of a surviving work. His perspective is expressly shaped by the judgement that Ezekiel's prophethood amounted to a 'decline of the spirit', leaving the psychopathologist to interpret the morbid process with all due precaution as a possible reason for this spiritual decline.

How does Jaspers go about this in detail? At the beginning of the relatively short essay, various passages from biblical texts are quoted which, as Jaspers claims, researchers have ascribed to Ezekiel with more or less certainty and in which the author depicts 'visions in abnormal conditions'. Speaking in abstract clinical terms, Jaspers cites 'elementary visual, acoustic and haptic phenomena', 'scene-like perceptions', 'extreme excitation', and quasi 'cataleptic attack[s] of motionlessness and dumbness;' this all combines to make the impression of a schizophrenic process (Jaspers 1951: 96–99). Jaspers also founds this diagnosis on the astounding prominence of 'sexual elements with a scope and directness which is unusual despite the uninhibitedness with which antiquity encountered sexuality'. From this he concludes: 'This is a state of affairs not infrequently found among schizophrenics' (Jaspers 1951: 99). It is also remarkable how closely Jaspers connects the levels of fact and value judgement when he describes the principle 'style and atmosphere' of this book of the Bible. He speaks of a 'manner of sensualizing the spiritual which is not only crude but also without feeling and shameless, or a change from abstract rational understanding and from caprice'. This résumé on the figure of the prophet is sketchy and wrought with ambivalence. Jaspers writes: 'For all his passion a coldness, an inhuman strangeness can be felt. And yet, like in schizophrenic art, peculiar, unforgettable, grand and terrifying images occur' (Jaspers 1951: 100).

As fascinating as it is to see how Jaspers attempts to grasp the psychopathological foundation of the impressive visions depicted by this prophet, the temptation which lies therein seems dangerous to an equal degree, particularly since the narrow empirical basis upon which such tendencies are described as diseased and degenerate does not conform to the author's own intellectual standards and ideals. The subjectivity of the interpreter plays a large, perhaps a too large role. Jaspers must have been aware of this problem while writing the text since he refrains from speaking of provable statements. He relativized his psychopathological ascriptions by using subjunctive phrases, making them appear as conjectures expressed in the mode of possibility. This subjunctive gesture of precaution manifests itself most tangibly in the résumé of the pointed comparison with other prophets who correspond more closely to Jaspers' ideal notion. In summary he finds:

> Ezekiel has many superb aspects. His seriousness is compelling but bitter. He approaches the limits of the ridiculous. Fundamental thoughts on prophethood take on an extreme shape in his writings. But he lacks the sublimity of Isaiah, the grandeur which lies in simple limitation, the depth and the power of the heart demonstrated by Jeremiah. It could be that what is lacking as well as what is impressive, what makes you awestruck is determined by the schizophrenic element. (Jaspers 1951: 101)

Nevertheless: Jaspers demonstrates quite a pronounced sense of self-criticism when he designates his ascriptions as 'hypothetical attempts' which endeavour, despite the sparse material provided by the surviving text, to find sufficient indications for the diagnosis of a schizophrenic process psychosis: 'With such a small amount of material, no answers can be provided with compelling certainty', he writes (Jaspers 1951: 103).

Jaspers, van Gogh, and Weimar art

Let us return in summary to his first pathography entitled *Strindberg and van Gogh* in which Jaspers anticipated his existence-philosophical critique of modernity. This is inconceivable without the profound influence exerted on Jaspers by Max Weber, not only in terms of methodological considerations.

So it is not surprising that the first inspiration to take personally interest in the works of the painter was given by Max Weber, who was himself fascinated by van Gogh. As Marianne Weber wrote in her biography, among the modern painters Weber had had a particular appreciation for this one: 'Van Gogh was difficult to grasp and unsettled the most' (Weber 1984: 507). Following Weber's lead, Jaspers undertook a journey to Paris in spring 1912, reporting in a letter to his mother from May of his lukewarm enthusiasm for the Impressionists Manet, Monet, Pissaro, Renoir, and Sisley (German Archive of Literature, Jaspers Papers). To be sure, he remarked in a letter to his sister eight days later, they stood out from the 'boring academic painting' but they were not capable of arousing the unsettling effect of a painter like van Gogh (German Archive of Literature, Jaspers Papers). For the realm of art this meant that he acknowledged Impressionism and realistic Naturalism as possessing the potential for providing the 'serenity of intuition'. Although, as Jaspers says, van Gogh's fragmentary art did not match the 'closed, perfected art works' of the tradition, he nevertheless obtained a 'singular height'—expressed in his body of correspondence as well—with his intellectual intentions: 'The absolute, his high aspiration, the religiously penetrated realism, the complete truthfulness have an effect on his entire existence' (Jaspers 1926: 128). Jaspers speaks of the 'identity of the religious, ethical and artistic impulse' one finds in van Gogh: 'With his art he wants to console' (Jaspers 1926: 129). The fact that the painter had succeeded in doing this was attributed to the transcendental horizon of his artistic production, which was authorized and sanctioned by his psychic history of affliction. To be sure, this was only possible by virtue of the exceptional talent shared with the poet Friedrich Hölderlin: 'The formative and disciplining power is capable of dissolving the trepidation. Van Gogh experiences his work on his paintings as "lightning rods," and Hölderlin sees poetic forming as a similar kind of salvation' (Jaspers 1926: 112).

Whereas Weber became open to the modern experience of an irreconcilable plurality later on, Jaspers took only partly an interest in its intriguing value pluralism calling at the same time for a standpoint above and beyond time. Although he experienced the decline of the bourgeois world as an unescapable 'boundary situation', he saw certain possibilities for solving this 'crisis' by making an existential decision in the personal realm. Jaspers applied the measure of a supraconventional metaphysics to artistic production as well. As he said, 'today as always, [it must] unintentionally make transcendence perceptible in the figuration which is really believed at the current point in time' (Jaspers 1931: 130). For Jaspers, the religious horizon invested this artist's work with an existential depth which made the other painters of Classic Modernism appear flat; thus is the pointedly polemical sentiment expressed in *Man in the Modern Age* in any case.: 'Today the arts appear as if whipped through existence; there is no altar where they find peace, where they find themselves, where their substance fulfils them' (Jaspers 1931: 129).

Jaspers articulates his polarizing reflections on modern aesthetics systematically a year later in his *Philosophy* (Jaspers 1932). In the name of existence philosophy he distinguishes between a deep and a superficial form of art: 'A divide separates all things referred to as works of art insofar as they fulfil the external feature of being man-made: some constitute the language of the cipher of transcendence while the others are without ground and depth'. According to Jaspers, only those inaugurated into existence philosophy are capable of making this distinction: 'It is in metaphysical thought that human beings perceive this divide consciously and believe they are approaching art with seriousness' (Jaspers 1932: 194).

The last section of the pathography makes it completely clear that what Jaspers meant by restless modernist art devoid of transcendence was in fact primarily Expressionist art of his day. This chapter, which bears the heading 'Schizophrenia and Culture of the Times', takes a critical look at the phenomenon that the epoch drew an exceedingly positive connection between art and mental illness. Never before had schizophrenic psychosis played such a culturally dominating role, Jaspers observes, to the effect that 'today a number of persons of high rank who have become schizophrenic have [had an impact] through works from the schizophrenic period' (Jaspers 1926: 148).

At the same time Jaspers calls attention to the phenomenon that interest was being taken not only in exceptional artists but also in the 'art of madmen'. Here Jaspers is alluding to the well-received appearance of the so-called 'Prinzhorn Collection' which the younger psychiatrist had published in 1922. Hans Prinzhorn's 'Picture-making of the mentally ill' was conceived of as a medical, but also cross disciplinary 'Contribution to the psychology and psychopathology of figuration', the intention being to open up a new field of insight for the study of artistic creativity through the analysis of patients' art (Prinzhorn 1922). For Jaspers the 'merit' of this work consisted in the fact that Prinzhorn had gathered together some 5,000 sheets from around 300 patients 'with painstaking care and perseverance', a selection of which was compiled to make the book; as was ascertained, the scientific conclusiveness of the material was yet to be explored (Jaspers 1926: 144).

Jaspers cites the publicly propagated, generally made association between art and psychiatry as an indication of the 'problematic situation', this being, in his eye, that 'the last foundations of existence had been loosened' (Jaspers 1926: 150). The pathograph polemically demonstrates his disdain for Expressionism when he interprets it derisively as 'screaming, mere making, violence, selfintoxication and enrapturement, as shallow immediacy and a stupid will to primitivity' (Jaspers 1926: 151). He distinguishes the 'broad mass of poetizing, drawing, painting and wood-cutting schizophrenics' from the few ill persons who possessed a 'disposition of genius' (Jaspers 1926: 97): 'Only original talent can become significant even in psychosis and create a visible expression for what are otherwise purely subjective experiences' (Jaspers 1926: 96). Thus in view of the revered artist van Gogh he writes: 'At the 1912 exhibition in Cologne, where strangely monotonist Expressionist art from all over Europe was on view in the vicinity of the wonderful art of van Gogh, I sometimes had the feeling that he was the only truly great and unwillingly "insane" one among so many who wanted to be insane but were really all too normal' (Jaspers 1926: 150).

For Jaspers, the impossibility of creating a schizophrenic condition—unlike states of hysteria, viewed as the mark of a profound spirit, which individuals had been capable of working themselves into artificially in earlier times—constituted protection against 'inauthenticity'. For Jaspers asks while making rhetorical allusions to the pluralism of modernism: 'Could it be that in such times schizophrenia is the condition for authenticity in spheres which can be experienced and represented as possessing authenticity without schizophrenia in times characterized by commitment?' (Jaspers 1926: 151). In closing, Jaspers concedes that for the most part, his considerations had been of a speculative and purely subjective nature, constituting merely a possibility of conceiving the cultural situation: 'May the reader himself reduce [the lines of connections] to the measure they deserve' (Jaspers 1926: 151).

The emphatic and critical view which Jaspers developed in regard to schizophrenia as a leading cultural aspect of the times has been confirmed from a present-day cultural-historical perspective. Doris Kaufmann underscores the fact that during the Weimar Republic, schizophrenia was the mental illness which drew the primary attention of psychiatric research and that moreover, other scientific disciplines such as art history concentrated on it as a 'pivotal concept for the discussion on general psychic structures, modes of thoughts and images of the world'. In addition, what is of importance in connection with Jaspers is the observation that during these years the concept of schizophrenia acted as the 'description of a condition perceived of as disrupted in societal and individual terms in the cultural discourse as well' (Kaufmann 2003: 119).

One can sum up that in keeping with the 'subjective reflection' which Jaspers engages in as an existence-philosophical pathograph, van Gogh had been 'beneficial' as a metaphysical painter. As Jaspers contends, it was in his psychotic disorder that he searched for the perennially '[concealed] absolute' in the relative. From the perspective of the religious-psychological *topos* of *fascinosum and tremendum* Jaspers writes:

> It is as if a last source of existence would become visible temporarily, as if concealed grounds of existence had a direct impact here. But for us this is a trepidation which cannot be endured for very long, which we would like to withdraw from again. [...] It is a trepidation which does not lead to an assimilation of the foreign aspect but rather one which urges us to convert it into another figuration suitable for us. It is formidable, exciting, but not our own world; a questioning emanates from there, an appeal to our own existence which has a beneficent effect insofar as a transformation begins. (Jaspers 1926: 150)

In his eye, van Gogh was a fascinating and terrifying artist alike whose differentness had the capacity to convey existential impetuses. The pedestal of disease had allowed him to see further but it had also excused the public from having to participate in the vision of the artist. Jaspers founds this assertion by quoting a verse by Hölderlin: 'A weak vessel cannot hold them forever; humans can endure the fullness of the gods only at times'. In his commentary he writes: 'Such experience, truly genuine, truly dangerous, is only given in schizophrenia' (Jaspers 1926: 112).

Jaspers advocated this 'subjective' view, which shaped his pathographic analysis in the later existence philosophy, with the institutional authority and self-assurance of his professorship. Psychiatric casuistic had done its service as maid of the philosophical statement. But as Jaspers contended, it had only been capable of leading the 'discussion of incomprehensible causal connections, for example those between the outbreak of a mental illness and the creative work of an artist' to the limits of plausible knowledge. Ultimately the artist was, for better or worse, a mystery unfathomable by any science. In pathological as in existential terms, the pathograph remained restricted to an external view barred from understanding on the other side of the border, focusing not on 'presumable, dominating insights which allowed one to "get behind" the mystery' but rather on insights used 'as a means of adopting those standpoints on which true mysteries are seen and cognized' (Jaspers 1926: 1).

With his postulate of a twofold limit to understanding Jaspers withdrew the justification for the attempt to interpret the 'art of madmen' as an understandable and significant reaction to the modern world we live in. As he concluded, psychoses remain biologically; they only intensify the capacity for perception and figuration in the case of very exceptional individuals. As mysteries, these appear hermetically closed while at the same time being representative in terms of the necessary search for the concealed absolute. Thus van Gogh becomes a projection of Jaspers' pathographic and existence-philosophical religion of art. The seeming deficiencies in painterly figuration bore witness to inevitable worldly failure. As Jaspers contended, van Gogh expressed his 'religious impulse' by turning his attention to 'the simplest objects' (Jaspers 1926: 129). In doing so the painter had adopted the motif of the incarnation of the godly which expresses itself in the suffering of the servant figure Jesus Christ. As Jaspers argued, this 'paradoxical main antithesis of Christian doctrine', i.e. being 'man and god, common and sublime' alike, corresponded to the impact which the writings of the New Testament, put into simple words, must have had on noble Rome (Auerbach 1958: 36). As an erudite psychiatrist and philosopher, Jaspers viewed van Gogh as a secularized mediator of this Christian paradox. His pathography helped to heighten the general public's appreciation for the coarse simplicity of his brushstroke. This, he observed, was no disqualified expression of anything pathological; indeed, as he contended, van Gogh's manner of painting invested the religious paradox of incarnation with new expression—one which shaped the painterly style of artists to come (Bluhm 2003: 19).

References

Auerbach, E. (1958). *Literatursprache und Publikum in der Lateinischen Spätantike und im Mittelalter.* Bern: Francke-Verlag.

Bluhm, A., Sassen, J.H., Verhoeven M. (2003). 'Van Gogh and Modern Art and the Influence of Modern Art on Van Gogh', in A. Bluhm, J.H. Sassen, M. Verhoeven (eds), *Gogh Modern. Vincent van Gogh and Contemporary Art.* Amsterdam: NAI Publisher, 13–25.

Bormuth, M. (2006). *Life Conduct in Modern Times. Karl Jaspers and Psychoanalysis.* Dordrecht: Springer-Publishing.

Bormuth, M. (2010). 'Psychiatrie als Kulturwissenschaft. Überlegungen nach Max Weber', *Nervenarzt,* **81**: 1246–1253.

Bormuth, M., Podoll K., Spitzer, C. (2007). *Kunst und Krankheit. Studien zur Pathographie.* Göttingen: Wallstein-Verlag.

Engelhardt, D. (1991). *Medizin in der Literatur der Neuzeit. Darstellung und Deutung.* Hürtgenwald: Pressler-Verlag.

German Archive of Literature. (n.d.). Jaspers' Papers. Marbech: German Archive of Literature.

Glatzel, J. (1986). 'Die Psychopathologie Karl Jaspers, in der Kritik', in J. Hersch, J.M. Lochman, R. Wiehl (eds) (1986), *Karl Jaspers. Philosoph, Arzt, politischer Denker.* Munich: Piper-Verlag, 161–178.

Gockel, B. (2010). *Die Pathologisierung des Künstlers. Künstlerlegenden der Moderne.* Berlin: Akademie-Verlag.

Häfner, H. (1963). 'Prozeß und Entwicklung als Grundbegriffe der Psychopathologie', *Fortschritte der Neurologie und Psychiatrie,* **31**: 393–438.

Hilken, S. (1993). *Wege und Probleme der psychiatrischen Pathographie.* Aachen: Fischer-Verlag.

James, W. (1929). *The Varieties of Religious Experience. A Study in Human Nature.* New York, NY: Random House.

Janzarik, W. (1974). *Themen und Tendenzen der deutschsprachigen Psychiatrie.* Berlin: Springer-Verlag.

Jaspers, K. (1913). *Allgemeine Psychopathologie.* Berlin: Springer-Verlag.

Jaspers, K. (1919). *Psychologie der Weltanschauungen.* Berlin: Springer-Verlag.

Jaspers, K. (1922). *Strindberg und van Gogh. Versuch einer pathographischen Analyse unter vergleichender Heranziehung von Swedenborg und Hölderlin.* Bern: Bircher-Verlag.

Jaspers, K. (1926). *Strindberg und van Gogh. Versuch einer pathographischen Analyse unter vergleichender Heranziehung von Swedenborg und Hölderlin.* Berlin: Springer-Verlag.

Jaspers, K. (1931). *Die geistige Situation der Zeit* (5th edn). Berlin: Gruyter-Verlag.

Jaspers, K. (1932). *Philosophie,* Vol. 3 (3rd edn). Berlin: Springer-Verlag.

Jaspers, K. (1936). *Nietzsche. Einführung in das Verständnis seines Philosophierens* (3rd edn). Berlin: Gruyter-Verlag.

Jaspers, K. (1947). *Vernunft und Existenz.* Fünf Vorlesungen, Bremen: Storm-Verlag.

Jaspers, K. (1951). 'Der Prophet Ezechiel', in *Rechenschaft und Ausblick.* München: Piper-Verlag, 95–106.

Jaspers, K. (1960). *Psychologie der Weltanschauungen* (5th edn). Berlin: Springer Verlag.

Jaspers, K. (1968). 'The Phenomenological Approach in Psychopathology', *The British Journal of Psychiatry*, **114**: 1313–1323.

Jaspers, K. (1997). *General Psychopathology* (7th edn) (J. Hoenig, M.W. Hamilton, trans.). Baltimore, MD: Johns Hopkins University Press.

Kaufmann, D. (2003). 'Eugenische Utopie und wissenschaftliche Praxis im Nationalsozialismus', in W. Hardtwig (ed), *Utopie und politische Herrschaft im Europa der Zwischenkriegszeit*. Munich: Oldenbourg-Verlag, 309–325.

Lange-Eichbaum, W. (1946). *Nietzsche: Krankheit und Wirkung*. Hamburg: Lettenbauer-Verlag.

Lange-Eichbaum W., Kurth, W. (1967). *Genie, Irrsinn und Ruhm. Genie-Mythos und Pathographie des Genies* (6th edn). Munich: Reinhard-Verlag.

Lombroso, C. (1987). *Genie und Irrsinn: in ihren Beziehungen zum Gesetz, zur Kritik und zur Geschichte*. Leipzig: Reclam-Verlag.

Möbius, P.J. (2000). *Nietzsche. Krankheit und Philosophie*. Schutterwald: Wissenschaftlicher Verlag.

Nietzsche, F. (1986). *Sämtliche Briefe. Kritische Studienausgabe*, Vol. 8 (G. Colli, M. Montinari, eds). Munich: Gruyter-Verlag.

Nordau, M. (1892). *Entartung*. 2 Vol.: Berlin: Carl Duncker-Verlag.

Prinzhorn, H. (1922). 'Bildnerei der Geisteskranken', in *Beitrag zur Psychologie und Psychopathologie der Gestaltung*. Berlin: Springer-Verlag.

Schneider, K. (1922). *Der Dichter und der Psychopathologe*. Cologne: Rheinland-Verlag.

Weber, M. (1984). *Max Weber. Ein Lebensbild*. München: Piper-Verlag.

Weber, M. (1998). *Max Weber Gesamtausgabe, II/7. Briefe 1911–12*, Vol. 2 (M.R. Lepsius, W.J. Mommsen, eds). Tübingen: Mohr-Verlag.

Chapter 11

Karl Jaspers' existential concept of psychotherapy

Jann E. Schlimme

Introduction

Karl Jaspers developed and portrayed his existential understanding of psychotherapy in a number of papers (e.g. *Zur Kritik der Psychotherapie*, 1950/1986c) and in the different editions of his *General Psychopathology* (*Allgemeine Psychopathologie*; 1913, 1920, 1923, 1946/1973). It has often been complained that Jaspers did not say more about an existential psychotherapy. In this chapter I would like to shed some light on this claim. In order to adequately do so I will first describe Jaspers' own understanding of psychotherapy as he delivered it in his writings. Then I will briefly demonstrate that from Jaspers' point of view it is crucial to recognize that we, as human beings, need to philosophize with respect to our style of life-conduct. Existential questions, like questions about the super-personal sense of life, need to be addressed philosophically, as they cannot be tackled in a scientific manner. Furthermore this entails that there is a gap between the two kinds of liberty which can be achieved through a psychotherapeutic modulation of our behaviour, on the one hand, and which can be grasped as existence in a Jaspersian sense, on the other hand. In other words, freedom cannot be achieved at a lower price, whether one suffers from a mental illness or not. Accordingly I will argue that due to methodological reasons, Jaspers did not intend to develop an existential form of psychotherapy, but an existential understanding of psychotherapy. I will demonstrate that his writings offer a rich framework for such an understanding and will further develop this framework drawing on Jaspers' own concepts of *Gehäuse*, *Grenzsituation*, and *Wille*.

Jaspers on psychotherapy in the early editions of *General Psychopathology*

In the first edition of *General Psychopathology* (1913) Jaspers basically distinguishes between those psychotherapeutic means which address and appeal to the patient as a person and those which do not (1913: 322). This basic differentiation can and will be found in all his writings on psychotherapy and is of crucial importance for Jaspers' existential understanding of psychotherapy, as will become clearer later on. In this he follows the German psychiatrist Max Isserlin, who addressed psychotherapeutic topics from a psychiatric, more or less Kraepelinian perspective (Isserlin 1910; Peters 2002b). In the first edition of *General Psychopathology*, Isserlin is Jaspers' major point of reference with respect to psychotherapeutic issues. From Isserlin's point of view psychotherapy calls upon the patient as a rational person: 'In a "Socratic dialogue" the psychotherapist tries to evoke an understanding in the patient for the problems that derive from his situation and personality. This kind of therapy avoids addressing the feelings and emotions and, especially, the unconscious' (Peters 2002b: 22; see Isserlin 1910). Isserlin's perspective was deeply influenced by the concept of a *psychothérapie rationnelle*, or *psychagogik*, as proposed by Paul Charles Dubois, one of the three pioneers of psychotherapy besides Pierre Janet and Sigmund Freud. Following Dubois, a threefold order of possible psychotherapeutic means can be proposed, basically identical with Jaspers' own distinction in the first three editions of his *General Psychopathology* (see Table 11.1; for Dubois, Müller 2002; for Dubois' influence on Isserlin, Peters 2002b). However, in the years before the First World War, Isserlin was publishing methodologically critical reviews on psychoanalysis and was well known to clinical psychiatrists from university departments in German-speaking countries. On the one hand for his pointed critique, claiming that psychoanalysis did not apply a scientific method, on the other hand for the so-called 'Isserlin scandal' in 1910. The latter was triggered by Carl Gustav Jung who disinvited Isserlin from the *Zweite Internationale Psychoanalytische Kongress* (Second International Psychoanalytical Congress) that took place on 30 to 31 March 1910 in Nürnberg. Jung disinvited Isserlin due to his critical position towards psychoanalysis. Eugen Bleuler as well as Emil Kraepelin, the two leading figures in German-speaking psychiatry during that decade, supported Isserlin in this confrontation, claiming pro–con debates to be a basic achievement and element of all sciences. Bleuler, who had been in conflict with Jung in 1909 after many years of prosperous co-working at the Burghölzli, complained about Jung's unscientific behaviour in his letters to Freud (Peters 2002a). In these letters he called it an example only adequate for religion or political parties. The 'Isserlin scandal' seems to be the starting point for the break-up between Bleuler and Freud, and, to a lesser degree, fuelled the disharmony between Freud and Jung. In any case, mentioning Isserlin as the major reference for psychotherapy during those days already entailed a psychoanalytically critical attitude in itself and mirrored the psychiatry-based perspective of the pertinent author.

In the first edition of *General Psychopathology* Jaspers distinguishes, besides the formerly described basic differentiation, three different ways of psychotherapeutic means (see Table 11.1). Besides methods of suggestion (i.e. hypnosis) he mentions techniques relying on faith and superstition as psychotherapeutic methods that do not call upon the patient as a person, 'It is irrelevant whether one administers sugared or blue-tinted water or a tonic pill, or whether one truly sends the electricity through the body or simply attracts this intuition by way of displaying big apparatuses. The patient needs to be convinced of the activity's significance; this alone is of importance' ('Es ist dabei gleichgültig, ob man Zuckerwasser, blaugefärbtes Wasser, eine tonische Pille verordnet, ob man den elektrischen Strom wirklich durch den Körper schickt oder durch großen Apparatenaufbau bloß den Schein hervorruft. Der Patient muß von der Bedeutung der Maßnahme überzeugt sein, das allein ist das Wichtige') (Jaspers 1913: 322). As a second kind of method not calling upon the patient as a person, Jaspers names talking cures and abreaction, which he compares with confessions (Jaspers 1913: 322–323).

Lastly, and perhaps most importantly, Jaspers talks about those methods that do address the patient as a person. These methods aim to convince of a healthier life-conduct for the afflicted person via offering new information and insights. As Jaspers points out, an improved (self) understanding of the person in its conscious and pre-conscious unity,

Table 11.1 The different kinds of psychotherapeutic methods in Jaspers' works

	General Psychopathology	
	First (1913), second (1920), and third (1923) edition	**Fourth edition (1941/1942)**
Methods not addressing the patient as a person	Suggestion	Methods of suggestion
	Means relying on superstition	Cathartic methods
	Confession, abreaction talking cure (possibly offering *Selbsterhellung* in a psychological sense, second and third edition)	Exercise (e.g. gymnastics, autogenic training) Methods of education (Co-working necessary)
Methods addressing the patient as a person	Effort of will Self-control (Self-)education Conduct of life	Sharing medical knowledge with the patient Justifying claims and convincing the patient Calling upon the will of the patient *Selbsterhellung*

especially with respect to mental operations on the pre-conscious level, can only be a first step. The second step implies an effort of will in order to conduct one's life according to the newly gained insights (Jaspers 1913: 323–324). In the first edition, Jaspers points out that crucial questions regarding this third dimension of psychotherapeutic means cannot be sufficiently answered with scientific methods alone, since 'the essential qualities depend, on the one hand, on the artistry of the psychiatrist's personality, and, on the other hand, on his *Weltanschauung*' ('das Wesentliche hängt ab von der Kunst der nervenärztlichen Persönlichkeit einerseits, von seiner Weltanschauung andererseits') (Jaspers 1913: 324). In the second edition, Jaspers strongly recommend consulting philosophy or theology with respect to these crucial questions. Here he will also insert two small paragraphs into his short explanations on psychotherapy, in which he will quote the Hippocratic saying, *iatros philosophos isotheos* (Jaspers 1920: 401). It is this quote which can be claimed to be of special importance for Jaspers, as will become clear later in this chapter. In this context it is interesting to note that Jaspers distinguishes between four types of patients with respect to their different concepts of health and well-being. He explicitly names three types: (1) an unreflecting, optimistic, and sober sentiment of life; (2) a religious sentiment of life, combined with an atmosphere of confidence and a presence of God; (3) a sentiment of life in which one deceives oneself and lives a lie (Jaspers 1913: 324, 1920: 399). Jaspers also describes a fourth type, even though he does not directly include it in his typification. This type would be interested in an enlightened, educated, and reflected sentiment of life. It is only indirectly addressed within an extensive quote of Nietzsche, and could be understood as precursor of an 'existential sentiment of life' which Jaspers later developed in his *Philosophy* (1932). Anyway, one's own concept of health and well-being in relation to one's life-conduct is of outstanding impact and importance from Jaspers' point of view. As he already claims in the first edition, they give each single psychotherapy a goal and a direction by answering the patient's personal question: what does health mean? (Jaspers 1913: 324; see Table 11.2).

Jaspers' understanding of psychotherapy differs from Isserlin's concept in some aspects for methodological reasons. Isserlin's point of view may be considered the most elaborate and methodologically critical position of a clinical and Kraepelinian psychiatrist regarding psychotherapy of his days. Jaspers' introduction of a hermeneutical approach to psychopathology and to psychotherapy as the practical side of psychopathological understanding also increases the possibilities of integrating psychotherapeutic means into clinical psychiatry. Isserlin, however, builds his methodological critique of psychoanalysis upon his positivistic understanding of science as natural science. From this attitude he compares psychoanalysis with a religion which has apparently influenced Jaspers' own point of view (see Rossi Monti, Chapter 3, this volume). Apart from the mentioned increments of the second edition, Jaspers is also more mindful of possible educational qualities of those means which call upon the patient as a person. He notes that these qualities could be more pronounced if the patient is voluntarily subordinating himself to his psychiatrist (Jaspers 1920: 398). He furthermore enlarges his understanding of the talking cures and concedes them to be an ability of possible *Selbsterhellung* (self-elucidation; Jaspers 1920: 397–398). Interestingly, there are no further changes in the third edition of the *General Psychopathology* within the paragraphs on psychotherapy (Jaspers 1923: 430–439). Substantial changes can be found, however, in the fourth edition. They are, as I will argue subsequently, also drawing on his detailed explanations on psychotherapy and medical practice in his *Philosophy* (Jaspers 1932/1994: 121–129; see Table 11.1).

Jaspers on psychotherapy in the fourth edition of *General Psychopathology*

Within the fourth edition, which Jaspers reworked during the years of his ban from publishing by the Nazi regime in Germany between 1941 and 1942, he extensively revised, among other things, his sections on psychotherapy. They are now subdivided into two larger sections instead of only one section within the epilogue (Jaspers 1946/1973: 661–686, 695–699). Jaspers now generally determines psychotherapy as a 'therapeutic mean which effect one's mind or body via one's mind' (Jaspers 1946/1973: 695). All psychotherapeutic methods require, as he emphasizes, that the patient co-works, although they do not necessarily call upon him as a person (see Table 11.1). He is now overly precise in distinguishing different methods and overly critical regarding psychoanalysis and other 'cathartic methods' (for this critique, the personal reasons of its background and Jaspers' important arguments regarding the 'psychoanalytic training as evidence of the authoritarian and sectarian trait of psychoanalysis', see Rossi Monti, Chapter 3, this volume; Schlimme et al. 2012). His writings in this fourth edition are, however, very clear when it comes to the limits and tasks of psychotherapy. His former distinction between four different types of life-sentiments seems no longer sufficient in order to capture his basic idea, although he still mentions this typology (see Table 11.2). He now explicitly states his basic and existential claim concerning medical practice: 'I can treat life, but freedom I can only appeal to' (Jaspers 1946/1973: 669: 'Das Leben kann ich behandeln, an die Freiheit kann ich nur appellieren')

Accordingly, beginning with the fourth edition and drawing on the explanations in his *Philosophy* (Jaspers 1932/1994, Vol. I: 121–129), Jaspers distinguishes four levels of medical therapy instead of simply opposing physical and mental practice (Table 11.2; Jaspers 1946/1973: 665). He argues a consecutive relation between these stages. The first and most

Table 11.2 Stages of medical practice in Jaspers' *General Psychopathology*

	General Psychopathology		
	First (1913) and second edition (1920)	**Third edition (1923)**	**Fourth edition (1941/1942)**
Stages of medical practice, methodologically founded	Somatic therapy e.g. direct bodily practice, dietetic practice	Somatic therapy e.g. direct bodily practice, dietetic practice	Technical/causal means Direct bodily practice e.g. surgery, medication
	Mental therapy e.g. mental care, psychotherapy	Mental therapy e.g. social and empowering care, psychotherapy	Dietetic rules Encouraging self-help Education
			Information Claiming life-conduct
			Psychotherapy
Framing stage of medical practice surmounting methodological foundations	What does health mean? sentiments of life		What is healing? Existential communication philosophy

fundamental stage includes technical and causal means, like surgery, substituting medication or direct bodily actions (i.e. putting plasters or physical restrictions). Founded upon this very basic level is the second stage consisting of dietetic rules as well as all self-help encouraging means (many modern medications which are merely modulating bodily functions would surely be ordered here (see Jaspers 1932/1994, Vol. I: 122)). A third stage comprises education and information and, drawing on them, calls for an adequate way of life-conduct. Of course, this resembles those psychotherapeutic means appealing to the patient as a person. Nonetheless, Jaspers distinguishes a further stage of medical practice that can be trained methodologically and is based on scientific methods. This highest, methodologically underpinned stage is psychotherapy: 'Psychotherapy is the attempt to help the sick person via psychic communication, exploring his inner self down to the utmost depths, in order to find an approach to guide him on the way of healing' ('Psychotherapie [ist] der Versuch, dem Kranken durch seelische Kommunikation zu helfen, sein Inneres bis in die letzten Tiefen zu erforschen, um die Ansätze zu einer Führung auf den Weg der Heilung zu finden' Jaspers 1946/1973: 665). From Jaspers' point of view successful (psycho-) therapy is a cathartic process leading to the 'philosophizing self-development of man' (Jaspers 1946/1973: 668) that takes place within an 'existential communication' between humans as fellow sufferers. This is the highest and framing stage of medical practice (see Table 11.2). It cannot be studied methodologically as it is not founded upon scientific methods. Instead, it is based on the fact that the psychiatrist himself is a person. It can therefore be refined by (existential) philosophizing or theologizing, as Jaspers describes in his *Philosophy* (1932/1994, Vol. I: 126). Jaspers will later emphasize this aspect in his oral presentations and writings of the 1950s (Jaspers 1950/1986c: 65). To summarize, Jaspers argues that the '*weltanschaulichen* foundations of setting out one's goals' cannot be lost. They should therefore not be denied in medical practice, since the patients as well as the medical doctor carry them into a situation, both of them being subjects (Jaspers 1946/1973: 671).

The crucial boundaries and limitations of all methodologically founded and derived practice are fuelled by the fact that human beings are transcending their bodily and mental embedment towards their freedom as existence (*Freiheit als Existenz*). Although certain qualities of our embedment cannot be changed or altered, human beings strive for personal freedom according to Jaspers (1946/1973: 667). From Jaspers' point of view, it is therefore necessary to recognize and accept one's '*ursprüngliche(s) Sosein*' (Jaspers 1946/1973: 672; fundamental being-as-it-is) and, accordingly, to find a way of conducting one's life that offers personal freedom. His existential understanding of medical practice and psychotherapy has an obviously methodologically critical background, as I have argued elsewhere in greater detail (Schlimme et al. 2012). Between 1913 and 1941 to 1942, Jaspers radicalizes his methodological attitude, emphasizing the limitations of all methodologically derived understanding and practice. The methodologically critical attitude in his later works resembles the transcendental-phenomenological attitude as introduced by Edmund Husserl. It is important to note that significant differences between Jaspers' and Husserl's methodological approaches do remain (for details on this, see Luft 2008; Rinofner-Kreidl 2008; Wiggins and Schwartz 1997, Chapter 2, this volume). Jaspers addresses the unresolvable difference between intuition and analysis, which can be considered a crucial phenomenological insight: while experienced objects are fully disclosed to me in an intuitive way, every analysis requires at least a minimal reflective quality.

To summarize, Jaspers conceptualizes psychotherapeutic means, except those relying on superstition, as effective, independent of the patient's and the therapist's *Weltanschauung*. In other words, the psychiatrist and psychotherapist can apply them freely within any framing context of a *Weltanschauung*, but he and the patient need to personally frame them nonetheless. The framing depends basically on the life-goals and life-conduct of the patient, and, to a lesser degree, on those of the psychotherapist. Accordingly Jaspers calls upon the medical doctors or psychotherapists to philosophize. Since Jaspers expects them to be methodologically critical persons, he argues that they cannot frame their practice and knowledge (justified beliefs) within their medical or psychotherapeutic practice and discourse exhaustively. Instead they need to explicitly and reflectively re-link their practice to the wholeness of their being and their possibility of 'being an existence'. This allows them to accept and admit the indeterminable quality of freedom and transcendence. Both can, as Jaspers doesn't tire of averring, neither be made nor scientifically addressed, but need to be experienced. They can be articulated philosophically within existential communication and can be called upon in the relation between patient and medical doctor or therapist (Jaspers 1932/1994, Vol. I: 122–126; see also Jaspers 1958/1986b: 47–57) (see Table 11.3). In other words, the subjectivity of man need not be introduced into medical practice, as Jaspers argues in *Arzt und Patient* (1953/1986a), because it is already always an inherent building block due to the patient's and therapist's subjectivity. It needs to be respected nevertheless (Jaspers 1953/1986a: 27–29).

Adopting an existential and methodologically critical attitude radicalizes the questions which Jaspers already addressed in the early editions of his *General Psychopathology* in terms of life-sentiments. He here asks in explicit terms: 'What is healing? What are the boundaries for psychotherapeutic means?' (Jaspers 1946/1973: 671). In the previous two sections I tried to offer some clarifications regarding Jaspers' existential concept of psychotherapy. In the

Table 11.3 The three Jaspersian aspects of understanding psychotherapy

Psychotherapy gains in scientific quality through methodological strictness. This implies that its effectiveness is independent of the therapist's interpretation of this effectiveness, including his 'generic *Weltanschauung*'
Psychotherapeutic processes operate, at least in some of their forms and brands such as, for example, psychoanalysis, as a 'hermeneutical' method of self-enlightenment. Hence these psychotherapies can offer some guidance for one's life-conduct
Psychotherapy would gain the status of a *Weltanschauung*, and overstep its epistemological limits, if it claims that it can allow us to answer those existential questions which are at the heart of our conduct of life. Jaspers repetitively highlights our need as psychotherapists to be aware of the limits of our respective psychotherapeutic approaches

Adapted from Schlimme, J.E., Paprotny, T., Brückner, B., 'Karl Jaspers: Aufgaben und Grenzen der Psychotherapie', *Der Nervenarzt*, 83(1): 84–91 © 2012, Springer Verlarg, with permission.

following three sections I will address what this offers for psychotherapy today, drawing on Jaspers' terms *Grenzsituation*, *Gehäuse*, and *Wille* and *Wollen*.

Jaspers' existential concept of psychotherapy: *Grenzsituation*

In his *Psychologie der Weltanschauungen* (1919) Jaspers develops the concept of the *Grenzsituation* (limit-situation, border-situation). In 1919 he determines suffering, fight, death (mortality), contingency, and guilt as situations that cannot easily be accepted as belonging to one's being (Jaspers 1919: 226–228). On the contrary, they pose a challenge for oneself. Nonetheless, as Jaspers underlines, their occurrence is not only unavoidable during one's life course, but can also be a chance for becoming an existence (Jaspers 1919: 202–251). Illnesses, physical as well as mental ones, often entail that the concerned persons face *Grenzsituationen*. In his *Philosophy*, Jaspers determines death (mortality), suffering, guilt, fight, and historicity as *Grenzsituationen*, whereby he slightly develops the list of these special situations (Jaspers 1932/1994, Vol. II: 232).

Grenzsituationen call for restitution and restructuring, or in other words, they call for a new *Gehäuse* (see later section). They furthermore give rise to existential questions; questions that are intimately connected to one's way of life-conduct. As Jaspers explains in his *Philosophy*, existence is a possible option for every human being and derives from itself. Or more precisely, it comes into being when a human being grasps itself *as* existence (*Existenz*) in a *Grenzsituation* (Jaspers 1932/1994, Vol. II: 232). To grasp the *Grenzsituation* as a situation which cannot be changed in a structural manner enables oneself to assimilate its limits as fundamentally belonging to oneself as a human being. Herewith 'potential existence rises itself up to an experience of *Sicheinswissen* (knowledge of being-in-unity) with its transcendence within a single source; this source is imagined in the *Grenzsituation*'. ('[…] schwingt sich in der Grenzsituation mögliche Existenz auf zur Erfahrung im Sicheinswissen mit ihrer Transzendenz in einem *Ursprung*, der in der Grenzsituation des Seins gedacht wird' Jaspers 1932/1994, Vol. II: 232). To grasp, accept, and assimilate this 'antinomic structure of *Dasein*' (Jaspers 1919: 204–210) means to exist in the Jaspersian sense (Jaspers 1919: 250–252). Accordingly, as Jaspers points out, existence affords a special kind of alienation, splitting or divisiveness (*Entzweiung*) from one's own being, because it requires taking the limits of one's own human being into account (Jaspers 1919: 284–285). This special form of divisiveness could well be named a 'wailing wall of existence' (Rombach 1987/1993: 327).

This situation is often found when a person suffers from a mental illness. Such persons typically recognize that they cannot shape their life according to their expectations even though they want to and continue to try to give their very best. Of course, the job of a psychotherapist is not to lure someone into desperation so that he can recognize the limits of being human. On the contrary, the afflicted person already knows that limitation. However, the psychotherapist should be open-minded with respect to this antinomic structure of *Dasein* and should at least recognize the bigger questions which are inevitably brought up due to such a *Grenzsituation*. In Jaspers' words, he should recognize and accept that philosophizing is required. This does not imply that philosophizing is a necessity for psychotherapy. Jaspers is well aware of the fact that a psychotherapist's task is not primarily to philosophize with patients during therapeutic sessions. As every trained psychotherapist knows all too well, therapeutic goals should be fixed early in the therapeutic process, and they should be 'smart': specific and simple, measurable and manageable, attainable and attractive, relevant and realistic, and also time-bound. Nonetheless, a certain amount of philosophizing cannot be circumvented in all psychotherapy, especially because the question regarding the meaning of therapy itself is present at times. It is indicating the existential dimension of this special relationship. It can be learned from Jaspers that it is thoughtful to be open-minded for this dimension too. And, it can be conceptualized with Jaspers that these questions are important for the patient, since they are linked to questions concerning his life-conduct.

If we accept this Jaspers' notion, the question remains: where does the capacity that is required in order to grasp and accept the *Grenzsituation* as belonging to one's existence come from? The pure recognition of one's limitations as a human being does not in itself entail that one can accept and assimilate these limitations (Fuchs 2008). As every person suffering from a mental illness knows all too well, it can indeed not be taken for granted that one's intentions effectively guide one's behaviour.

Jaspers' existential concept of psychotherapy: *Gehäuse*

In his *Psychologie der Weltanschauungen* Jaspers develops yet another concept of outstanding interest to a Jaspersian-existential understanding of psychotherapy. It is the concept of the *Gehäuse* (shell, housings). Essentially, Jaspers introduces this term for describing fixed *Weltanschauungen* (Jaspers 1919: 269; a general discussion in Paprotny 2003). People tend to fix their *Weltanschauungen*, as Jaspers assumes, because they wish that 'something shall be "right," a way of living, a picture of the world, an order of values' (Jaspers 1919: 269). Nonetheless, a *Gehäuse* need not be fixed and static, but it can be in constant flux. As Jaspers points out, a *Gehäuse* can be under way and in correction, as each *Gehäuse* entails a reflective element, and because people tend to get into *Grenzsituationen* (Jaspers 1919: 270–273). There is, however, a tendency in every *Gehäuse* to assimilate unfamiliar aspects and to rationalize irritating aspects of one's experience (Jaspers 1919: 271–274). Accordingly, fixed *Weltanschauungen* can offer possibilities to defuse those challenging aspects of *Grenzsituationen* which Jaspers highlights as being important for grasping oneself as existence. Beside this tendency to fix one's explicit understanding of the world or the super-personal sense of life, it cannot be denied that human beings are unable to live permanently outside of a *Gehäuse*. In Jaspers' words, 'human beings can experience a specific purpose only in an element of a *Gehäuse*' (Jaspers 1919: 273). Drawing on Jaspers, we can conclude that our lifeworld as an experiential workspace, as a world in which specific action-properties are directly presented within the perceived objects disclosed to us (so-called *Zuhandenheit* (Heidegger 1927/1993: 68–76)), necessarily entails a mental superstructure which could be called *Gehäuse*.

Jaspers' concept of the *Gehäuse* offers an existential analysis of psychotherapeutic processes. Drawing on this concept we can conclude that mental illnesses inform and influence the *Weltanschauung* of the pertinent person. The mentally ill person adjusts, rearranges, and basically builds a *Gehäuse* as the person who suffers from a specific illness. In other words, her mental illness is, at least usually, a more or less substantial part and building block of her *Gehäuse*. This *Gehäuse* can have specific advantages, however small they might be. For example, it might offer some fairly good explanations for things going disturbingly wrong or being irritatingly weird in one's lifeworld. Or it might offer a more or less rational interpretation of those alterations and symptoms caused by one's mental illness. It might also be protecting against other, perhaps even more hazardous influences. And it might offer certain options of living one's life. The latter could be addressed as a more or less successful integration, or assimilation of the mental illness into one's *Gehäuse*. Accordingly, we can suspect that psychotherapeutic processes should enable the mentally ill person to develop a kind of *Gehäuse* which allows the pertinent person to tackle unavoidable challenges of her *Grenzsituationen* and to find an adequate and satisfying style of life-conduct. This might even afford to leave one's *Gehäuse* behind and to build a new one from the very ground. But, usually, it should simply imply rearranging certain aspects of one's housings so that one's *Weltanschauung* becomes more open-minded.

The question remains, however, where the capacity to grasp and accept the *Grenzsituation* as belonging to one's existence comes from, but it is this capacity that enables one to develop a new kind of *Gehäuse*. It is an already addressed fact that one's intentions are not necessarily strong enough to guide one's behaviour effectively. Jaspers' existential concept of the *Gehäuse* does not explain this sufficiently with respect to mental illnesses, because it is very much located on a reflective and conative level. It takes neither pre-reflective levels of mental life nor perceptive or affective layers adequately into account. Nonetheless, it might be possible to develop this concept if the prescriptive level of our habitualities is taken into consideration.

Jaspers' existential concept of psychotherapy: *Wille* and *Wollen*

To discuss questions regarding the sense of life is, to say the least, challenging in psychotherapeutic sessions. Nonetheless, it cannot be avoided that these questions are, at least superficially addressed. On the one hand, such questions are necessarily given if people reflect on themselves. On the other hand, therapy should be meaningful in itself. To accept these insights and recalling our existential analysis of psychotherapy, drawing on Jaspers' terms of *Grenzsituation* and *Gehäuse*, we are challenged by the task of an existential analysis in Jaspers' terms regarding the issue of capacity. This seems, from Jaspers' vantage point, to match the topic of the will, or *Wille* and *Wollen*.

Recalling Jaspers' distinction between psychotherapeutic methods which address the patient as a person, lack of will and especially lack of effort of will seem to be the most common reasons why people are unable to grasp themselves as existence. It seems, for example, sensible to argue that people with severe neuropsychological impairments like fronto-temporal dementia, entailing anosognosia, are unable to grasp themselves as existence and develop an adequate *Gehäuse* due to missing capacities of self-recognition. There may, however, be other reasons rendering one's effort of will ineffective. For example, Jaspers (1913: 322, 1920: 399, 1923: 433, 1946/1973: 701) is convinced that psychotherapeutic efforts concerning people suffering from schizophrenia are 'ridiculous'. This seems to be a fundamental misinterpretation, which is most probably fuelled by Jaspers' conception of schizophrenia as primarily an (neuro-)organic process that is therefore basically incomprehensible, even though he muses whether it could be possible to sensibly comprehend this process in his early work on 'Delusions of Jealousy' (*Eifersuchtswahn*) in 1910 (Jaspers 1963: 116; see Brückner 2009).

In his *General Psychopathology*, Jaspers (1913: 242–244) describes the will as the active pole and as a 'gathered effluence' (*Sammelausfluss*) of the personality. It is the will that allows the person to use all her other mental or physical functions for certain purposes, goals, or goods (Jaspers 1913: 180). In this description Jaspers draws heavily on the work of Else Wentscher, whom he mentions as an important source for his own debate on this topic. She describes the conscious will by a three-stepped-concept of 'Weighing—Approving—Deciding' (Wentscher 1910: 44–45). On the one hand, Jaspers adopts this concept; on the other hand, he highlights features like the inner fight, mastery, and capability of resistance often being associated with self-conscious decision-making (Jaspers 1913: 246–248). Accordingly, he distinguishes three aspects of will: an 'awareness of voluntariness' (*Willkürbewußtsein*) that is especially characterized in weighing pros and cons in decision-making; the experience of a drive that can be valued as belonging to one's personality or not; and, importantly, a divisiveness (*Entzweiung*) that refers to the very moment of reflection between the experienced drive and the voluntary behaviour (Jaspers 1913: 68). Jaspers describes this divisiveness in terms of an inner fight that takes place in instances of conflicting motivations, a fight that may have two different outcomes: 'either with the feeling of asserting one's personality and the consciousness of freedom or with the feeling of being defeated and the consciousness of coercion' ('entweder mit dem Gefühl der Behauptung der Persönlichkeit und dem Bewußtsein der Freiheit oder mit dem Gefühl des Unterliegens und dem Bewußtsein des Zwanges' Jaspers 1913: 69). Apparently, Jaspers is aware of possible impairments of one's effort of the will in the sense of being constrained or even helpless (Jaspers 1913: 70–72). Summing it up one could say that Jaspers underscores the aspects of reflection, of resistance and reasoning, and of an internal locus of control (Schlimme 2008). Living one's life in a meaningful and healthy way requires, from Jaspers' point of view, self-consciousness and self-control. Accordingly, both can be described as crucial features of his existence-philosophy. As Jaspers argues in his *Philosophy*, the will is the 'original power of the human being in its existence' (1932/1994, Vol. II: 157) and is gained, because it is wanted (Jaspers 1932/1994: 162). Or in other words, the will is not purpose-oriented, but aims at transcendence or freedom and grows in power if one's aims at existence. Nonetheless, self-consciousness and self-control are required as first steps for this higher, existential form of *Wille* and *Wollen*.

Jaspers neither introduced the existential concepts of *Gehäuse* or *Grenzsituation* in his writings on psychotherapy, nor did he explicitly address his concept of the will and its crucial importance for those psychotherapeutic means which call upon the patient as a person. The latter is, however, of outstanding merit, because it allows us to describe more precisely the difficulties that arise if one transposed the existential concepts of *Gehäuse* and *Grenzsituation* into a psychotherapeutic context. Since both self-consciousness and self-control can be impaired by, or sometimes even be lacking due to mental illness, this allows us to pinpoint the limits of an existential concept of psychotherapy. Or, more precisely, it allows us to understand why Jaspers basically argued for an existential understanding of psychotherapy and an existence-philosophy. The latter might be called a sophisticated way of existential counselling. Nonetheless, Jaspers did explicitly not argue, at least not in the end, for an existential psychotherapy.

Limits of Jaspers' existential concept of psychotherapy

Jaspers argues that many persons might be unable to imagine that they live in a *Gehäuse* instead of a strong and indestructible castle. In these cases it is even more crucial that the professional therapist hands the control over to the patient, at least with respect to existential questions. Jaspers refers to Ibsen's ingenious statement presented by Dr Relling in *Vildanden* (*The Wild Duck*), who explains that healing an 'average person' means to take care that his life-long illusion is maintained (already mentioned in the first edition of 1913: 324; see also the fourth edition of 1946/73: 671). Such life-long illusions could be called a *Gehäuse*, but Jaspers does not offer this transposition. The question remains why Jaspers did not apply his own concepts of *Grenzsituation* and *Gehäuse* to an improved existential analysis of psychotherapy? A clear answer to this question has, as far as I know, never been provided by Jaspers himself. However, two kinds of answers seem to be possible: firstly, methodological reasons might have prevented this kind of application; secondly, personal reasons might have fuelled resentments against it. Jaspers was, after all, no psychotherapist.

The idea that personal reasons could be a crucial factor for the directions of Jaspers' work might appear highly speculative; furthermore, such speculations might be deemed to be bad taste. Therefore I want to apologize for the speculation that follows; it might be of interest nonetheless. It is well known that Jaspers made some attempts in the field of psychotherapy in the 1910s when affiliated with the department of psychiatry in Heidelberg. As Schultz-Hencke reports, these attempts failed (Schultz-Hencke 1951). Drawing on our profound reconstruction of Jaspers' existential concept of psychotherapy, Jaspers' first psychotherapeutic steps would have most probably been based upon his ideas of psychotherapy in its highest form, maybe in a style of the *psychothérapie rationnelle* as proposed by Dubois (Dubois 1913). This would, most probably, entail the suggestion to gain insight into one's *Grenzsituation* and *Gehäuse* as possible backgrounds for one's suffering and for one's inability to grasp one's being-as-it-is as existence. Admittedly, this ought to be a successful way of coaching a person through a kind of crisis which is not rendering this person incapable of behaving according to her intentions. Situations would be completely different if exactly this kind of capability would be lost. This is, unfortunately, the usual problem in persons suffering from a mental illness. In this way Jaspers' psychotherapeutic attempts should have gone completely wrong, if he would really have tried to directly address people suffering from mental illnesses in a sense of 'please grasp your situation as a *Grenzsituation*'. To achieve a level in psychotherapeutic communication that allows fruitfully addressing these issues requires a long time of preparation, as Arthur Kronfeld, Jaspers' ingenious counterpart in Berlin, himself being deeply influenced by Dubois' concept of *psychagogik*, pointed out in his influential work on *Psychotherapie* (Kronfeld 1924: 239–243). By such preparation, the patient might gain a distanced attitude concerning his own situation, primarily via a psychological attitude towards his own experiences and situations. Hence existential issues are, as Kronfeld argues, usually addressed indirectly in the long run and, in the best case, solved by the patient himself as a last step of healing. In other words, to grasp one's distressing situation as a *Grenzsituation* might be a goal of psychotherapy. It may even indicate that one doesn't need psychotherapy any more. However, it does not seem plausible to expect the capacity to actually grasp one's situation as a *Grenzsituation* as the starting point of the psychotherapeutic process. But, has Jaspers really been this naïve? Did Jaspers really overestimate the direct influence of one's will that grossly? This does not seem very probable, as could, for example, be argued referring to Jaspers' Dr Relling quote by Ibsen. Still, the question remains: why did he not use his insights for the sake of an even deeper existential analysis of mental illnesses, addressing, for example, the pre-reflective qualities and the habitualities of mental life? Or did he try exactly this in his pathographical analysis *Strindberg and van Gogh* (Jaspers 1922; see Schlimme 2010, 2011), which might not be very convincing from the vantage point of comprehensive psychology, but which seems to be ingenious from a cultural perspective and challenging for the meta-discourse about psychiatry? These questions might remain unanswered. Nonetheless, I would like to summarize with the conclusion that personal reasons were not primarily responsible for Jaspers' abstention of transposing his existential terms into a psychotherapeutic discourse.

However, methodological reasons for his abstention can also be claimed. These reasons imply, whether fuelled by unsuccessful psychotherapeutic baby-steps or not, a clear insight into the limits of one's voluntary influence on oneself. Jaspers did not, after all, try to develop an existential psychotherapy, but headed for an existence-philosophy and an existential comprehension of psychotherapy instead. And he was apparently aware of important limits, as his reference to Ibsen's Dr Relling demonstrates. As Sonja Rinofner-Kreidl showed in her meticulous and brilliant study on Jaspers' methodological development, his methodological reflections aimed more and more at the most fundamental difference between 'intuition and analysis' (Rinofner-Kreidl 2008: 86). It has to be admitted, however, that Jaspers' earliest methodological reflections, as displayed in his first editions of the *General Psychopathology*, remained insufficient with respect to the necessary pre-structure of understanding. This pre-structure of understanding is of crucial importance for interpersonal communication, hermeneutical methods, and, accordingly, for psychiatry and psychotherapy (Straus 1963: 940). However, already in the first edition of his *General Psychopathology* Jaspers offers, due to his introduction of a hermeneutical method as a valuable scientific method for psychiatry, an understanding of psychotherapy that steps beyond the standard position of clinical psychiatry in the wake of Isserlin and Kraepelin. This holds true, even if psychotherapy is performed in the way of Dubois' *psychothérapie rationnelle*, and even if this kind of psychotherapy is judged to be the highest form of psychotherapy, as Jaspers himself obviously did. Nonetheless, exactly those fundamental methodological reflections demonstrate why it is indeed impossible to analyse freedom, and why it is necessary to call upon freedom instead. Calling upon freedom cannot be done other than by philosophizing personally. Jaspers was well aware of the impossibility to entirely comprehend mental life: 'Comprehensive psychology needs to be modest' (Jaspers 1932/1994, Vol. II: 312).

Taking these methodological reflections into account, I would like to argue that Jaspers transfers his fundamental distinction between intuition and analysis to the domain of activity. In other words, he aims in his subsequent paragraphs and writings on psychotherapy and medical practice towards a fundamental distinction between purpose- and freedom-oriented behaviour. When Jaspers claims that freedom cannot be made, this does not entail that freedom cannot be the goal of one's behaviour, but that no clear and proven rules can be named that guarantee the outcome of one's struggle to be free (Paprotny 2003: 39). While purpose-oriented behaviour can only be performed within a *Gehäuse*, and while it can and should be tested with respect to its affectivity, in other words, with respect to wanted and unwanted effects, freedom-oriented behaviour cannot be founded on scientific methods. It requires, from Jaspers' vantage point, that a person philosophizes herself (these methodological reflections fuel also Jaspers' critique of 'training psychoanalysis' as a serious attack to freedom (see Rossi Monti, Chapter 3, this volume)).

Accordingly, and because Jaspers assumes freedom to be the ultimate goal of any human life-conduct, psychotherapy reaches its limits in the inextricable connection between the style of one's life-conduct and one's experience able (super-personal) sense of life (e.g. freedom in the case of Jaspers or an 'existential life-conduct'). In other words, he believed super-personal sense of life refers also to one's lived experience which is, of course, not completely independent from one's life-conduct. This linkage, which cannot be disrupted by any kind of justifiable belief or falsifiable knowledge, can be addressed and thematized through existentially philosophizing. For this, it is essential for medical doctors, psychotherapists, and all kinds of professional therapists, to recall from time to time the simple Hippocratic truth: 'Therapy cannot substitute what alone life can give' (Jaspers 1946/1973: 672). For Jaspers this implies, whether a person might suffer from a mental illness or not, she will always remain on the way towards freedom. In order to advance on this way it is necessary to philosophically reflect on this 'being-on-the-way' (Jaspers 1976: 109). In other words, to understand existential concepts like *Gehäuse* and *Grenzsituation* in a fruitful way already requires both self-consciousness and self-control, or *Wille* and *Wollen* to a certain extent. Psychiatrists as well as psychotherapists need to be aware of these requirements if becoming engaged in existential communication with their patients.

Drawing on these methodological reflections, we can claim methodological reasons as motives for Jaspers not even trying to transpose terms from his existential philosophy into a comprehensive psychology or vice versa. Following Jaspers, it should be more beneficial, for patients, psychiatrists, and psychotherapists, to be aware of the dangers and difficulties that arise when transposing terms from existential philosophy into psychology. In other words, it is better to achieve an existential concept of psychotherapy, than encumbering psychotherapy with existential counselling or philosophizing in the first place.

Conclusion

Psychotherapy is, from Jaspers' vantage point, a therapeutic mean founded on scientific methods and performed by actors displaying a methodologically critical attitude. This should entail explicit recognition of fundamental limits. Since psychotherapy deals with real persons and is performed by real persons, these limits call upon the engaged persons to philosophize and, at least from a Jaspers point of view, to grasp oneself as existence. In the latter sense, psychotherapy might be offering self-elucidation, but it is not, at least not necessarily, elucidating one's potentiality of being an existence. To recognize this potentiality and to grasp oneself as existence is the prerogative of existential communication. In existential communication the patient and the psychiatrist or psychotherapist disclose themselves to each other as fellow sufferers. This is simply founded on the fact that this patient is 'my patient', and this psychiatrist or psychotherapist is 'my therapist' or 'my medical doctor'. These 'my' indicate a fundamental quality of the relationship that can neither be denied, nor be arbitrary or valid for anyone else. This quality concerns only these two individual persons in their relation to each other. Existential communication in medical or psychotherapeutic practice is furthermore based upon a certain, at least minimal independence of these questions concerning the meaning of life from one's pre-reflective levels of mental life. Even if one's habitualities are deeply altered by a mental illness, such questions concerning the (super-personal) meaning of one's life can only be answered if actually reflecting on oneself, one's lifeworld and life-history as well as one's life-goals. Accordingly, it is important for the psychiatrist or psychotherapist to adopt an existential perspective on their relation to their patient from time to time. In this adoption Jaspers' existential terms *Gehäuse*, *Grenzsituation*, and *Wille* can be of interest, as argued in this chapter.

Furthermore, to adopt a framing perspective on our medical or therapeutic practice seems to be of importance, because our patients' way of pursuing happiness and their style of life-conduct challenge our own understanding of these essential topics. In other words, they force us to reflect on our own way of life-conduct as well as our own normative and common-sense habituality. Obviously we can learn from our patients if we are open for existential communication in our relation with them. Although such a level of existential communication can be achieved within this relationship, and is persistently present in the background, it is neither a principal nor a common task of psychotherapy (Jaspers 1946/1973: 667, 683). As Jaspers argues in *Der Arzt im technischen Zeitalter* (1958/1986b: 47–57), it is necessary to accept the simple fact that freedom cannot be addressed scientifically. Freedom can only be called upon within the relation between patient and medical doctor or professional therapist. And it calls upon both of them to philosophize.

Acknowledgements

The author would like to thank Sonja Rinofner-Kreidl, Graz, and Catharina Bonnemann, Hannover, for discussing a preliminary version of this paper. All translations of the quotes of Karl Jaspers are by the author and Christoph Bonnemann, Freiburg.

References

Brückner, B. (2009). 'Geschichtlichkeit und Aktualität der Theorie des Wahns in der "Allgemeinen Psychopathologie" von Karl Jaspers', *Journal für Philosophie & Psychiatrie*, 2, available at: <http://www.jfpp.org/jfpp-2-2009-03.html> (accessed 17 November 2011).

Dubois, P. (1913). 'Rationelle Psychotherapie', *Jahreskurse für ärztliche Fortbildung*, 5: 25–32.

Fuchs, T. (2008). 'Ansätze zu einer Psychopathologie der Grenzsituation', in S. Rinofner-Kreidl, H.A. Wiltsche (eds), *Karl Jaspers' Allgemeine Psychopathologie zwischen Wissenschaft, Philosophie und Praxis*. Würzburg: Königshausen & Neumann, 95–107.

Heidegger, M. (1993). *Sein und Zeit* (17th unaltered edn). Tübingen: Max Niemeyer. (Original work published in German in 1927.)

Isserlin, M. (1910). 'Die psychoanalytische Methode Freuds', *Zeitschrift für die gesamte Neurologie und Psychiatrie*, **1**: 52–80.

Jaspers, K. (1913). *Allgemeine Psychopathologie* (1st edn). Berlin: Springer.

Jaspers, K. (1919). *Psychologie der Weltanschauungen*. Berlin: Springer.

Jaspers, K. (1920). *Allgemeine Psychopathologie* (2nd edn). Berlin: Springer.

Jaspers, K. (1922). *Strindberg und van Gogh. Versuch einer pathographischen Analyse unter vergleichender Heranziehung von Swedenborg und Hölderlin*. Bern: Piper.

Jaspers, K. (1923). *Allgemeine Psychopathologie* (3rd edn). Berlin: Springer.

Jaspers, K. (1963). *Gesammelte Schriften zur Psychopathologie*. Berlin: Springer.

Jaspers, K. (1973). *Allgemeine Psychopathologie* (9th edn). Heidelberg: Springer. (Original work published in German 1946.)

Jaspers, K. (1976). 'Grundfragen der Philosophie (12 Radiovorträge von 1949)', in K. Jaspers, *Was ist Philosophie?*. München: Deutscher Taschenbuch Verlag, 33–120.

Jaspers, K. (1986a). 'Arzt und Patient', in *Der Arzt im technischen Zeitalter*. München: Piper, 19–38. (Original work published in German 1953.)

Jaspers, K. (1986b). 'Der Arzt im technischen Zeitalter', in *Der Arzt im technischen Zeitalter*. München: Piper, 39–58. (Original work published in German 1958.)

Jaspers, K. (1986c). 'Zur Kritik der Psychoanalyse', in *Der Arzt im technischen Zeitalter*. München: Piper, 59–68. (Original work published in German 1950.)

Jaspers, K. (1994). *Philosophie*, Vol. 3. München: Piper. (Original work published in German in 1932.)

Kronfeld, A. (1924). *Psychotherapie. Charakterlehre, Psychoanalyse, Hypnose, Psychagogik*. Berlin: Springer.

Luft, S. (2008). 'Zur phänomenologischen Methode in Karl Jaspers' Allgemeine Psychopathologie', in S. Rinofner-Kreidl, H.A. Wiltsche (eds), *Karl Jaspers' Allgemeine Psychopathologie zwischen Wissenschaft, Philosophie und Praxis*. Würzburg: Königshausen & Neumann, 31–51.

Müller, C. (2002). *"Sie müssen an Ihre Heilung glauben!" Paul Dubois (1848–1918). Ein vergessener Pionier der Psychotherapie*. Basel: Schwabe.

Paprotny, T. (2003). *Das Wagnis der Philosophie. Denkwege und Diskurse bei Karl Jaspers*. Freiburg/Breisgau: Karl Alber.

Peters, U.H. (2002a). 'Die Isserlin-Affäre. Ein Stellvertreter-Disput zwischen Kraepelin und Freud', *Fortschritte der Neurologie und Psychiatrie*, **70**: 27–33.

Peters, U.H. (2002b). 'Max Isserlin. Kantianer in Königsberg, Psychotherapeut bei Kraepelin, Begründer der Münchner Kinderpsychiatrie, Emigrant in England', *Fortschritte der Neurologie und Psychiatrie*, **70**: 18–26.

Rinofner-Kreidl, S. (2008). 'Zur Idee des Methodenpartikularismus in Jaspers' Allgemeiner Psychopathologie', in S. Rinofner-Kreidl, H.A. Wiltsche (eds), *Karl Jaspers' Allgemeine Psychopathologie zwischen Wissenschaft, Philosophie und Praxis*. Würzburg: Königshausen & Neumann, 75–94.

Rombach, H. (1993). *Strukturanthropologie. 'Der menschliche Mensch'* (2nd rev. edn). Freiburg/Breisgau: Karl Alber. (Original work published in German in 1987.)

Schlimme, J.E. (2008). 'Willensschwäche und Getriebensein. Zugänge zu Jaspers' Verständnis der Sucht', in S. Rinofner-Kreidl, H.A. Wiltsche (eds), *Karl Jaspers' Allgemeine Psychopathologie zwischen Wissenschaft, Philosophie und Praxis*. Würzburg: Königshausen & Neumann, 147–170.

Schlimme, J.E. (2010). 'Karl Jaspers. Pathographie zwischen "genetischem Verstehen" und Existenzerhellung', in U. Gonther, J.E. Schlimme (eds), *Hölderlin und die Psychiatrie: Schriften der Hölderlin-Gesellschaft*, Vol. 25 (2nd unaltered edn). Bonn: Edition Das Narrenschiff im Psychiatrie-Verlag, 177–193.

Schlimme, J.E. (2011). 'Psychiatrie und Psychotherapie im Denken Karl Jaspers', in H. Yousefi, W. Schüßler, R. Schulz, U. Diehl (eds), *Karl Jaspers. Eine Einführung*. Reinbek: Lau Verlag, 229–250.

Schlimme, J.E., Paprotny, T., Brückner, B. (2012). 'Karl Jaspers: Aufgaben und Grenzen der Psychotherapie', *Der Nervenarzt*, **83**(1): 84–91.

Schultz-Hencke, H. (1951). 'Zur Verteidigung der Psychoanalyse', *Der Monat*, **3**: 438–440.

Straus, E. (1963). 'Philosophische Grundfragen der Psychiatrie, II. Psychiatrie und Philosophie', in H.W. Gruhle, R. Jung, W. Mayer-Gross, M. Müller (eds), *Psychiatrie der Gegenwart*, Vol. I/2. Heidelberg and Berlin: Springer, 926–994.

Wentscher, E. (1910). *Der Wille*. Leipzig: B.G. Teubner.

Wiggins, O.P., Schwartz, M.A. (1997). 'Edmund Husserl's influence in Karl Jaspers' phenomenology', *Philosophy, Psychiatry, & Psychology*, **4**: 15–36.

Chapter 12

The ethics of incomprehensibility

Giovanni Stanghellini

Jaspers for clinicians

Jaspers' life as a clinician was like a meteor—short-lived and intensely bright. In January 1908 he began work as a medical trainee. In July 1911 Julius Springer commissioned him to write a compendium guide for medical students, doctors, and psychologists; he was a 28-year-old unpaid voluntary assistant who had spent more or less three years in Heidelberg Psychiatric Clinic, but apparently had enough clinical knowledge—or institutional naïveté—to be aware that psychiatry was in strong need of a systematic clarification of its concepts and methods. He was especially critical of the 'therapeutic nihilism' (quoted in Kirkbright 2004: 62) worshipped in the Heidelberg Clinic at that time, and argued for a renaissance of psychiatry founded on the clinician–patient relationship accepting the dignity and limitations of the partners concerned, thus on what he, as a philosopher, would later call 'existential communication' (Jaspers 1969–1971). When, in July 1913, *General Psychopathology* was published (Jaspers 1997), his career as a clinician virtually ended, but his influence on psychiatry lasted for a very long time (see Mundt, Chapter 4, this volume).

What can psychiatrists, especially young psychiatrists, one century after the publication of Jaspers' opus magnum, learn from a young inexperienced doctor who, due to his severe lung problems, was unable to complete his ward rounds? Can this young man be taken as an example by in-career trainees, who being told by his boss Franz Nissl (whom he admired) that there was not enough opportunity for him to continue working in the Clinic made this potential fiasco into an opportunity and felt free to attend philosophical seminars, thus attaining an original stance in his research? What can they share with this man who was grateful enough to Aesculapius and to Aesculapius' disciple Albert Fraenkel, the physician who so tactfully informed the young Jaspers of his illness and took care of him, to decide to devote himself to the 'investigation of the human body [as] the foundation of all other knowledge about the human psyche' (quoted in Kirkbright 2004: 22)? What can they learn from a medical doctor who held that the future of medicine was in 'binding philosophy to science' (Jaspers 1971: 11)?

And, above all, how can young psychiatrists, who are so hungry for handbook knowledge, structured interviews, decision-making criteria, therapeutic protocols, etc. be so patient as to listen to such a hybrid clinician-philosopher arguing for a kind of knowledge which is stubbornly aware of its limits, and breathlessly revolting against all sorts of dogmatism and objectification? How can those who are looking for 'expert knowledge' like current sociology, psychology, and anthropology (Jaspers 2010: 144) be satisfied with a kind of knowledge which conceives of itself as an 'unlimited task', a 'limitless movement' which takes place in the face-to-face, here-and-now encounter between two persons?

How can they be happy with a teacher who is convinced that the essence of knowledge is not the possession, but the *search for* truth, at the same time rejecting all epistemological nihilism and mysticism? Jaspers' main teaching can be condensed into one sentence: '[Q]uestions are more essential than answers, and every answer becomes a new question' (Jaspers 2003: 12). Where shall we find such intrepid young colleagues who, on the basis of this *on-the-way philosophy*, will follow Jaspers' medical credo: '[M]edical treatment must rely on un-understood life' (Jaspers 1971: 24)?

What do we need for a sound-enough clinical practice?

To answer these questions, we need to tackle another more fundamental one: what do we need for a sound-enough clinical practice? On what kind of knowledge can we rely to establish the foundations of psychiatry? Jaspers' explicit answer is very clear and can be condensed in one single word: *psychopathology*. What is psychopathology? A rather sketchy, but not incorrect, answer is that psycho-patho-logy is a discourse (*logos*) that endeavours to articulate the suffering (*pathos*) that troubles the human mind (*psyche*). Psychopathology is a *logos* for *pathos*—that is, a discourse about what troubles the human person. Psychopathology provides a language to talk and make sense of the phenomena that express the vulnerability of the human person.

According to Jaspers, psychopathology has two major aims. First, it offers 'clarification, order, formation' (Jaspers 1997: 38), that is, concrete descriptions, a suitable terminology, and methodical groupings that allow us to bring order into the chaos of disturbing mental phenomena. The main objects of descriptive psychopathology are the patients' experiences. The purpose is to rescue the subjective quality and the personal meaning of abnormal phenomena. The form in which these phenomena are presented is considered more significant than contents. Perceptions, ideas, judgements, feelings, drives, and self-awareness are all forms of psychic phenomena, denoting the particular mode of existence in which a content is experienced. Avoiding all theoretical prejudices is the quintessential methodological as well as ethical (i.e. maximally respecting the person as a subject of experience) prerequisite of Jaspers' psychopathology. Focusing on the phenomena that are present to the patient's consciousness, psychopathology is not concerned with any subsidiary speculations, psychological constructions, interpretations, or evaluations. It is essential to note that Jaspers' psychopathology does not aim to provide an all-encompassing theory of mental disorders, with an ambition of establishing nosological and aetiopathogenetical knowledge. Rather, more modestly and realistically, it supplies clinicians with a palette with different qualities and shades of colour that may allow them to recognize the kind, the tonality, and the intensity of abnormal experiences at play in the single individual (Stanghellini and Rosfort 2013). Jaspers acknowledges the clinicians' need to classify phenomena, but this classification, he suggests, must not be 'like an outline [*Entwurf*] of a continent but more like an outline of possible ways to explore it' (Jaspers 1997: 749).

This leads to the second, and perhaps more important, aim of *General Psychopathology*. Jaspers aims at 'a psychopathological education' (Jaspers 1997: 50), endowing clinicians with a valid and reliable methodology, i.e. providing a philosophically sound background for the encounter with their patients. The purpose is to make clinicians more epistemologically and ethically aware of the characteristics of the tools they use when trying to grasp, assess, and make sense of their patients' experiences and behaviours and of the limitations of these tools. The most famous example of this is Jaspers' discussion of empathic understanding and its boundaries. Empathy is a special kind of intentional experience through which a person tries to recreate in himself the subjective experience of another person to obtain a valid and reliable description of it. In Jaspers' sense, psychopathology is methodologically based on the intuitive presentation of the other person's mental life through first-person understanding of his experiences. Since we cannot directly perceive the psychic experiences of the other person, psychopathology attempts to make a representation of them based on the patients' own self-descriptions (Stanghellini 2007).

Thus, empathic understanding is one of the columns of Jaspers' psychopathology (see Hoerl, Chapter 8, this volume), the other one being establishing meaningful connections between mental abnormal phenomena (see Sass, Chapter 7, this volume). But in some cases, while performing this act of imaginative self-transposal, we experience the radical un-understandability of the other. What is at work here is Jaspers' notorious 'theorem of incomprehensibility' (Baeyer 1979). Jaspers' concept of 'incomprehensibility', I will argue, is not simply a methodological or epistemological principle but also an *ethical attitude*. I will put it very roughly: to develop the foundations for a sound-enough clinical practice we need, following Jaspers, an *ethics of incomprehensibility*. This ethics is based both on the idea that truth is not a possession but rather a being-on-the-way and on the rejection of all kind of absolute knowledge (Jaspers 2003: 12). This will be my point of departure as I set off to rescue the more implicit of Jaspers' answers to the question that entitles this paragraph.

An asymptotic kind of knowledge

Jaspers' concept of 'incomprehensibility' applies to two distinct areas. One is psychotic experience. The other is human existence as a whole.

Jaspers acknowledges that empathic understanding fails when it comes to certain kinds of abnormal phenomena such as, for instance, delusion proper. Jaspers maintains that the 'primary experiences', that is, the background metamorphosis of consciousness underlying delusions proper, are beyond the reach of empathic understanding. When faced with the patient's descriptions of the uncanny experiences of self- and world-transformation taking place during the initial phase of schizophrenia, we touch an unsurpassable limit as we encounter something radically unfamiliar: 'The environment is somehow different, not to a gross degree, perception is unaltered in itself but there is some change which envelops everything with subtle, pervasive and strangely uncertain light' (Jaspers 1997: 98). The patients feel 'as if they have lost their grip on things' and are invaded by a 'distrustful, uncomfortable, uncanny tension' (Jaspers 1997: 98).

Jaspers' famous attitude towards the incomprehensibility of schizophrenic delusions emphasizes a form of empathy that is immediate or spontaneous and essentially non-intellectual. This does not imply that this kind of empathy is unnecessary in such cases. On the contrary, while discovering the limits of empathy we realize that we need to adopt a different approach if we want to move towards and try to understand the patient's experiences. Jaspers describes in detail the changes in experience from which schizophrenic delusions arise. But, as argued by Sass (Chapter 7, this volume) and Ratcliffe (Chapter 15, this volume), he does not encourage the appreciation of general ontological or horizonal changes. He restricts his research to the phenomenal or experiential level, and does not investigate the fundamental mutations of the pre-reflective structure in which this metamorphosis of experience is inscribed (see Stanghellini and Rosfort 2013).

Sass and Ratcliffe, while trying to improve Jaspers' concept of 'empathic understanding', suggest that severe aberrations of experience such as those that can be met with in schizophrenia would seem to require a different, and more theoretical, kind of empathy than the one proposed by Jaspers. Understanding psychotic experiences like schizophrenic, or melancholic, or manic ones, requires a kind of training that goes beyond spontaneous and naïf empathic skills. The clinician's standard empathic capacities need some kind of education. I suggest that we name the achievement of this learning *second-order empathy*, the method required for grasping those experiences that are not understandable via simply transposing oneself into another person (Stanghellini, in press). To achieve second-order empathy, first of all I need to acknowledge that the lifeworld inhabited by the other person is not like my own. The supposition that the other person lives in a world like my own—that he experiences time, space, his own body, others, the materiality of objects, etc. just like I do—is often the source of serious misunderstanding. In order to empathize I must acknowledge the radical difference that separates me from the way of being in the world that characterizes the other. Any forgetting of this difference, paradigmatically between my own world and that of a schizophrenic patient (but I would say, also, *mutatis mutandis* between my own and an adolescent's or an old man's world), will be an obstacle to empathic understanding, since these people live in a life-world whose structure is (at least in part) different from my own (Stanghellini and Ballerini 2007). Achieving second-order empathy thus requires bracketing my own pre-reflexive, natural attitude (in which my first-order empathic capacities are rooted), and approaching the other's world as I would do while exploring an unknown country.

Jaspers acknowledges that in order to understand psychotic phenomena like delusion proper in persons with schizophrenia we need to grasp the metamorphosis of 'personality', i.e. the deep and implicit structures of existence. Grasping the intimate transformation of subjectivity underlying the manifold symptoms—to use Minkowski's words 'the way in which personality is situated, in normal as well as in pathological terms, in relation to lived time and lived space' (Minkowski 1993: 2)—is not part of Jaspers' agenda. He seems not to develop a proper method for grasping this transformation or for filling in the gap between my (the clinician's) ordinary and his (the patient's) aberrant experience. Why? I suggest that a reason is Jaspers' recalcitrance to all kinds of all-encompassing understanding of human existence. Jaspers may have seen in schizophrenic existence the paradigm of the irreducibility of a person's existence as a whole to any kind of all-embracing 'expert knowledge' (Jaspers 2010: 146). The case of the incomprehensibility of schizophrenic experience is a hyperbolic illustration of Jaspers' attitude towards knowledge in general: all knowledge must have an *asymptotic character*.[1] 'The humility of an enduring question is indispensable' (Jaspers 2003: 80).

---

[1] In geometry, an asymptote of a curve is a line such that the distance between the curve and the line approaches zero as they tend to infinity. The word asymptote is derived from the Greek ἀασυμπτοτος which means 'not falling together'. An asymptote is also defined as a line which is tangent to a curve *at infinity*. The asymptote tends to touch the curve but never reaches it.

The issue of understanding schizophrenic existence is also tied to another question: do people with schizophrenia always want to be understood? The answer is not as obvious as it may seem.

The philosophical roots of the theorem of incomprehensibility

This brings us to the second aspect of Jaspers' theorem of incomprehensibility, the one with which clinicians may be less familiar, that none the less has the paramount importance of rooting clinical practice in a sound-enough methodological and ethical ground.

In the Introduction I quoted this rather obscure and perplexing sentence from *Philosophy of Existence*:

> All practice on the basis of knowledge must rely on the unseen encompassing: medical treatment must rely on un-understood life. (Jaspers 1971: 24)

This sentence requires an interpretation that I will try to develop building on and extending Jaspers' reflections on what I called the ethics of incomprehensibility. For the sake of clarity, I will divide this paragraph into subsections each treating, with the help of quotes from Jaspers (mainly from his philosophical essays), the different aspect of the whole issue.

The link between medicine, philosophy, and science

First of all, the sentence brings together medicine ('medical treatment') and philosophy ('the unseen encompassing'). The unseen encompassing, a key concept in Jaspers' philosophy, is the limit of our objective knowledge, including medical knowledge and our knowledge of another person. To Jaspers, the comprehensible relies on the un-understood. The encompassing is not the horizon of our knowledge. Rather it is the source from which all new horizons emerge, without itself ever being visible as a horizon (Jaspers 1971: 17). Thus, all kind of knowledge is precariously based on what cannot be understood. If, and only if, we are aware of this, we grasp a new profundity (Jaspers 1971: 24). This ties in particular to the idea of a person as necessarily incompletely fathomable. The Other can be approximated, 'encircled but not reached' (Jaspers 2003: 41). The awareness that knowing another person is an unlimited task keeps us alert of the 'breadth' of the essence of being human (Jaspers 1971: 27).

That in this sentence Jaspers links philosophy with medicine is obviously not surprising, since for Jaspers medical practice is to be seen as 'concrete philosophy' (Jaspers' *Der Arzt im technischen Zeitalter* (Jaspers 1958). The question is about which kind of philosophy is needed to found medical (in general) and particularly psychiatric practice. Jaspers' answer

Indeed, they reject being assimilated by the other person, and understanding (as we will see in detail later) implies some kind of assimilation since, when I understand you, it is implied that what you feel is similar to what I myself can and would feel in your place. Now, the schizophrenic value system, which conveys an overall crisis of common sense, reflects the choice of taking an eccentric or *antagonomic* stand in the face of commonly shared assumptions and the here and now 'other'. Also, schizophrenic persons' *idionomia* reflects the feeling of the radical uniqueness and exceptionality of one's being with respect to common sense and other human beings (Stanghellini and Ballerini 2007). This suggests that persons with schizophrenia may sometimes be recalcitrant to feeling understood by other persons including clinicians.

is twofold. First, we need 'a life-grounding philosophy' (Jaspers 1971: 6), that is, a kind of philosophy that faces the real-world problems of human existence. Existence philosophy, in its dealing with the limit-situations (Jaspers 1919, 1971) of suffering, fight, mortality, contingency, and guilt as situations that pose a challenge for oneself, and that are often given when a person suffers from a mental illness, can serve this purpose.

Also, we need a kind of philosophy that helps science to understand itself. Science and philosophy are the two roots of psychiatry. Submission to science and rejection of science, writes Jaspers (Jaspers 2003: 149), spell the end of knowledge. We can say of psychiatry what Jaspers says about philosophy: '[w]hether it is the slave of science or whether it denies all science' (Jaspers 2003: 150), psychiatry has in either case ceased to be good psychiatry. Philosophy and science are intimately intertwined. The road to science is 'indispensable for philosophy, since only a knowledge of that road prevents philosophizing from again making unsound and subjective claims to factual knowledge that really belongs to methodologically exact research' (Jaspers 1971: 10). A similar claim can be found in *Way to Wisdom* (Jaspers 2003: 159): 'Any philosopher who is not trained in a scientific discipline and who fails to keep his scientific interest constantly alive will inevitably bungle and stumble and mistake uncritical rough drafts for definitive knowledge. Unless an idea is submitted to the coldly dispassionate test of scientific inquiry, it is rapidly consumed in the fire of emotions and passions, or else it withers into a dry and narrow fanaticism' (here, 'philosopher' could be altered to 'psychiatrist' and the sentence would not change its force). Conversely, philosophical clarity is indispensable to science since '[w]ithout philosophy science does not understand itself' (Jaspers 1971: 10)—that is, it does not understand its purpose and its limits.

Knowledge as the critical awareness of the limits of knowledge

Neither philosophy nor science can provide a full knowledge of man as a whole. All determinate knowledge shows its limitations when faced with the breadth of human existence. This is the case with any attempt to grasp the complexity of another person's concrete existence, as well as with all kinds of impersonal expert knowledge (see later). Jaspers, as we have seen, argues for an *asymptotic kind of knowledge*. Knowledge and truth are not possessions but rather a being-on-the-way. The essence of true knowledge is compared to a 'limitless movement' (Jaspers 1971: 24). Jaspers also illustrates this idea with an oxymoron borrowed from Schelling: philosophy here, coextensive with true knowledge, is an 'open secret'. In this scenario, questions are more essential than answers, and every answer must become a new question (Jaspers 2003: 12). Claiming to have fully understood something is '[t]he most devastating threat to truth' (Jaspers 2003: 70). It seems that the real purpose of the search for knowledge is not achieving knowledge but rather attaining an '*increasing lucidity of a sense of being* totally different from all determinate knowledge' (Jaspers 1971: 19). The final outcome of this unlimited striving for insight is 'a critical awareness of the quality and limit of every insight' (Jaspers 2003: 87). This applies, in the domain of medicine and psychiatry, to the attempt of understanding the life of another person. Through the knowledge we attain in our attempts, together with its relativization, we 'grasp a new profundity' (Jaspers 1971: 24) since the awareness that understanding another person is an unlimited task keeps us alert of the 'breadth' of the essence of being human (Jaspers 1971: 27).

Limitations of expert knowledge

As no clinician can attain a full understanding of his patient, no researcher can attain a full knowledge of Man. The sciences of mankind, including sociology, psychology, and anthropology, and all kind of 'expert knowledge' cannot achieve a full grasp of what man is. 'Man is always something more than what he knows about himself. He is not what he is simply once for all, but is a process' (Jaspers 2010: 146). When methods of inquiry such as ethnology, psychoanalysis, or Marxism 'lay claim to absolute knowledge of the whole man—and this they have all done—they lose sight of the real man' (Jaspers 2003: 66).

This is also the case with biomedical 'expert knowledge'. In the 'technical age', medicine makes three nefarious mistakes. First, it conceives of the patient as just the locus of a particular occurrence of a universal category (an illness), not as an individuum (Jaspers' *Arzt und Patient* (Jaspers 1983)). Second, in an inane effort to establish objectivity, it tends to focus exclusively on the clinical datum (a symptom) overlooking the meaning that the datum has for the patient who suffers for it (Jaspers' *Der Arzt im technischen Zeitalter* (Jaspers 1958). Third, it forgets that medical practice is based on two pillars: scientific knowledge as well as humanitarian ethos (Jaspers' *Die Idee des Arztes* (Jaspers 1953)). Humanitarian ethos means, here, proximity to the patient and the awareness of the character of approximation of our clinical knowledge. I will develop this issue in the section on communicative action.

'New' paradigms of medicine, like psychosomatic medicine, did not solve this problem—rather they exacerbated it. Jaspers is very critical towards what he calls 'pseudo-revolutionary' medicine such as von Weizsäcker's psychosomatics (see Rossi Monti, Chapter 3, this volume). While stigmatizing the objectification of the patient perpetrated by technical medicine, von Weizsäcker's psychoanalytically founded medicine uses the 'rediscovery of subjectivity' as a slogan and reduces the patient to an object by its own metaphysical and dogmatic understanding of the illness process and of human subjectivity (Jaspers' *Die Idee des Arztes* (Jaspers 1953/1983c)). It also distorts the traditional role of the clinician by turning her, unrealistically and almost fanatically, into a shepherd of souls.

Man's existence is in time

If Jaspers argues for the 'on-the-wayness' of knowledge and rejects all dogmatism, that is, rejects a 'body of didactic principles purporting to be definitive and complete', this is because man's destiny is in time (Jaspers 2003: 12).

This sentence can be seen from several different, and complementary, angles. The first considers the fact that, since *human existence develops in time*, one's knowledge of oneself is interminable practice of unfolding: 'Man is not a finished life which repeats itself from generation to generation, nor is he a manifest life which plainly reveals itself to him. He "breaks through" the passivity of perpetually renewed identical circles, and is dependent upon his activity, whereby the process of his life is carried on towards an unknown goal' (Jaspers 2010: 146). Being a person, as well as knowing oneself, is a work in progress. Self-knowledge is a process of unfolding, rather than a solid possession. A crystallized kind of self-knowledge bears the same relation to this process of unfolding as does 'the herbarium to living plants, or as does a collection of bones to living bodies' (Jaspers 2003: 49). There is an infinite dialectics between what someone has understood about himself and what he thinks of what he has understood. We do not only get some knowledge about ourselves, but take a position on what we have just come to know. The reason for this is that '[t]here is an inner cleavage in man's innermost nature' which implies that 'whatever he thinks of himself, he must think against himself and against what is not-himself' (Jaspers 2010: 146). The decisive point is that man must always be setting himself in a dialectical position with himself. The person can take a position (*Stellungsnahme*), react, take up an attitude towards what he has understood of himself and try to overcome it. This makes of self-knowledge a never-ending task. There is no human existence without cleavage. Yet man cannot rest content in this cleavage. 'The ways in which he overcomes it, the way in which he transcends it, reveals the conception he has of himself' (Jaspers 2010: 146).

Knowledge as approximation

The second angle is that *my knowledge about another man* is in time, it is not a-temporal; rather, it is given within a temporal and historical horizon. This horizon is that of the relationship with the other. Knowledge is not an ideal that can be fixed once and forever, but is 'an unlimited task' (Jaspers 1971: 27)[2]—the task to approximate the other. Knowledge can be given only in approximation. Although the structure of knowledge forces us to make whatever we want to know into a determinate object, another person should never become a fixed object. Knowledge of the other always *announces* itself. It may help, to clarify this point, to let Jaspers' thinking resonate with Levinas' philosophy of 'otherness':

> The Other is neither initially nor ultimately what we grasp or what we thematize. For truth is neither in seeing nor in grasping, which are modes of enjoyment, sensibility, and possession; it is in transcendence, in which absolute exteriority presents itself in expressing itself, in a movement at each instant recovering and deciphering the very signs it emits. (Levinas 1969: 172)

The way in which the other presents himself, exceeding the idea of the other in me, is what Levinas names 'face'. The face of the other is inscribed in the ethical impossibility of grasping him in his totality because he overflows every containing *idea* I can have of him. The other cannot and should not be reduced to the same—that is, to my knowledge of him. Rather, the other calls *me* into question. The deployment of this peaceful relation with the other is produced in language. Language 'is contact across a distance, relation with the non-touchable, across a void. It takes place in the dimension of absolute desire by which the same is in relation with another that was not simply lost by the same' (Levinas 1969: 172).

Crucial to man is his attitude to this failure, to the failure of grasping the totality of the other. 'The way man approaches his failure determines what he will become' (Jaspers 2003: 22). Instead of falling prey to the aphasia of scepticism, or to the impersonality of metaphysics, the blind alleys of positivistic or nihilistic fanaticism (Arendt 1948), he takes the risk of building, in the void that separates him from the other, provisional, fleeting constellations of meanings. 'The fall from absolutes which were after all illusory becomes an ability to soar; what seemed an abyss becomes space for freedom; apparent Nothingness is transformed into that from which authentic being speaks to us' (Jaspers 2003: 38). Here is an analogy between what Jaspers calls the 'leap to transcendence' (Jaspers 1971: 26)—that is,

---

[2] 'Actually, men are in the obscurity and this inquiry has served and serves more to train the intelligence that to find truth' ('in effetto gli uomini sono al buio delle cose, e questa indagazione ha servito e serve più a esercitare gli ingegni che a trovare la verità' (Guicciardini 1933: 125)).

the effort to 'detach oneself from all determinate knowledge of being, after I have appropriated its full portent' (Jaspers 1971)—and what we might call the *leap to the other*: deliberating striving to navigate the infinite space that separates me from the other.

Knowledge between description and interpretation

That man's destiny is in time has another significant implication that concerns the *meaning of personal experience* and its relation with time. Jaspers seems to appropriate Hamlet's motto (quoted in Jaspers 1952):

> The time is out of joint; o cursed spite, that ever I was born to set it right. (Shakespeare, *Hamlet*, I, 5: 188–189)

'Time is out of joint' means that the 'real' is not a set of organized events. The interconnections between events, from which events derive their meaning, are not a priori given. Events do not get their meaning from having taken place one after the other. Rather, they derive their meaning from the way we arrange them one next to the other in a structure. If we want to make sense of events in our existence, we need to construe a network of connections in which they take place. Knowledge always has the character of interpretation (Jaspers 2003: 79). Interpreting involves establishing meaningful connections. It is through meaningful connections that we establish an order in our experiences. Meaningful psychic connections (*Verstehende Psychologie*) are the topic of part two of *General Psychopathology* in which Jaspers attempts to answer the questions 'What might be the source?' of a given phenomenon and 'With what else it might be connected?' (Jaspers 1997: 301). Answering these questions depends primarily on gathering 'tangible facts' like the 'patients' expressive movements, acts, speech and self-descriptions' (Jaspers 1997: 303). At a given moment in the course of our inquiry, these psychic facts become meaningfully connected to each other and this strikes us as something self-evident, we see psychic phenomena emerge out of each other in a way that we can understand. Psychological or genetic understanding is 'the inner, subjective, direct grasp of psychic connectedness' (Jaspers 1997: 307). Two things must be clear: first, such conviction is gained on the occasion of the encounter with a concrete person, not acquired inductively through repetition of experience. Psychological understanding is the grasping of meaningful connections in a single individual: it must not lead to theories (and should not be guided by theories), but is limited to the concrete encounter with one person. When we come across a particular meaningful connection in an individual *we must refrain from generalizing* what we understand. 'Psychological understanding cannot be used mechanically as a sort of generalized knowledge but fresh, personal intuition is needed in every occasion' (Jaspers 1997: 313). Second, self-evidence does not prove that the connection we grasp is really there. Our understanding is always *more or less an interpretation*. The more phenomena we gather, the richer we are in connecting them, the less we need to interpret, the more subtle and correct will our analysis be (Jaspers 1997: 314). A 'thick description' (Geertz 1979) spontaneously generates meaningfulness. Meaningfulness ideally comes into sight and emerges via a spiral of approximations. The role of the knowing subject is that of letting the manifestation of meaningful connections happen.

The kind of order established by meaningful connections is not a chronological order in a strict sense (what might be the source or origin of these phenomena?). The point is not to provide an archaeology of phenomena, rescuing their historical antecedents. That kind of order would be, in the end, a *causal* order. Rather, what is looked for here is an order based on meaningfulness, that is, how one phenomenon is semantically connected with the others in a coherent pattern. The connections we establish between these phenomena need not be aetiological (that is based on causal relationships), but hermeneutical (based on meaningful relationships). To have a grasp of these phenomena is to establish the structural nexus that lend coherence and continuity to them (Stanghellini 2010).

The idea of an interpretative order is the antidote to the idea of disordered phenomena that dissolve the sick person into fragmented pieces of a self. Phenomena, as presented by patients, are first and foremost 'out of joint'. At face value, they may not show any order. The destiny, the purpose, and the vocation of the clinician is to 'set them right', that is interpreting them. Interpreting implies responsibility. The clinician, if he wants to approximate his patient, must take up the onus to see in the disorder of psychological phenomena the space for order and for meaning, being aware that what he grasps *may not* be really there and that no a priori knowledge can diminish his being responsible for the meaningful connections he established.

Knowing in cyphers

Jaspers' theory of knowledge is encapsulated in his concept of the 'cypher' (Jaspers 2003). Knowledge, writes Jaspers, is an 'unending movement' which 'finds a foothold through objectivity in which love has its fulfilment' (Jaspers 2003: 19). Here is another sentence that needs to be explained. Man's knowledge is not limited to the ways in which the world objectively displays itself. Empirical cognition is just one kind of knowledge. Empirical reality speaks to men also through another language: the language of cyphers. The encompassing, that is the limit of our knowledge, manifests itself through cyphers, which transcend all empirical knowledge. Cypher-reading is an essential character of being a man. 'Cypher-reading is the primary requisite of manhood' (Jaspers 2003: 50). In contrast to the definite, categorically secure, restricted particular empirical knowledge, through cyphers we become open to the unknown encompassing. Cyphers show what without them would remain implicit for us. They are like *symptoms*: a special kind of phenomenon through which the hidden, yet operative (and perplexing, or disturbing), dimension of our existence is made manifest. Like a patient's symptom, which is not accidental to that patient but is rather the manifestation of his or her true identity, cyphers are the contingent opportunity of a possible encounter between the person and the encompassing.

Obviously, if the cypher 'becomes fixed and definite and turns into an object, then it loses its essential force. It collapses into a sign' (Jaspers 2003: 49). The cypher must keep on an inexhaustible signification with which no definite interpretation is commensurate (Jaspers 2003: 42). Cyphers must not be crystallized into a kind of definite, categorical concept. The meaning(s) of the cypher must be kept 'in suspension' (Jaspers 2003: 38), remain *unsaturated*. The defection from the cypher to the pure concept (as it happens when from the cypher grows a single meaning), as well as the interpretation of a cypher as if it were a symbol (as it is the case when the cypher is interpreted through an 'other'), destroy the force of the cypher.

The need for a method rather than for systematic knowledge

'Anything really meaningful', Jaspers writes, 'tends to have a concrete form and generalization destroys it' (Jaspers 1997: 314). We expect systematic knowledge in science—and psychopathology is a science, although one of a peculiar kind—but we cannot systematize meaningful connections. The clinician needs to know his patient, but he also needs to avoid making him into an object. He should not look for a systematic design of human experience 'showing how everything we know has its place somewhere within this construct or as part of it' (Jaspers 1997: 748). What he needs is not systematic knowledge, rather *systematic awareness of the ways to gain such knowledge*, 'we can at least order our methods according to *principles of understanding*' (Jaspers 1997: 314). Jaspers' main purpose in *General Psychopathology* was to organize '*the way we gain such knowledge*' (Jaspers 1997: 748). What the clinician needs is a *method* rather than an 'ontological theory of human life' (Jaspers 1997: 749). Establishing a method to explore human subjectivity, Jaspers admits (Jaspers 1941), has been the principal aim of *General Psychopathology*.

Knowledge as communication

Jaspers' critical attitude towards all-encompassing expert knowledge, like ontological theories or any sort of impersonal metaphysics of human existence, does not lead him to nosological nihilism. Rather, he acknowledges the need to classify psychopathological phenomena. But this classification, he suggests, must not be 'like an outline [*Entwurf*] of a continent but more like an outline of possible ways to explore it' (Jaspers 1997: 749). Again and again Jaspers declares that the clinician's main preoccupation should be methodology, rather than taxonomy. None the less, Jaspers rejects irrational anti-nosological attitudes and does not fall prey to the mysticism of the encounter or the myths of romantic fusion of horizons between the clinician and his patient. Rather, he suggests adopting a rational attitude conducting, through the experience of the limitations of knowledge, to authentic communication.

Jaspers is light-years away from the jargon of authenticity (as Adorno would call it). Authentic communication, here, means a kind of dialogue enlightened by reason. 'Enlightenment is—in the words of Kant—"man's departure from the condition of immaturity for which he himself is responsible"' (Jaspers 2003: 88). Its values are equality, reciprocity, tolerance, freedom, rationality, responsibility. Knowledge is never a possession, rather being-on-the-way. *Philo*-sophy is longing for truth, not the possession of it. It's the very idea of true knowledge as on-the-wayness that binds the search for knowledge with communication.

The question, roughly speaking, is '*Where* is truth?'. Should we look for truth in the profundity of an object? Is it hidden in the depth of the object, beyond its appearance? Is the way to truth in the space that separates the mind from the object which it inquires? Is truth *adaequatio rei et intellectus*? Or is the place of truth between a mind and another mind, rather than between the mind and its object? Is truth an effect of communication, rather than of discovery? Is truth the agreement between persons, rather than the grasping of the essence or the totality of an object?

To Jaspers, *truth is what connects us* (Bormuth and Meyer-Bohlen 2008). The ultimate source of knowledge is 'the will to authentic communication' (Jaspers 2003: 26). Communication is the aim of philosophy (Jaspers 2003: 27) as well as of clinical care. 'The certainty of authentic being resides only in unreserved communication between men who live together and vie with one another in a free community, who regard their association with one another as but a preliminary stage, who take nothing for granted and question everything' (Jaspers 2003: 26). In this ideal conversation, informed by equality, reciprocity and tolerance, both the clinician and his patient gain a better understanding of themselves (Bormuth and Meyer-Bohlen 2008: 288–9). Through understanding, the clinician does not aim to obtain a specific effect, but rather to appeal to freedom (Jaspers' *Zur Kritik der Psychoanalyse* (Jaspers 1950). Freedom is the infinite space of clarification of what man can be (Jaspers' *Der Arzt im technischen Zeitalter* (Jaspers 1958). 'At the summit of freedom, upon which our activity seems necessary to us, not through the outward constraints of an inexorable process of natural law but as the inner consent that does not will otherwise, we are aware of ourselves as freely given to ourselves by transcendence' (Jaspers 2003: 64–65).

Jaspers' unspoken theory of clinical practice

With this overview of Jaspers' philosophy in place, I will now try to rescue Jaspers' implicit answers to the guiding question of this chapter: what do we need for a sound-enough clinical practice? The standard answer is that we need three basic ingredients. First, we need an anthropology, that is, a knowledge of Man, or at least a clinical anthropology, that is, a theoretical understanding of human existence able to guide clinical practice. Second, we need a theory of human vulnerability, which helps understanding how and why men get mentally sick. Third, we need a theory of care, or of clinical practice, which helps answering questions like 'How to treat a person affected by that given pathology?', and 'Why this kind of treatment should work?'

To answer these questions we must link psychiatry with philosophy and with science. Building on Jaspers' work we can find answers to each of these questions, although he explicitly stigmatizes all theories trying to reply to the first question, rejects all systematic approaches to the second problem, and criticizes all attempts available in his time to answer to the third issue. Nonetheless, hints are systematically scattered (so to speak) throughout his psychopathological, psychological, and philosophical essays. My purpose, in this last section, is to rescue a general theory for clinical practice from Jaspers' works.

Jaspers' anthropology of disunion

> Man is not a finished life which repeats itself from generation to generation, nor is he a manifest life which plainly reveals itself to him. He 'breaks through' the passivity of perpetually renewed identical circles, and is dependent upon his activity, whereby the process of his life is carried on towards an unknown goal.
>
> Consequently, there is an inner cleavage in man's innermost nature, whatever he thinks of himself, he must think against himself and against what is not-himself. He sees everything in conflict or in contradiction […]. The decisive point is that he must always be setting himself in opposition to himself. There is no human existence without cleavage. Yet he cannot rest content in this cleavage. The ways in which he overcomes it, the way in which he transcends it, reveals the conception he has of himself. (Jaspers 2010: 146)

This is (I suggest), in a nutshell, Jaspers' anthropology. There is an inner cleavage in man's innermost condition. Jaspers (as many others philosophers in the twentieth century) subscribes to an *anthropology of disunion*. Disunion does not amount merely to internal conflicts, in a strict psychoanalytical sense; rather, it is the ubiquitous presence of non-coincidence and eccentricity. Human existence constantly escapes any coinciding with an essence. This is the signature of the human condition: its perennial duality, otherness-haunting selfhood, complexity-challenging one-sided concepts, antithesis-troubling, so that we are condemned to perpetual self-becoming. This is coherently linked to Jaspers' ethics of incomprehensibility. Man cannot passively rely on an objective correlative to define itself. Whenever he thinks something of himself, he must think against this something he has thought, and against what he has thought against this something. This anthropology of disunion is also a theme that Jaspers takes up in his studies on tragedy (Jaspers 1952), epitomized in Iago's lament 'I am not what I am' (Shakespeare, *Othello*, I). Disunion also means that the human condition is one of radical homelessness, of diaspora, and of nostalgia. Man is away from himself. Man, Jaspers says, cannot rest content in his condition of separateness. He cannot find peace by simply defining himself an outcast, someone decentred, away from home. This awareness should not be a desperate and nihilistic acceptance.[3] He constantly sets himself the task of overcoming his condition of disunion. Domesticating disunion is a task in human existence. The way man faces this task reveals the conception he has of himself. Disunion, finally, means that man is called to take a position in front of himself, and more specifically in front of the otherness he experiences in his existence. Man does not coincide with his experience. There is a cleavage between man and his sufferings. Man is a self-interpreting animal thus he is compelled to make a *logos* of his *pathos*. To be human is to deal with this reflective duplicity by taking upon ourselves the responsibility for articulating, making sense of, coping with and appropriating of experiences—well aware that that the *logos* is always restless and fragile (Stanghellini and Rosfort 2013).

Jaspers' dialectical model of human vulnerability

Jaspers' model of human vulnerability can be derived from his anthropology of disunion. The central idea underpinning what we will call here the *dialectical model* in psychopathology is that there is an active interplay between the person and his basic abnormal experiences. The dialectical model of mental disorders draws attention to the active role that the person, as a self-interpreting agent or 'goal-directed being' engaged in a world shared with other persons, has in interacting with his or her basic disorder and in the shaping of psychopathological syndromes. This person-centred approach helps us to see patients as meaning-making rather than passive individuals, and their attempt at self-understanding as not necessarily pathological and potentially adaptive (Stanghellini et al. 2013).

Jaspers' discussion of the patient's attitude towards his illness develops out of his more widely cited account of the early stages of schizophrenia in *General Psychopathology*. Faced with the uncanny experiences characterizing the initial stage of the illness (*Wahnstimmung*), most patients' first reaction is what Jaspers calls 'perplexity'—a state whereby the patient's level of activity is falling and he is gradually becoming detached from external reality. Individual differences start to appear almost immediately afterwards as the patient tries to make sense of what is happening to him. The patient 'works through' his abnormal

[3] 'Accepting that we are flawed and our problems not fully soluble'—writes John Gray, an outstanding interpreter of human history—'need not be paralysing; it could make us more flexible and resourceful. […] Keat's negative capability—"being in uncertainties, mysteries, doubts, without any irritable reaching after fact and certainty"—seems to me a more interesting way to live, and more likely to yield glimpses of truth' (Gray 2010: 16–17). Jaspers would certainly subscribe to Gray's sober lucidity.

experiences, i.e. reflecting on his perplexity and other uncanny feelings and perceptions, he 'can *see* himself, *judge* himself, and *mould* himself' (Jaspers 1997: 424)· Thus we find patients for whom the *Wahnstimmung* introduces new significance into their life, others for whom the content of their abnormal experience is linked with their pre-onset personality, and yet others for whom the content of their incipient psychosis remains entirely alien and brings no added significance. Delusions are conceived as a top-down attempt to explain the aberrant experiences taking place during the initial pre-delusional stages of schizophrenia. One feature of this model is that it explains the diversity of the manifestations of psychopathological syndromes as a consequence of the different ways patients seek to make sense of the basic changes in self and world experiences. Whereas these basic changes are expressions of an underlying vulnerability, full-blown symptoms are the outcome of a sort of negotiation between the patient and her vulnerability. According to the dialectical model therefore, the individual person, with her unique strengths and resources as well as needs and difficulties, plays a central role in outcomes, course, and manifestations of the vulnerability afflicting her.

Jaspers' theory of care as authentic communication

We could say that, being the self-interpreting animals that we are, we are compelled to make a *logos* of our *pathos*. To be human is articulating, making sense of, coping with, and appropriating our vulnerability—well aware that the *logos* is always restless and fragile. To be human is to acknowledge our vulnerability, that is, to recognize the ambiguity of our feelings and the fact that conflicts, in the city as in the soul, cannot be avoided. To be human is taking upon ourselves the personal responsibility for dealing with these ambiguities and conflicts avoiding relying on external authorities, or on impersonal formula and solutions—as well as rejecting scepticism, subjectivism, and relativism.

'Reason'—writes Gray (2010: 23)—'can enlighten us as to our ethical conflicts. Often, it shows them to be deeper than we thought, and leaves us in the lurch as to how to resolve them'. Conflicts are a normal part of our life. What reason can do is neither reconcile conflicting parts of oneself, nor reconcile individuals embodying conflicting values by finding a consensus between them. What reason can do is facilitate communication by acknowledging the intrinsically conflictual nature of human existence and the limitations of human understanding. Inherent to reason, and to its awareness of its own frailty, is the value of tolerance. 'What is toleration?', writes Voltaire (1928) in the *Philosophical Dictionary*.[4] It is the appurtenance of humanity. We are all full of weakness and errors; let us mutually pardon each other for our follies'. Care, Jaspers argues, is authentic communication. Authentic communication is based on tolerance, that is, on the acceptance of a plurality of values, of world-views and of ways of life. At the summit of authentic communication between clinician and his patient there is the enlightenment of both as responsible agents who cannot, and must not, rely on any definite, absolute, impersonal, all-encompassing, metaphysical knowledge, to set forth good life, but only on the mature awareness of the 'un-understood life'. This is the import of Jaspers' theorem of incomprehensibility. The ultimate ground for the action of the clinician and his patient is their shared consent to a kind of truth that is

[4] Quoted in Gray (2010: 22–23).

based on communication. The final goal is communication itself, since truth is not simply the effect of communication—it *is* communication itself.

Conclusion

There is no general consensus about Jaspers' concept of incomprehensibility. Most students of Jaspers, however, see it as a methodological principle setting the boundaries of what can grasped and made sense of in another person's existence. I have argued that this understanding of this concept is imperfect. To have a better interpretation of Jaspers' incomprehensibility we must see from the angle of *ethics*, not of epistemology. As a merely methodological principle, Jaspers' theorem of incomprehensibility is flawed; it was an innovative product of an intellectual debate that took place one century ago and has been surpassed in more recent times. It is not true that schizophrenic phenomena cannot be understood. It is true that they cannot be understood from the first-person perspective, that is, via standard or naïf empathic capacities, trying to transpose oneself into the schizophrenic person's experience. But schizophrenic experiences can instead be understood adopting second-order empathic stance. To achieve second-order empathy I need to acknowledge that the lifeworld inhabited by the other person is not like my own, to bracket my own pre-reflexive natural attitude, and to explore the other's world as an alien country.

A better way to see Jaspers' incomprehensibility as a clinically useful concept is to link it with ethics. In this light, it sets the agenda for a kind of clinical care based on the practice of approximation. This applies to understanding schizophrenic existence, as well as to human existence as a whole. Crucial to this practice is the clinician's attitude to the inevitable failure of grasping the totality of his patient's existence; and to the failure of reducing the otherness of the other to the same, that is, understanding the other by analogy to myself. The other is not like me; rather he calls *me* into question. This relation of *coexistence,* not of identity, analogy, or consensus, with the other is produced in language, which is contact across a distance. Instead of falling prey to scepticism, or of an impersonal and metaphysical knowledge of the other, Jaspers exhorts clinicians to navigate the infinite space that separates them from their patients.

References

Arendt, H. (1948). 'Was ist Existenzphilosohie?', in *Sechs Essays*. Heidelberg: L. Schneider, 48–80.

Baeyer, W.R.V. (1979). *Wähnen und Wahn*. Stuttgart: Enke.

Bormuth, M., Meyer-Bohlen M. (eds) (2008). *Truth is What Connects Us*. Bremen: Hauschild.

Geertz, C. (1979). *The Interpretation of Cultures*. New York, NY: Basic Books.

Gray, J. (2010). *Gray's Anatomy*. London: Penguin.

Guicciardini, F. (1933). *Ricordi*. Bari: Laterza.

Jaspers, K. (1919). *Psychologie der Weltanschauungen*. Heidelberg: Springer.

Jaspers, K. (1941). 'La filosofia dell'esistenza nel mio sviluppo spirituale', *Logos*, **24**(5): 217–259.

Jaspers, K. (1952). *Ueber das Tragische*. Munchen: Piper & Co.

Jaspers, K. (1956). *Von der Warheit* (Partial English translation in *Truth and Symbol* (2003). Munchen: Piper & Co.)

Jaspers, K. (1969–1971). *Philosophy, 'Existential Elucidation'*, Vol. 2. Chicago, IL: Chicago University Press.

Jaspers, K. (1971). *Philosophy of Existence*. Philadelphia, PA: University of Pennsylvania Press.

Jaspers, K. (1958). 'Der Arzt im techischen Zeitalter', *Klinische Wochenschrift*, **36**: 1037–1143.

Jaspers, K.(1983). 'Arzt und Patient', in *Wahrheit und Bewährung*. Munich: Piper & Co., 59–78. (Original work published in 1953.)

Jaspers, K. (1953). 'Die Idee desArztes', *Schweizerische Ärztezeitung*, **34**(27): 253–257.

Jaspers, K.(1950). 'Zur Kritikder Psychoanalyse', *Der Nervenarzt*, **21**: 465–468.

Jaspers, K. (1997). *General Psychopathology* (7th edn) (J. Hoenig, M.W. Hamilton, trans.). Baltimore, MD: Johns Hopkins University Press.

Jaspers, K. (2003). *Truth and Symbol*. Lanham, MD: Rowman & Littlefield.

Jaspers, K. (2003). *Way to Wisdom*. New Haven, CT: Yale University Press.

Jaspers, K. (2010). *Man in the Modern Age*. London: Routledge.

Kirkbright, S. (2004). *Karl Jaspers. A Biography. Navigations in Truth*. New Haven, CT: Yale University Press.

Levinas, E. (1969). *Totality and Infinity* (A. Lingis, trans.). Pittsburgh, PA: Duquesne University Press.

Minkowski, E. (1993). *Structure des depressions*. Paris: Nouvel Object.

Stanghellini, G. (2007). 'The Grammar of Psychiatric Interview', *Psychopathology*, 40: 69–74.

Stanghellini, G. (2010). 'A Hermeneutic Framework for Psychopathology', *Psychopathology*, 43: 319–326.

Stanghellini, G. (in press). 'Philosophical Resources for the Psychiatric Interview', in K.W.M. Fulford, M. Davies, R.G.T.Gipps, G. Graham, J.Z. Sadler, G. Stanghellini, et al. (eds), *Oxford Handbook of Philosophy and Psychiatry*. Oxford: Oxford University Press.

Stanghellini, G., Ballerini, M. (2007). 'Values in Persons with Schizophrenia'. *Schizophrenia Bulletin*, **33**(1): 131–141.

Stanghellini, G., Fulford, K.W.M., Bolton, D. (2013). 'Person-Centered Psychopathology of Schizophrenia. Building on Karl Jaspers' understanding of the patient's attitude towards his illness', *Schizophrenia Bulletin*, 39(2): 287–294.

Stanghellini, G., Rosfort, R. (2013). *Emotions and Personhood*. Oxford: Oxford University Press.

Voltaire (1928). *Philosophical Dictionary*. New York, NY: Knopf.

Section 3

Clinical concepts

Chapter 13

Karl Jaspers' hierarchical principle and current psychiatric classification

Henning Sass and Umberto Volpe

> We would be in a poor position indeed if empirical science were the only kind of science possible.
> *Edmund Husserl, 1917*

> The diagnostic schema has the most scientific interest where it shows discrepancies.
> *Karl Jaspers, 1913*

Introduction

Although the current classification systems of mental disorders have been significantly and implicitly influenced by the diagnostic concepts formulated by Karl Jaspers in his *Allgemeine Psychopathologie* (*General Psychopathology*), the scientific debate concerning diagnosis in psychiatry over the last decades apparently tended to underestimate the contribution of the phenomenological psychopathology and of the subjective approaches to the clinical method in psychiatry. Powerful trends in contemporary psychiatry, neglecting the approach of Jaspers, are linked with a significant loss in research and practice of our discipline (Huber 2002).

Phenomenological psychopathology has been significantly advanced by Karl Jaspers, since he first provided a convincing general theoretical framework along with a clear, concise, and complete clinical method (Gross and Huber 2000). With Karl Jaspers, psychopathology stemmed from empirical clinical descriptions and flourished as an autonomous discipline. It is not by chance that Jaspers' textbook *General Psychopathology* has been often considered as the 'most important single book on the aims and logic of psychological medicine' (Shepherd 1990).

However, while until a few decades ago most trainees in psychiatry used *General Psychopathology* as one of their main conceptual frameworks by which to observe and understand mental phenomena, in these days (with very few exceptions) they tend to have their first conceptual approach to mental illnesses through standardized operational criteria, often collapsed to mere check-lists, of international diagnostic manuals. Although the 1913 publication of *Allgemeine Psychopathologie* made Jaspers immediately known to the scientific community of his time, it did not grant its author a large consensus, especially in the Anglophone countries. As Gruhle (1947) wittily summarized, Jaspers' general psychopathology was often not only retained more as a theory than a true clinical method but also a rather complicated one, which required an extensive study of terms and concepts which might not have been the true concern of psychiatrists. Since the phenomenological clinical attitude is not easily learned, it may be associated with a risk of achieving unverifiable interpretations or complex hermeneutic understandings, the Jaspers' clinical method had been often deemed not easily applicable in routine clinical settings. Furthermore, Jaspers overtly criticized psychoanalysis (deeming that Freud radically confused meaningful inner experiences with causal explanation of mental phenomena) and, as noted by Shepherd (1990), the term 'psychopathology' was entrenched in a psychoanalytical *milieu*, at the time; the negative attitude developed by the powerful psychoanalytical lobby against their former detractor probably did not help to spread Jaspers' ideas in the psychiatric community. It is not surprising that an English translation of the *Allgemeine Psychopathologie* appeared only 50 years after its original publication in German. Finally, it has to be considered that the reader of Jaspers' *General Psychopathology* has to become familiar with the structure of a very dense and complex text, being aware of its many sources and of the areas of related knowledge, in order to thoroughly understand his work (Gross and Huber 2000).

However, the fading interest in introspective psychopathology and its methods might also be related to a more general criticism which began to spread, in the first half of the twentieth century, towards subjective methods in science. After having entered the era of the discovery of DNA, medicine began to transform itself 'from a practicing art into a scientific discipline' (Pauling et al. 1949); also, due to the constantly growing scientific and technical knowledge and to the greater availability of diagnostic and therapeutic tools, doctors probably tended to think they had to provide their patients with the 'scientific' and 'objective' truth about their subjective symptoms (usually disregarded as unreliable and potentially false matter). Psychiatry, although with some delay, was no exception and despite being the medical discipline with the strongest links to the humanities (such as, at least, philosophy, social sciences and psychology), utterly adopted the famous Griesinger motto (1845) 'mental diseases being diseases of the brain' and forced itself to enter into the mainstream of objective medicine and to privilege rigidly bio-scientific models of practice.

As noted by Healy (2002), the discovery of psychotropic drugs characterized by an apparent specificity in the 1950s (the use of chlorpromazine for schizophrenia, lithium for mania, and imipramine for depression was validated by the first clinical trials at the time) clearly pushed forward the use of a simpler and more clear-cut (i.e. categorical) diagnostic system, such as that proposed by Kraepelin, a contemporary opponent of Jaspers' phenomenological approach. The evolving administrative pressure created by the need to organize and regulate the healthcare system expenditures (together with the issues of regulatory approval and marketing of psychotropic drugs) clearly made Kraepelin's descriptive schema 'quite serviceable' (Ghaemi 2009) and probably, at the same time, disfavoured Jaspers' diagnostic conceptions.

Also, due to the need to 'standardize' a discipline classically depicted as too subjective and unreliable, to the anti-psychiatric and socio-political trends, and to the considerable amount of biological evidence produced in the second half of the twentieth century (Sass 1987), psychiatry radically directed its diagnostic and clinical attitudes away from subjective phenomena, trying 'to be as scientific, impersonal and objective as possible towards what is most personal and subjective', as Laing (1985) elegantly noted.

Provided this general framework, it might not be surprising that Jaspers' nosological method has been disregarded in favour of simpler and more immediate diagnostic classifications. Although current versions of international diagnostic manuals are still influenced by Jaspers' nosological conception, this probably happened partially and at a subtle and often under-recognized level. Thus, in order to properly trace Jaspersian nosological elements within current diagnostic approaches and to correctly identify commonalities and differences between international classification systems and Jaspers' nosology, a brief account of the latter appears necessary.

Jaspers' phenomenological method

Karl Jaspers was probably the first psychiatrist to provide a convincing general reference along with a clear, complete, and precise method for psychopathology of practical relevance. In chapter XII of his *General Psychopathology* (Jaspers 1913, 1997), he specifically deals with the 'synthesis of disease entities', providing his personal view of psychiatric nosology.

Jaspers' clinical method is characterized by a particular style of gathering information, which groups related phenomena clearly differentiable by patients' self-descriptions, excluding any preconceived notion or theory and focusing on the modes in which the experience comes to expression. Jaspers was the first psychiatrist to explicitly realize, as revealed in the chapter on the 'Scientific Analysis of Connections' (Jaspers 1913, 1997), the fundamental significance and the cogent implications for psychiatry of the dichotomy between (causal) explanation and understanding (see Figure 13.1). Jaspers systematically divided the issues that can be understood from those that can be explained, within the psychiatric context. Wilhelm Dilthey (1894/1961) first emphasized the distinction between explanation (as the method and aim of natural sciences) and understanding (as the aim and method of the human sciences or *Geisteswissenschaften*) in philosophy, by his famous phrase: 'nature is what we explain; mental life is what we understand'. Jaspers elucidated more precisely that three levels of understanding do exist, an objective understanding (aiming to record only objective symptoms), a 'static' understanding (aiming to assess subjective symptoms), and a 'genetic' understanding (aimed at comprehending the events narrated by the patient from an inner perspective, through the analysis of one's meaningful connections). Such levels have to be integrated in a pluralistic fashion into the phenomenological methodology, which has to be applied to different settings and under different circumstances.

In Jaspers' view, a psychiatrist can never be a pure natural scientist (*Naturwissenschaftler*), as he would be constantly engaged in understanding/interpreting activities: in psychiatry, there can be no choice between explanation and understanding, since it is indeed the junction of such opposite conceptual polarities which creates the phenomenal world as it is. Patients, having both mind and brain, have to be considered both as agents and organisms. Because of the junction between mind and brain, the phenomenal world must be viewed from several different perspectives if it is to be fully appreciated (Slavney and McHugh 1985). Jaspers affirmed the relevance of this part of phenomenological differentiation by the distinction between objective and subjective symptoms. The latter are emotions, inner processes, and sensory manifestations like fear, grief, or cheerfulness. They cannot be perceived by sensory organs but only by putting ourselves into another's soul, by empathy—the

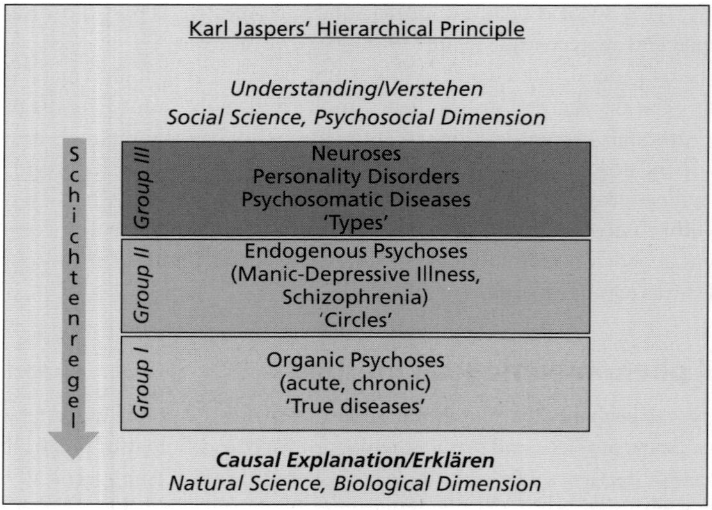

Figure 13.1 Graphical depiction of Jaspers' nosological schema, based on a hierarchical principle (*Schichtenregel*). The heterogeneous nature of psychopathological phenomena is taken into account by a scheme encompassing biologically based diseases (which might be explored by means of biological investigations and pertain to the field of natural science), 'circles' (which can be clearly demarcated from normality, but without clear boundaries among themselves), and 'types' (which have no clear boundaries among themselves nor with normality, and might be better explained in the sense of social sciences and humanities).

only clinical method which allows depicting as clearly as possible the various inner psychological conditions as they are experienced by the patient. Such subjective symptoms can be easily differentiated from the objective symptoms which are all the processes that can be perceived with the senses (e.g. reflexes, visible movements, the photographable face, motor agitation, speech utterances, written products, actions, lifestyle, etc.). These phenomena can only be understood by thinking rationally. The phenomenological approach gives a special emphasis to introspection, via an interactive and empathic process between the clinician and the patient, aimed to clarify mental phenomena 'from inside'. For Jaspers, the good clinician should try to abandon his preconceived ideas about the patient, to enter into his/her inner world by means of an attitude of neutral empathy; he has to accept the only possible truth of the individual's subjective experience and base his judgement on an *epoché* (i.e. a suspension of any judgement) on the true nature of reality. According to Husserl (1929), the philosophical foundations of science (the so-called 'phenomenology of reason') require that all claims to real knowledge should be grounded in 'evidence'. Jaspers, although not being a phenomenology radical, thought that the hermeneutic interpretation of a patient's inner experiences was the only meaningful and adequate source of psychopathological evidence.

Jaspers remarked in his philosophical autobiography that anyone speaking about the mind must know 'what one knows, how one knows it, and what one does not know' (Jaspers 1957). There is no single 'optimal method' for the study of mind and brain and the empirical method of enquiry is maintained solely by the patient's communications. The crucial methodological question for Jaspersian phenomenology thus becomes the following: by what scientific method can the psychiatrist achieve a valid knowledge of the subjective experiences of another person, namely, the experiences of his or her patient? This method of one person experiencing another person's experiences will require a special 'phenomenological attitude' (*'phänomenologische Einstellung'*) and also some form of empathy (Wiggins et al. 1992), and empathy should be regarded as an especially valuable and indispensable tool for human relationships, out of which the patient–doctor relationship is just a special case.

A psychopathological approach, in Jaspers' view, has to deal with 'isolated phenomena', which in turn show a great variety of 'nuances', depending on the different diseases in which they are seen. Jaspers believed that such clinical nuances can be 'felt', but not 'formulated precisely'. Descending from this view, the conceptualization of disease-entities as 'mosaic-like structures, composed from a variety of individual and identical pieces' seemed to Jaspers a very 'superficial method', which he named 'the method of the living mosaic' (Jaspers 1913, 1997).

Jaspers' hierarchical principle and the classification of psychiatric disorders

As for nosology itself, Jaspers admits the clinical need of coordinating all the clinical viewpoints within a single diagnostic schema but he also believes not to have sufficient knowledge to provide disease-entities with a 'final significance', deeming that complex disease entities (such as mental diseases) remain an 'endless, inextricable web'. He recognizes that doctors dealing with 'special psychiatry' and those who have to make statistical investigations might need to continue developing and using diagnostic schemata; but, on the other hand, he mainly questions 'what do we diagnose' as a mental disorder and invites his readers to abandon the concept of disease-entity. To Jaspers, classifying mental disorders is just drawing 'the line where none exists' and every classification should have a 'provisional value' only. The main scope of such classification 'fiction' should be to make doctors aware of the 'actual state of their knowledge', by controlling what the various disease-entities have "*achieved in respect of the overall picture of existing psychic disorders*" (Jaspers 1913, 1997: 604; italics in the original text).

Jaspers proposed three distinct 'Groups' of diseases (see Figure 13.1), which later became the famous 'triadic system' (*Triadisches System*) in the clinical psychopathology of Kurt Schneider and Gert Huber (Huber 2002). The first is made of the 'known somatic illnesses with psychic disturbances', which includes infections, poisonings, head traumas, cerebral tumours, cerebrovascular diseases, and other organic diseases associated with somatic or psychic symptoms. The second group refers to the 'major psychoses' and encompassed, besides idiopathic epilepsy, the Kraepelinian dichotomy between the manic-depressive illness and schizophrenia (with its hebephrenic, catatonic, and paranoid subtypes). The last group includes the 'personality-disorders' or abnormal personalities, the neurotic syndromes, and all the abnormal reactions that do not belong to Groups I and II. Jaspers also suggested that only 'true diseases' (included in Group I) have clear boundaries among themselves and with normality, whereas the so-called 'circles' belonging to Group II only have clear boundaries with normality, but not among themselves. Finally, 'types' included in Group III do not have clear boundaries either among themselves or with normality and Jaspers thought that these clinical phenomena continuously keep merging into each other; consequently, they are the disorders with the least classification agreement.

Jaspers clarified that an exact and proper diagnosis was possible only for true diseases of Group I, whereas the classification of Group II cannot be clearly delineated and 'basic concepts regarding the extent and limits of the psychoses vary' and depends on 'the consensus of contemporary psychiatric opinion' (Jaspers 1913, 1997). For Group III, Jaspers thought that diagnosis was just 'an impossibility' and, in these cases, he recommended rather a delineation of general typology by a multidimensional approach.

In the third paragraph of chapter XII, Jaspers (1913, 1997) reveals to the reader how to cope with unavoidable coexistence of different clinical phenomena within one single diagnosis, enunciating his 'hierarchical principle' (*Schichtenregel*), according to which one phenomenon should be considered the most relevant for diagnostic purposes and the remaining clinical phenomena should be regarded as 'secondary' or 'accidental'. In his diagnostic view, Jaspers recommended that, within the triadic system, the preceding group always had preference over the following one, giving higher weight to 'organic diseases', investigable by means of natural science and for which a causal explanation was possible; the 'psychopathies', i.e. the 'personality disorders' of current terminology, had, on the contrary, the lowest importance in his diagnostic scheme since they were embedded in a psychosocial rather than a neurobiological dimension and they could have been only understood, but not scientifically explained.

Within the Jaspersian nosology scheme, every diagnosis excludes the presence of symptoms of all diseases ranking higher in hierarchy, whereas the symptoms of all lower ranked diseases are included. Again according to Jaspers' view, the hierarchy of disease symptoms might have been illustrated pictorially, in terms of three different superimposed planes or layers (see Figure 13.1): at the top of such schema Jaspers posed neurotic and psychosomatic symptoms, then the 'process symptoms' of manic-depressive illness and schizophrenia, and finally the organic (both psychic and somatic) symptoms of true diseases. The hierarchical diagnostic process consisted, in Jaspers' view, of a 'narrowing down in significance of what is diagnosed' since the lowest plane reached by the examination of each individual case will decide the diagnosis. In any case, the lowest layer is the crucial one for the final diagnosis.

In synthesis, Jaspers had a profound refusal of any rationalistic or reductionistic view and his epistemological fundaments were close to the Kantian concept of ideas, which, applied to psychiatric diagnosis, resulted in a basic premise that no actual 'disease entity' really exists and that any nosological schema should be discharged in its function when it will not be able to prove itself to be the most 'apt for the time' anymore. Jaspers strongly believed that no natural schema would accommodate every case. The ultimate subject of the Jaspers' clinical investigation is the entire human being and not a mere cluster of symptoms. Furthermore, Jaspers was very much aware that psychiatry had limited knowledge concerning both mental phenomena and brain processes and he deemed any nosological schema to be clinically useful and not necessarily oriented to the understanding of the etiological causes of psychiatric illnesses.

The 'living mosaics': current diagnostic manuals and classifications of mental disorders

In the early days of the development of psychiatry as a scientific discipline, diagnostic entities were empirically derived on descriptive 'primary' sources of data (i.e. the clinician's account of psychopathological constructs) and did not have the declared presumption of being directly connected to the pathophysiology of disease entities. In these days, on the contrary, although clear clues concerning the real aetiopathogenesis of mental disorders are still not available, current diagnostic concepts tend to go beyond the imperfect ontological status of psychiatric diagnosis and aim to be as objective as possible. Thus, younger generations of psychiatrists have to deal with reductive conceptualizations of psychiatric diseases and clinicians with non-realistic descriptions of mental disorders, whose diagnostic criteria are dangerously elusive and shallow. It is not surprising that the complex set of current diagnostic criteria for mental disorders is rarely used in routine conditions. However, diagnostic manuals serve many purposes, ranging from their use in clinical practice to guidance in neurobiological research, from grouping for statistical analyses to creating categories for public health surveys, and are thus supposed to be used in routine psychiatric practice.

Although the influence of Karl Jaspers and his phenomenological method on contemporary psychiatric operationalized diagnostic systems may be seen in many ways (mainly, the evidence-based attitude towards clinical diagnosis, the use of a descriptive approach, and an aetiological neutrality; see Table 13.1), over the last century, some theoretical underpinnings of the diagnostic process are somehow opposite of that of Jaspers concerning psychiatric diagnosis. While Jaspers was convinced of the nomological irreducibility of the pathological mental phenomena, psychiatry as a discipline, instead of being aware of the limitations of nosology in psychiatry, clearly tended to the reification of rather arbitrary diagnostic concepts and possibly to its own reductionistic impoverishment. As an example, one should consider that the Jaspersian conception of diagnosis has been practically translated in a mechanical, simplicistic and elementaristic application of a merely criteriological approach. Such a diagnostic-nosological attitude might introduce a significant risk of losing one of the fundamental elements of the Jaspers' diagnostic approach (i.e. the patient's biographical and situational background, his 'wholeness' or *Ganzheit*), and of excessively simplifying the whole diagnostic process, determining a lack of that methodological pluralism, originally advocated for psychiatry by Jaspers. Furthermore, according to Jaspers, although psychopathology could not be reduced to a pure philosophical methodology (as in the case of Husserl's transcendental phenomenology), it can neither be totally detached by a philosophical system behind clinical practice. The pretention of international classification manuals not to have any explicit ideological orientation is clearly not realistic.

Finally, the true essence of Jaspers' nosological approach has got probably lost since a true hierarchical order in both the *Diagnostic and Statistical Manual of Mental Disorders* (DSM) and the International Classification of Diseases (ICD) for mental disorders seems to be missing. Although some hierarchical elements are still present in current diagnostic systems, these are mostly used to exclude medical conditions or substance abuse, whereas

Table 13.1 Basic characteristics of operational psychiatric diagnostic systems

Descriptive approach
Explicit inclusion- and exclusion-criteria
Algorithms for the criteriology of every single diagnosis
Nominalistic understanding of psychiatric diagnoses
Aetiological neutrality (questionable 'atheoretical approach')
Multiaxiality (mainly in the DSM system)
Focus on severity ('quantitative approach')

the coexistence of different mental disorders and superimposed personality disorders is the new rule.

In the following paragraphs, an attempt will be made to describe the reasons why operationalism took over the Jaspersian nosological approach to psychiatric disease entities and which might be the relevant caveats for the evolution of the contemporary psychiatric diagnostic process.

The influence of operationalism

The two major current diagnostic systems differ significantly in one aspect: while ICD tends to use a more prototypical approach to psychiatric diagnosis, DSM has moved more rigidly towards an operationalization of the psychiatric diagnostic process.

Prototypical diagnosis relies mainly on the degree of similarity the single clinical case shows with respect to a defined clinical concept and includes the case within a certain category if the case is more similar to that prototype rather than to prototypes of competing categories (Wakefield 2012); this diagnostic process is substantially based on the Wittgenstein's 'family resemblance' concept (i.e. concepts consist of necessary-and-sufficient criteria for category membership), leaves the clinician with more clinical flexibility, does not imply the use of complicated algorithms nor long lists of criteria (Westen 2012), and might be closer to the idea of a fuzzier and less rigidly defined classification of mental disorders, as hypothesized by Jaspers for the most of non-organic psychiatric syndromes.

With the third edition of DSM, a conceptual change happened in psychiatric diagnosis and nosology since empirical descriptions intended to depict the phenomenology of clinical entities were disregarded in favour of a fully operationalized approach to diagnosis. According to the basic principles of operationalism in science, each concept should be defined by and correspond to the set of operations by which they were to be observed and measured (Bridgman 1982). Applying operationalism in psychiatric diagnosis was initially thought to avoid diagnostic misconstructions, based on misleading concepts and not on measureable observations; diagnoses would have thus been rooted in operations and no longer in concepts, defined by their apparent properties (McHugh and Slavney 1982). In 'hard sciences', the spread of a logical and positivistic attitude, stemming from the scientific and philosophical tradition of empiricism, was saluted as a necessary attempt to avoid misconstructions and subjective concepts, defined by their apparent properties and without reference to anything external (McHugh and Slavney 1998). The lead taken by operational diagnostic approaches to mental disorders in the second part of the twentieth century over other nosological approaches to mental disorders was probably a response to the many concerns raised against the low reliability of psychiatric diagnosis (Robins and Guze 1970).

While the introduction of operationalized and simplified diagnosis in psychiatry was deemed a very useful accomplishment for the initial research purposes, such a diagnostic approach subsequently became a sort of unavoidable nosological reference, being used not only by highly trained researchers but also in ordinary practice by the average clinician or in teaching by educators and psychiatric trainees; however, this happened even if very little research has really investigated if a method of diagnosing patients designed for research purposes really achieved a more clinically useful and valid diagnosis at all (Westen 2012) and in spite of the evidence that satisfactory diagnostic reliability could be achieved even without using rigid criteria and relying on standardized empirical descriptions (Sartorius et al. 1993).

Furthermore, the rigid diagnostic categories introduced by recent editions of the DSM are far from being reliable and seem more and more artificial. As Cloninger (1999) firmly stated more than ten years ago, there is no empirical evidence at all for natural boundaries between major syndromes and yet 'no one has ever found a set of symptoms, signs, or tests that separate mental disorders fully into non-overlapping categories' (1999: 176). When DSM-III-R was introduced, the use of simplified and objective operational diagnosis was presented as one of the main advantage for its use in clinical and biological research. However, after decades of psychiatric research, we are now facing a reality different from that expected to come having mapped the entire human genome, we now know that multiple genes regulate/underlie many diagnostic psychiatric patterns and that different environmental factors (e.g. childhood sexual abuse and psychological traumas) are common to many mental illnesses (Banzato 2004), but no clear clues concerning genetic/environmental causes of psychiatric disorders are yet available. Despite many proposed candidates, no single biological marker has been found to be specific for any DSM-defined syndrome; also pharmacological trials proved, over the years, that psychotropic drugs are largely unspecific and that their action 'cuts across the DSM-defined categories' (Moeller 2008). Actually, the advances of neuroscience and genetics have taught us a great deal about the normal functioning of the brain but also left us with the ineluctable complexity of mental disorders and, in most of the cases, clearly challenged the theoretical underpinnings of current classifications (Kendell and Jablensky 2003), leaving the elusive riddles of psychopathology unsolved (Frances 2012).

After Griesinger's idea of identifying definite psychiatric 'disease units' and Kahlbaum's first proposal to establish a scientifically grounded 'clinical method' in psychiatry, psychiatric research and practice have probably always struggled to subsume aetiology, neurobiology, diagnosis, prognosis, course, outcome, and treatment indications of mental disorders, under a unifying nosological umbrella. However, after more than 100 years of continuous research in the field, this original task is still largely unachieved, as we are still in search of basic criteria which may provide a link to causal factors, a reliable assignation of individual cases, and a good correlation with response to therapeutic procedures (Moeller 2008); more relevantly, current criteria do not allow any reliable forecast of outcome/prognosis of diagnostic categories, although according to Woodruff et al. (1974), the link between diagnostic categories and the outcome of the defined disease remains the most crucial one ('diagnosis is prognosis'). On the other hand, the tendency to create and use simplified, fuzzy, and unreliable psychiatric diagnostic categories has largely spread, probably due to historical, social, cultural, and pragmatic issues, rather than for scientifically sound reasons.

Forerunners of modern nosology

As Zilboorg (1967) effectively stated, the late nineteenth and early twentieth centuries can be regarded as the 'era of systems', since this period of time witnessed a proliferation of many nosology systems put forward by experts throughout medicine. Psychiatry was no exception: eminent and influential clinicians brought into psychiatric classifications their wide experience, but also a large range of personal assumptions about what constituted the core features of psychiatric diseases.

Currently available diagnostic manuals (both the ICD and DSM) are just the final result of such a general process. The DSM of the American Psychiatric Association surely did not begin with a 'blank slate', but substantially incorporated the major diagnostic categories of psychiatric illnesses as articulated by European psychiatrists from the late eighteenth century onward. As noted by Kendler (2009), each creation and revision of the DSM is 'firmly entrenched in a particular historical context', and what we consider today 'first-rank' symptoms to make one of the more characteristic psychiatric diagnosis (i.e. schizophrenia), might be just less crucial if Robert Spitzer had not been so impressed by John Wing's work, who in turn was deeply influenced by what Kurt Schneider, Hans W. Gruhle, Willy Mayer-Gross, and the other main representatives of the Heidelberg School thought schizophrenia really was. What if these eminent psychiatrists had not moved to the Anglo-Saxon countries during the Second World War? If history had been different, would have these concepts become so readily available to the Anglophone scientific communities anyway? If the context had not been the actual one, would the Heidelberg School concept of schizophrenia been operationalized in current international diagnostic systems? Probably not, since every nosology is affected by consensus-procedures, political influences, by publishing strategies, and even by certain imperialism in science.

After the 'UK-US Diagnostic Project' (Cooper et al. 1972), it became widely accepted by the psychiatric scientific community that using standardized diagnostic criteria greatly reduced the risk of misdiagnosis. Following this general idea, standardized and operationalized diagnosis became the rule in clinical psychiatry and DSM-III developed standardized and fully operationalized criteria for the psychiatric diagnosis, substantially relying on earlier criteria sets (Feighner et al. 1972; Spitzer et al. 1975, 1978). The advantages in terms of higher diagnostic reliability and reproducibility have probably made the authors of the DSM lean more towards operationalized diagnostic processes. Probably for the same reason, although the DSM criteria were designed to be of transitional nature and aimed essentially to gather research data, there has been a push to adopt them also in clinical practice.

Even the tenth version of the ICD, although preserving some European psychopathological tradition in its clinical descriptions (a sort of *Gestalt* imprint of the different disorders) and creating a more flexible approach to diagnosis with a more user-friendly format, basically followed the same general orientation after the 1970s and the successful DSM approach of III. Unfortunately, over the last decades, the revision processes of DSM and ICD refined the criteria and diagnostic categories but did not focus on the diagnostic process itself, and especially not on their epistemological premises.

According to Jaspers (1913, 1997), the rigid and precise definition of some psychiatric disorders is just not possible and refining one criterion or another would implicitly perpetuate the same basic nosological error. While DSM-5 will yet provide categorical diagnosis with operational criteria, the 11th revision of ICD will hopefully remain based on narrative descriptions of the mental disorders (Maj 2011).

Although the definition and use of categorical diagnostic systems was critical in the *zeitgeist* in which it was developed, its limitations and conceptual conundrums are now well documented (Krueger and Markon 2012) and a critical reappraisal of their advantages and disadvantages is now probably unavoidable.

Advantages and disadvantages of modern diagnostic systems

The introduction of operationalized psychiatric classifications had some advantages: it improved the diagnostic reliability in routine settings, it greatly contributed to the generation of common psychiatric procedures (at least, in terms of diagnostic algorithms), and allowed an unprecedented ability to compare findings in therapy, research, administration, and quality control in psychiatric settings (Mundt and Spitzer 2000).

Actually, Karl Jaspers had already advised 100 years ago that diagnostic schemas might indeed be useful to 'make statistical investigations of a large case materials' (Jaspers 1913, 1997) or to present scientific data to other researchers. But Jaspers also warned that, for its intrinsic fictional and arbitrary nature, any classification never quite 'squares with the facts' and that it should be dropped as soon as it is no longer proves to be optimal for the tasks at issue. He also foresaw that such a 'mosaic' diagnostic approach may turn 'psychopathological investigation and diagnosis into something mechanical' and 'petrifies discovery', but also that 'many beginners tend to favour it because it is so easy to grasp and can be learned relatively quickly' (Jaspers 1913, 1997: 573).

Today, still we have to admit that Jaspers was indeed right: several shortcomings of current psychiatric diagnostic systems (tentatively listed in Table 13.2) are not distant from many of the possible dangers already foreseen by the thoughtful psychiatrist and philosopher 100 years ago.

Although the limitations of nosological approaches, based on the prominence of a simplified set of symptoms were criticized by Kraepelin himself (Kendler and Jablensky 2010), categorical/operationalized diagnoses are still widely used in clinical settings. However, despite having shown advantages in many respects, over the last decades of the twentieth century, critical objections began to prevail towards the use of operational diagnoses in psychiatry.

In this respect, it should be considered that the supposed higher reliability of the DSM criteria-based diagnosis was probably 'oversold', since it can be achieved in research settings with highly trained interviewers and structured instrument on selected patients, but it might easily disappear when applied in real-world contexts, in which clinicians have only minutes to do their evaluations on unselected patients (Frances 2012).

Besides the lack of advantages, the use of operational criteria also has many disadvantages. Mainly, psychiatric operationalism may dangerously be also translated into the

Table 13.2 Shortcomings of modern psychiatric diagnostic classification

Reductionism in conceptualization of psychopathology and its assessment
Inflation of diagnostic categories (DSM-III 229 ⇒ DSM-IV 395)
Consensus-politics and 'scientific imperialism'
Rarification of psychopathological differentiations
Danger of reification of verbalized syndromes based on conventions
Abandoning crucial psychopathological concepts (neurosis, psychosis, endogenous depression)
Abandoning conceptual history and psychopathological traditions
Abandoning psychodynamic and psychostructural factors
Disregarding aspects of subjective experience and biography
Lack of predictive validity, e.g. therapeutic response and course
Restriction to observable behaviour
Horizontalization of clinical diagnosis by the concept of comorbidity

transformation of an abstract and arbitrary concept into something artificially made 'concrete' (in order to be easily observed and measured). In turn, such an attitude may imply the risk of inducing the elimination of subjectivity and inner aspects and of privileging objective and demonstrable symptoms, which do not need co-experience and empathy to be perceived by the observer. Other possible significant risks of an improper use of operationalism in psychiatry, which in reality is often condensed to a mere 'checklist approach', range from the possible loss of the inner/subjective perspective in psychiatry and its implications for psychiatric research, to the problem of psychiatric boundaries and the related issue of psychiatric comorbidity.

Implications for clinical practice

The simplification of the diagnostic process may leave undetected many relevant psychopathological aspects of the clinical picture, just because they are not listed within arbitrary and seemingly objective diagnostic criteria. The mental experiences (as described by the patient) their consequences, and their inherent associations are probably not really relevant to the current diagnostic process, which seeks rather to standardize and objectify the psychiatric diagnosis by eliminating the 'background noise', represented by subjectivity. However, such 'background noise' not only represents a possible source of bias, but rather a virtual space filled up with shared thoughts and feelings, accessible only through non-standardized empathic processes. Modern classification manuals represent a mean by which the basic element of psychiatry, psychopathology, is restricted to a technical aid for distinctions in biological psychiatry, with the consequent loss of the notion of a 'pure psychopathology', i.e. methodologically reflected thinking about structural and functional connections of the normal and abnormal mental life, and especially the inner experiences (Janzarik 1976, 1988; Sass 1987, 2001). Psychodynamic and psychostructural factors are completely set aside, with a strong tendency towards thinking along objective criteria and disregarding aspects of subjective experience and biography. Such a reductionistic approach should not be considered a satisfying end-point for a scientific discipline, definitely implying a substantial impoverishment.

Losing this part of the psychiatric clinical process, the proper study of the inner experiences, may jeopardize the real understanding of patients' problems and needs, as well as the quality of doctor–patient relationships and that of psychiatric care itself. In addition, psychiatrists trained only to assess symptoms by checklists and rating scales, mainly directed to observable behaviours, might be just focused on the most obvious aspects of psychiatric daily practice. This may force psychiatry into clinical oversimplification.

The purpose of the average clinician is indeed not to enhance reliability of their sequential assessments, but rather to comprehensively describe the complex inner reality of the patient sitting in front of him/her, and not only to describe, but also to try to communicate with him/her in these phenomena. For such purposes, operational criteria probably cannot be regarded as a crucial reference. Whereas, over the last decades, general medicine in particular started to rethink its attitude towards patients, by estimating the risk of oversimplifying the doctor–patient relationship and of reducing it to a dehumanizing approach (Lown 1997), psychiatry is still reluctant to dismiss a strictly categorical/operational approach with its reductionistic tendencies. Although Saunders (2000) pointed out that the practice of medicine should indeed be conceived both as an 'art' as well as a 'science' and that evidence-based models, even if correct in principle, might show significant limits in clinical practice, psychiatry still struggles in trying to objectify its clinical object. On the contrary, psychiatry's epistemological foundations should by definition be broad since its 'object' (i.e. the human mind) is complex by nature. A complex discipline has to have a proper 'philosophical system' behind the method of clinical practice, in order to allow a true multidimensional approach to a multidimensional entity.

Psychopathology and research

Beyond the clear implications that an excessive reductionism and objectification may have on psychiatric clinical practice, there is also a more subtle risk for the entire discipline: a diagnosis rising only from observable behaviours might be easily detached from aetiology, especially from psychological determinants of mental illnesses. Where would such a 'restricted psychiatry' end? What would be the meaningfulness of psychiatric research if it is not led by meaningful models? The recent trend of privileging a neurobiological approach has to be balanced by the awareness that the mind cannot simply be reduced to an epiphenomenon of the brain. Even the best designed and most technically sophisticated neuroimaging study would fail to catch the neurobiological basis of a mental illness if no satisfying model of that illness lies at the basis of the experiment.

In addition, the 'reification' of DSM entities to the point that they are considered equivalent to diseases is more likely to obscure than elucidate research findings (Moeller 2008). At least at the present moment, we have insufficient knowledge to build meaningful clinical categories and logical/empirical classifications tend to resemble an artificial rather than a natural one. Thus, it is no surprise that current nosology is challenged from many viewpoints and that several respected authors recently used the adjective 'chaotic' to define late twentieth-century psychiatric nosology (Kraam 2008) or the word 'chaos' to refer to the current diagnostic process in psychiatry (Maj 2011). A simplicistic approach to diagnosis may have strong implications for psychiatric research: as already advised some years ago, biological research in psychiatry would clearly represent a 'sterile and fruitless effort' (Andreasen 1998), if other psychiatric fields are left aside, and especially if psychiatry neglects its psychopathological foundation. The 'Tower of Babel' that psychiatric research resembles these days, is probably not unconnected to the use of oversimplified clinical diagnoses, built upon highly replicable lists of easily identifiable symptoms, which—on the other hand—may easily fail to focus on crucial psychopathological details when standing in front of a patient. When enrolling a patient into a clinical trial, do researchers really ask themselves 'What do we want to study?'. A superficial diagnostic attitude may well end up with no more than a general outline of the patient's true psychopathology, a sort of 'draft diagnosis', rather than a really meaningful one, bearing the same risk that one would run if looking at 'a painting by Vermeer in which the blues have been left out' and feeling that it might look 'Vermeer-like, but it is not a Vermeer' (Van Praag 1992: 266).

The problem of boundaries

At the present moment, the current concepts of psychiatric disorders are merely 'working hypotheses' (Jablensky 2012), defined by 'pseudoprecise criteria' (First 2012) whose value is nothing more than 'provisional' (Jablensly 2012) and which describe rather 'crisscross patterns' (Banzato 2004). No 'points' (nor 'zones') of rarity are currently available to really distinguish between DSM categories, which rather seem 'arbitrary loci in a multidimensional space' (Kendell and Jablensky 2003). The lack of a clear, objective and independent 'splitting strategy' in psychiatric disorders makes mental disorders appear like 'fuzzy constructs' that may easily shift from one to another conceptualization when viewed in different ways (Kendler 2009) and forcing us to face the high non-specificity of current diagnostic categories, which in turn may heavily influence the search for causal factors (Moeller 2008). Decades-spanning scientific literature made available many examples of how the empirical evidence concerning the nosological distinctions reported in international diagnostic manuals in use are questionable at different levels.

First, as Jaspers pointed out decades ago, there are no clear boundaries to properly define crucial psychopathological entities. One prominent example of such fundamental nosological ambiguity is the current diagnosis of schizophrenia: its current formulation within the DSM-IV holds few traces of the Kraepelinian, Bleulerian, and Schneiderian concepts, while it is made mainly by exclusion of other medical and mental diseases (Maj 1998). Unsurprisingly the current diagnosis of schizophrenia significantly lacks stability: in a paradigmatic two-year follow-up evaluation, only 19% of diagnosed schizophrenics retained such diagnosis (Naz et al. 2003). As recently pointed out by Kapur (2011), to date, there is no reliable biological test to identify any clinical subtype of schizophrenia; neither are any of them able to orient effective treatment strategies for this mental disease (Cannon 2011). After 100 years of using the Kraepelinian definition of schizophrenia, psychiatrists are still in search of pathophysiological findings and proper theoretical models which might allow a proper clinical handling and a real understanding of the illness (Lawrie et al. 2011; Strik 2011).

Second, not even basic psychiatric symptoms are clearly designated within current diagnostic systems. Classical psychopathological concepts have simply been abandoned, leaving the clinician without valid alternatives to characterize psychiatric symptoms. For example, anguish is presented, within the diagnostic glossary of DSM, as a sort of homogeneous concept whereas it may express very different meanings (e.g. fear of failure, fear for external threats or anxiety); similarly, aggression may be aroused, according to such glossary, by humiliation, external threats, need to defend own territory or ideas; but, in most cases, the qualitative heterogeneity of such symptoms is just missed. Some essential psychiatric symptoms have apparently been just 'emptied out' in current diagnostic manuals. Thus, how could a contemporary psychiatrist fit the subtle psychopathological nuances of the *depressio sine depressione* into strict diagnostic criteria? Usually the early stages of the 'vital depression' (Borgna 1969) would just be missed in an excessively standardized setting; should a patient with no marked sadness but covertly feeling spiritless, down-hearted, or irritable, and with persistent bodily 'hang-over-like' sensations be helped by a psychiatrist? Probably yes, if only such a psychiatrist would be interested and trained to recognize such a specific affective state in the person sitting in front of them.

Third, current diagnostic systems only attempt to (but do not succeed to) define boundaries between abnormal and normal mental functioning: the absence of clear thresholds of clinical significance simply bears the risk of under-detection of clinically meaningful sub-threshold syndromes. As an example, some distress syndromes, which would be recognized on a subjective level of investigation but would probably not easily fit any categorical diagnosis, have been demonstrated to be associated with high levels of disability in primary care settings, sometimes comparable to full-fledged disorders (Rucci et al. 2003). The presence of a high number of exclusion criteria to make a psychiatric diagnosis surely has the scope to avoid misdiagnosis, but it also contains the risk to just leave symptoms unrecorded; furthermore, these criteria have been reported to be rarely used in practice, not to have a solid empirical basis, and to leave high proportions of undetected or 'not otherwise specified' cases (Maj 2011).

This is particularly relevant when considering delicate symptoms, which lie at the 'interface' between objective and subjective, being 'quasi-subjective' in nature. As an example, German psychiatrists trained in Jaspersian psychopathology identify a specific pre-delusional state, called *Wahnstimmung*, a special mood state in which a patient's experiences might become delusional but are not clearly of that nature yet, as they are still modifiable and correctable. Would a purely objective evaluator really be able to grasp the patient's inner turmoil, if such a condition is not readily observable nor can be easily verbalized, thus not completing the listed criteria needed to fulfil a diagnostic algorithm? Probably asking few standardized questions in a limited amount of time would not represent the ideal strategy to get access to and understand the patient's suffering.

On the whole, the requirement of higher reliability naturally implies the tendency to concentrate on observable behaviours during the diagnostic process, whereas the inner experiences of the patient get less attention. Standardized questionnaires may generate subjective estimates (and not real objective measures), since they are implicitly affected by two relevant potential sources of bias. First, a severity score on a rating scale still represents the interviewer's 'translation' of a patient's subjective symptom into a presumably objective statement: this process might imply a significant bias due to the rater's ability to understand what the individual is communicating. Second, another unavoidable source of bias for 'objective assessments' lies in the subjective variations of a patient's ability and/or will to recognize and correctly verbalize their own inner experiences. As a third problematic issue related to current nosological systems, it should be noted that within such systems there are often no clear boundaries 'within' disorders. For example, according to the DSM system, chronic depression should be viewed as a single 'broad' condition with many possible 'specifiers': although some of them carry relevant clinical information (e.g. 'atypical depression' seems really to be a different syndrome), others do not seem to distinguish specific features (e.g. besides its occurrence after delivery, how is postpartum depression different from any other depression, in phenomenological terms?).

A fourth level of nosological ambiguity in current classification schemata can be traced in the absence of clear boundaries 'between' different disorders. As an example, let's consider the most common diagnosis among affective disorders: the mixed anxiety-depression diagnosis. It has only survived in ICD whereas in the DSM system (although the text of the manual acknowledges that patients with major depression frequently present with anxiety) the two clinical phenomena are categorized as different nosological entities. However, the separation between depression and anxiety has been criticized on many grounds: besides the fact that these two supposedly different diagnostic entities share many common aetiological factors and represent therapeutic targets for the very same classes of drugs, mixed anxiety-depression has a greater diagnostic long-term stability than the two disorders alone (Merikangas et al. 2003).

The problematic concept of comorbidity

The problems of boundaries are directly related to the recent phenomenon of the inflation of psychiatric comorbidity. Feinstein (1970) first defined comorbidity as the co-occurrence of two (or more) different diagnoses in medicine. Initially, the term was used in psychiatry to designate patients who received both a psychiatric and a general medical diagnosis, which seems to be quite plausible, but subsequently in psychiatry it has become very frequently used also for cases in which more than one psychiatric diagnosis was present ('psychiatric comorbidity'; see Maj 2005). The use of the term comorbidity in psychiatry should thus designate the coexistence of two different clinical entities. However, comorbidity lately represents the norm rather than the exception in clinical practice and thus many authors questioned the use of such a term since it might rather designate two different manifestations of a single disease, with different manifestations which we erroneously tend to fit in artificial diagnostic boxes. Given the high proliferation of diagnostic categories within recent diagnostic systems, psychiatric comorbidity seems to represent more their 'by-product' rather than a real and frequent clinical phenomenon. The reason for such proliferation probably lies in the implicit assumption of 'disease entities' when speaking about different clinical syndromes. Although major diagnostic categories are an obvious and natural part of our clinical view, the so-called 'essentialist' approaches are based on top-down/a priori specifications of key add hyphen traits on which current classification depends (Kendler 2009). However, we should bear in mind that current diagnostic categories are nothing more than artificial 'concepts', which should be justified only if they provide a useful framework for organizing and exploring the complexity of clinical experience, in order to derive inferences about outcome and guide decisions about treatment (Kendell and Jablensky 2003). Diagnoses are merely conventions, shared ways of perceiving. Plus, the current diagnostic categories are still 'wildly heterogeneous' in their underlying causes and constitute only 'very rough first approximations' to the real-world psychiatric diseases (Frances 2012).

There is, in this phase of the evolution of the psychiatric discipline, a diagnostic trend towards horizontalization, via the comorbidity principle, which leads to sometimes curious results (e.g. when diagnosing a multitude of personality disorders for the same individual). On this specific topic, Jaspers' ideas (1913, 1997) might be of the opposite advice, self-explicative and enlightening: while describing the principles for his 'synthesis of diseases' he deals with the '*types of personality*', defining them as 'shifting phenomena ... which continuously keep merging into each other'; thus, according to Jaspers, for personality disorders and neuroses no clear boundaries do exist and the diagnostic process for the syndromes belonging to his 'Group III' should remain 'typological and multidimensional', especially (or 'at least') for the different kinds of personality. Reading Jasper's own words, in the light of the clinical evidence of an 'apparent comorbidity' of DSM axis-II disorders (Tyrer et al. 1997), shows that some aspects of mental life are probably irreducible to discrete entities and that current diagnostic categories are just more likely to introduce some artificial heterogeneity in nosological systems.

False dichotomies in the intellectual framework of psychiatry

The relevance of 'subjective psychiatry' is not only a scholarly issue of interest for research, but it has clear implications for the clinician since it directly affects pharmacological treatments as well as psychological interventions delivered to psychiatric patients. For example, the presence of a Freudian 'character neurosis' has been demonstrated to exert influence over the response to psychotropic drugs, although being a non-standardized condition

(Van Praag 1992); similarly, a psychiatrist who would just ignore 'subjective feelings' (since, again, they might not be easily standardizable) is simply more prone to miss subtle changes in symptomatology and probably to worsen the final outcome of any pharmacological treatment. This issue is relevant also for non-pharmacological treatments: panic attacks are described, within the DSM-IV, as the rise of anxiety symptoms 'developed abruptly' (i.e. without any apparent or demonstrable cause); most psychotherapists would not agree to the absence of a connection between life events and panic attacks (although non-immediate and probably covert), and their work would indeed concentrate on such subjective experiences and on the hidden relationships with the symptoms.

Phenomenologically-oriented psychopathology is, in most of the cases, neglected in contemporary training in psychiatry, due to the great relevance of neuroscience and neuropharmacology in psychiatric research on pathophysiology and therapy. The implicit assumption of contemporary psychiatry is that the latter approaches are alternative to the empathic and subjective approaches to psychiatric patients (Beveridge 2002). However, as Damasio (1994) correctly pointed out, referring to it as the 'Descartes' error', such a dichotomy is probably an artificial divide. It is simply not true that a greater attention to existential factors and first-person perspective will lead to neglect bioscientific knowledge. In turn, the integration of different thoughts and clinical schemes is necessary for the growth of the discipline, whereas privileging just one or the other of the earlier mentioned two approaches would probably result in its impoverishment.

The differentiated methods of understanding a patient's inner perspective in the sense of Jaspers still represents the *via regia* for establishing a close relationship between patient and physician, and it is crucial for a personalized psychiatry. Understanding the subjective experience of the patient and the relationship between patient and physician cannot be fully replaced by concentrating on observational behaviours and data from neuroscience or biological psychiatry. All techniques together support each other and are connected in an integrated approach to find a diagnostic formulation and design a multimodal treatment strategy using psychotherapeutic, psychopharmacological, and psychosocial methodology.

However, in order to translate such methods in everyday clinical practice some steps have yet to be taken. Probably there is still the need to develop more reliable instruments to access and describe the patient's inner world. Subjective psychopathology is usually conceived as impossible to measure by definition, but it is probably just not well measured by currently available rating and diagnostic tools. Although psychopathologically informed empirical studies are paying more attention to subjective experiences (especially for psychotic disorders; see: Parnas 2005), a special effort should be devoted in the upcoming years to develop new evaluation and rating instruments, which may integrate objective and subjective approaches to psychiatric diagnosis. The use of oriented but yet 'free' (rather than structured) interviews or (already available) projective psychological tests might represent a valuable add-on to standardized rating scales, in order to achieve an acceptable degree of reliability without losing subjective information.

Eisenberg (2000), more than ten years ago, already claimed the need of a more balanced attitude in psychiatry to avoid the risk of making our discipline either 'brainless' or 'mindless'. Fulford (1999) argued that, psychiatrists need to operate both in the 'world of facts' (represented by science) but also in the world of values (represented by the humanities). Psychiatric practice truly lies at that peculiar interface between the biological, psychological, and social factors, which are currently thought to represent the true determinants of mental illnesses.

Of course, such an integration is not easily achievable, but probably represents the only way out from the possible danger of a scientific and clinical stagnation of our discipline.

Actually Griesinger (1845: 5), over 100 years ago, wrote in his famous textbook:

> Even if we knew all the things going on in the brain, all chemical electrical processes in detail—what would it be good for? All oscillations and vibrations, everything electrical and mechanical is still no mental state, no visualization. How it can become like that—this riddle will remain unsolved till the end of time, and I believe if an angel would be coming down from heaven and would explain everything to us, our intellect would not be able to comprehend.

The brain–mind dilemma is not only a philosophical issue of scholarly interest, but it directly affects psychiatric teaching and epistemology as well as clinical theory and practice (Kendell and Jablensky 2003).

Conclusions

Kandel (1998), while attempting to define a 'new intellectual framework for psychiatry' at the turning point of the new millennium, already foresaw that psychiatry in the future should have a sort of 'double role', both asking questions on its own level (i.e. how to diagnose and treat mental disorders, including the patient's perspective) and posing questions regarding human behaviour and higher mental processes (to answer to which, biology is definitely needed).

A possible escape of the critical diagnostic situation, as described earlier, might be the use of 'epistemic iterations' as proposed by Kendler (2009): subsequent revisions of diagnostic systems should have a cumulative nature and provide increasingly accurate estimation of a desired parameter, with respect to its predecessors. However, up to now, subsequent editions of diagnostic manuals did not really improve on their predecessors and the idea of increasing accuracy in describing the clinical 'truth' seems more and more unrealistic. It seems rather that the attempt to objectively describe the supposed truth has reached its asymptote, without providing a reliable estimate.

The recent developments in composing DSM-5 showed some relative efforts to come to a harmonization with ICD-10. Axes I, II, and III of DSM-IV might be collapsed into one axis containing all psychiatric and general medical diagnoses. This would bring DSM-5 into greater harmony with the single-axis approach of ICD. Axis IV does currently contain psychosocial and environmental problems; the working group on this axis is examining codes that are comparable to ICD-10. Axis V will allow clinicians to rate a patient's level of functioning so that disability and distress should be better assessed in DSM-5 and follow more closely the outlines of the World Health Organization (WHO).

All these changes, however, would be more or less technical and stay within the limitations of the existing systems. A move towards more fundamental changes acknowledging the phenomenological analysis of inner experiences and subjectivity as a highway to an empathetic understanding does not seem to be timely. Of special interest for such perspectives could have been the tendencies in the discussion process for ICD-11 to reach a more 'personalized' approach. Laín-Entralgo (1982) cogently pointed out that diagnosis is more than just identifying a disorder and distinguishing one disorder from another: beyond nosological and differential diagnoses, lies the real understanding of the mind–body uniqueness of individual presenting for care seeking. Developing a person-centred integrative diagnosis as a theoretical model as well as a practical guide and designing the best possible classification of mental disorders has been the goal of the WHO/World Psychiatric Association (ICD-11) and American Psychiatric Association (DSM-5) and other national and regional psychiatric associations in the past years (Mezzich and Salloum 2007). Unfortunately, however, it seems to be abandoned during the ongoing process of finalization of diagnostic psychiatric manuals.

Phenomenological-descriptive psychopathology, as it has recently been characterized (Stanghellini 2009), still has the aim of sorting out, defining, differentiating, and describing specific psychic phenomena, which are thereby actualized and are regularly described in specific terms. It represents a style and method of information gathering, which groups related phenomena clearly differentiable by patients' self-descriptions, excluding any preconceived notion or theory and focusing on the modes in which the experience comes to expression. Since this approach gives a special emphasis to introspection via an interactive and empathic process between the clinician and the patient, it may allow clarification of mental phenomena 'from inside' and represent a clinical method of interest for contemporary clinical psychiatrists. Jaspers in such a modern approach may refocus the view of psychiatrists: not only concentrating on pathological constructs (categories, disorders) and instead focusing once again on the whole person (Musalek et al. 2010).

The fascination and risks in psychiatric thinking lies in the complex nature of psychiatric disorders, which is characterized by an intricate interplay of somatic functions, learning processes, attitudes acquired during biography, and situation-specific influences (Sass 2001). Mental disorders mostly occur in the 'inner perspective' of the patients. They suffer from changes due to their disorder in their self-experience, feelings, emotions, intentions, hopes, expectations, plans, self-estimation, and estimation of other persons; thus, they suffer from modifications of subjectivity and inter-personality. These human qualities correlate indeed with brain processes and disordered functioning, but they do have also an autonomy that goes beyond and is nevertheless natural (Maier et al. 2005).

Finally, it should be considered that, to date, no single optimal method for the study of the mind and brain exists and that, in most of the cases, several methods will have to be used in concert such that their respective strengths are combined and their respective weaknesses compensated for. Also in clinical practice the problem of classification probably cannot be solved by choosing just one model or another: preferring classes (i.e. a pure categorical approach aimed to produce a unifying system, as anticipated mainly by Kahlbaum and Kraepelin), prototypes (i.e. typological classification, based on clinical impressions about extreme/accumulations types), or dimensional models (based on Eysenk's theories of behavioural patterns and pharmacological evidence, oriented towards syndromes and not nosological entities). This would probably end up in not meaningful conclusions, since—as Jaspers advised 100 years ago—any classification of non-organic psychiatric disorders would probably not be flawless. But any of them may be useful depending on its characteristics and its range of application, provided that there is awareness of its limitations.

In this sense, the most practical solution to the problems concerning diagnosis and classification in psychiatry probably lies in an open and holistic attitude to our discipline, with phenomenological psychopathology, as it was developed by Karl Jaspers a century ago, still as a conceptual foundation of the discipline itself, although being oriented at constantly adapting current nosological systems to the growing body of clinical and research knowledge. When the philosopher Jaques Derrida, a fervid criticizer of Husserl's phenomenology, attempted to explain the relationship between philosophy and science he had to warn his reader of an ineludible 'originary complexity' and of its multiple consequences in many fields, by saying that 'we are all translators, mediators' of such complexity (Derrida 1995). This philosophical position might also fit well the complexity of the brain/mind issue and should probably be kept in mind when attempting to create the definitive nosology for psychiatry.

References

Andreasen, N. (1998). 'Understanding Schizophrenia: A Silent Spring?', *American Journal of Psychiatry*, **155**: 1657–1659.

Banzato, C.E. (2004). 'Classification in Psychiatry: The Move Towards ICD-11 and DSM-V.', *Current Opinion in Psychiatry*, **17**: 497–591.

Beveridge, A. (2002). 'Time to Abandon the Subjective-Objective Divide?', *The Psychiatrist*, **26**: 101–103.

Borgna, E. (1969). 'Psychopathology and Clinical Aspects of Depression sine Depressione', *Rivista Sperimentale di Freniatria e Medicina Legale delle Alienazioni Mentali*, **93**: 1276–1290.

Bridgman, P.W. (1982). 'Einstein's Theories and the Operational Point of View', in P.A. Schilpp (ed), *Albert Einstein: Philosopher-Scientist*, Vol. 2. La Salle, IL: Open Court, 335–354.

Cannon, T.D. (2011). 'Objective Tests for Schizophrenia: Window to the Future', *World Psychiatry*, **10**(1): 36–37.

Cloninger, C.R. (1999). 'A New Conceptual Paradigm from Genetics and Psychobiology for the Science of Mental Health', *Australian and New Zealand Journal of Psychiatry*, **33**: 174–186.

Cooper, J.E., Kendell, R.E., Gurland, B.J., Sharpe, L., Copeland, J.R.M., Simon, R. (1972). *Psychiatric Diagnosis in New York and London*. Maudsley Monograph 20. Oxford: Oxford University Press.

Damasio, A. (1994). *Descartes' Error*. New York, NY: Avon Books.

Derrida, J. (1995). 'Unsealing ("the Old New Language")', in E. Weber (ed), *Point: Interviews 1974–1994*. Stanford, CA: Stanford University Press, 115–117.

Dilthey, W. (1894). 'Ideen über eine beschreibende und zergliedernde Psychologie', in H. Nohl (1961), *Wilhelm Dilthey—Eine Auswahl aus seinen Schriften*. Teubner, Stuttgart, 131–229.

Eisenberg, L. (2000). 'Is Psychiatry More Mindful or Brainer than it was a Decade Ago?', *British Journal of Psychiatry*, **176**: 1–5.

Feighner, J.P., Robins, E., Guze, S.B., Woodruff, R.A. Jr, Winokur, G., Munoz, R. (1972). 'Diagnostic Criteria for Use in Psychiatric Research', *Archives of General Psychiatry*, **26**: 57–63.

Feinstein, A.R. (1970). 'The Pre-Therapeutic Classification of Co-Morbidity in Chronic Disease', *Journal of Chronic Disease*, **23**: 455–468.

First, M.B. (2012). 'A Practical Prototypic System for Psychiatric Diagnosis: the ICD-11 Clinical Descriptions and Diagnostic Guidelines', *World Psychiatry*, **11**(1): 24–25.

Frances, A. (2012). 'Prototypal Diagnosis: Will this Relic From the Past Become the wave of the Future?', *World Psychiatry*, **11**(1): 26.

Fulford, W. (1999). 'Analytic Philosophy, Brain Science, and the Concept of Disorder', in S. Bloch, P. Chodoff, S. Green (eds), *Psychiatric Ethics*. Oxford: Oxford University Press, 161–192.

Ghaemi, N.S. (2009). 'Nosologomania: DSM & Karl Jaspers' Critique of Kraepelin', *Philosophy, Ethics, and Humanities in Medicine*, **4**: 10.

Griesinger, W. (1845). *Die Pathologie und Therapie der psychischen Krankheiten*. Stuttgart: Krabbe.

Gross, G., Huber, G. (2000). 'The Relevance of Jaspersian-Schneiderian Psychopathology for Today's Psychiatry', *Neurology Psychiatry and Brain Research*, **8**: 53–68.

Gruhle, H.W. (1947). Karl Jaspers: Allgemeine Psychopathologie. *Nervenarzt* **18**, 380–383.

Healy, D. (2002). *The Creation of Psychopharmacology*. Cambridge, MA: Harvard University Press.

Huber, G. (2002). 'The Psychopathology of K. Jaspers and K. Schneider as a Fundamental Method in Psychiatry', *World Journal of Biological Psychiatry*, **3**: 50–57.

Jablensky, A. (2012). 'Proptotypes, Syndromes and Dimensions of Psychopathology: An Open Agenda for Research', *World Psychiatry*, **11**(1): 22–23.

Janzarik, W. (1976). 'Die Krise der Psychopathologie', *Nervenarzt*, **47**: 73–80.

Janzarik, W. (1988). *Die strukturdynamischen Grundlagen der Psychiatrie*. Stuttgart: Enke.

Jaspers, K. (1913). *Allgemeine Psychopathologie* (1st edn). Berlin: Springer.

Jaspers, K. (1957). *The Philosophy of Karl Jaspers* (P.A. Schilpp, ed). New York, NY: Tudor.

Jaspers, K. (1997). *General Psychopathology* (7th edn) (J. Hoenig, M.W. Hamilton, trans.). Baltimore, MD: Johns Hopkins University Press.

Kandel, E. (1998). 'A New Intellectual Framework for Psychiatry', *American Journal of Psychiatry*, **155**: 457–469.

Kapur, S. (2011). 'Looking for a "Biological Test" to Diagnose "Schizophrenia": Are We Chasing Red Herrings?', *World Psychiatry*, **10**(1): 32.

Kendell, R., Jablensky, A. (2003). 'Distinguishing Between the Validity and Utility of Psychiatric Diagnoses', *American Journal of Psychiatry*, **160**: 4–12.

Kendler, K.S. (2009). 'An Historical Framework for Psychiatric Nosology', *Psychological Medicine*, **39**(12): 1935–1941.

Kendler, K.S., Jablensky A. (2010). 'Kraepelin's Concept of Psychiatric Illness', *Psychological Medicine*, **1**: 1–8.

Kraam, A. (2008). 'Karl Ludwig Kahlbaum by Dr. Ewald Hecker (1899)', *History of Psychiatry*, **19**: 77–80.

Krueger, R.F., Markon, K.E. (2012). 'Toward a Clinically Useful and Empirically Based Dimensional Model of Psychopathology', *World Psychiatry*, **11**(1): 23–24.

Laín-Entralgo, P. (1982). *El Diagnóstico Médico: Historia y Teoría*. Barcelona: Salvat.

Laing, R.D. (1985). *Wisdom, Madness and Folly*. London: Macmillan.

Lawrie, S.M., Olabi, B., Hall, J., McIntosh, A.M. (2011). 'Do We Have Any Solid Evidence of Clinical Utility About the Pathophysiology of Schizophrenia?', *World Psychiatry*, **10**(1): 19–31.

Lown, B. (1997). *The Lost Art of Healing*. Boston, MA: Houghton Mifflin.

Maier, W., Helmchen, H., Sass, H. (2005). 'Hirnforschung und Menschenbild in 21 Jahrhundert', *Nervenarzt*, **76**: 543–545.

Maj, M. (1998). 'Critique of the DSM-IV Operational Diagnostic Criteria for Schizophrenia', *British Journal of Psychiatry*, **172**: 458–460.

Maj, M. (2005). '"Psychiatric Comorbidity": An Artefact of Current Diagnostic Systems?', *British Journal of Psychiatry*, **186**: 182–184.

Maj, M. (2011). 'Psychiatric Diagnosis: Pros and Cons of Prototypes vs. Operational Criteria', *World Psychiatry*, **10**(2): 81–82.

McHugh, P.R., Slavney, P.R. (1982). 'Methods of Reasoning in Psychopathology: Conflict and Resolution', *Comprehensive Psychiatry*, 23(3): 197–215.

McHugh, P.R., Slavney, P.R. (1998). *The Perspectives of Psychiatry* (2nd edn). Baltimore, MD: Johns Hopkins University Press.

Merikangas, K.R., Zhang, H., Avenevoli, S., Acharyya, S., Neuenschwander, M., Angst J., *et al.* (2003). 'Zurich Cohort Study. Longitudinal Trajectories of Depression and Anxiety in a Prospective Community Study: the Zurich Cohort Study', *Archives of General Psychiatry*, **60**(10): 993–1000.

Mezzich, J.E., Salloum, I.M. (2007). 'Towards Innovative International Classification and Diagnostic Systems: ICD-11 and Person-Centered Integrative Diagnosis', *Acta Psychiatrica Scandinava*, **116**(1): 1–5.

Moeller, H.J. (2008). 'Systematic of Psychiatric Disorders Between Categorical and Dimensional Approaches—Kraepelin's Dichotomy and Beyond', *European Archives of Psychiatry and Clinical Neuroscience*, **258**(Suppl. 2): 48–73.

Mundt, C., Spitzer, M. (2000). 'Psychopathology Today', in F.G. Henn, N. Sartorius, H. Helmchen, H. Lauter (eds), *Contemporary Psychiatry*, Vol. 3, Part 1. Berlin: Springer, 161–193.

Musalek, M., Larach-Walters, V., Lépine, J.P., Millet, B., Gaebel, W.; WFSBP Task Force on Nosology and Psychopathology. (2010). 'Task Force on Nosology and Psychopathology. Psychopathology in the 21st century', *World Journal of Biological Psychiatry*, **11**: 844–851.

Naz, B., Bromet, E.J., Mojtabai, R. (2003). 'Distinguishing Between First-Admission Schizophreniform Disorder and Schizophrenia', *Schizophrenia Research*, **62**: 51–58.

Parnas, J. (2005). 'Clinical Detection of Schizophrenia-Prone Individuals: Critical Appraisal', *British Journal of Psychiatry*, **48**: 111–112.

Pauling, L., Itana, H.A., Singer, S.J., Wells, I.C. (1949). 'Sickle Cell Anemia: A Molecular Disease', *Science*, **110**: 543–548.

Robins, E., Guze, S.B. (1970). 'Establishment of Diagnostic Validity in Psychiatric Illness: Its Application to Schizophrenia', *American Journal of Psychiatry*, **126**: 983–987.

Rucci, P., Gherardi, S., Tansella, M., Piccinelli, M., Berardi, D., Bisoffi, G., *et al.* (2003). 'Subthreshold Psychiatric Disorders in Primary Care: Prevalence and Associated Characteristics', *Journal of Affective Disorders*, **76**(1–3): 171–181.

Sartorius, N., Kaelber, C.T., Cooper, J.E., Roper, M.T., Rae, D.S., Gulbinat, W., *et al.* (1993). 'Progress Toward Achieving a Common Language in Psychiatry. Results from the Field Trial of the Clinical Guidelines Accompanying the WHO Classification of Mental and Behavioral Disorders in ICD-10', *Archives General Psychiatry*, **50**: 115–124.

Sass, H. (1987). 'Die Krise der psychiatrischen Diagnostik', *Fortschritte der Neurologie-Psychiatrie*, **55**: 355–360.

Sass, H. (2001). 'Personality Disorders', in F. Henn, N. Sartorius, H. Helmchen, H. Lauter (eds), *Contemporary Psychiatry*. Berlin: Springer, 161–193.

Saunders, J. (2000). 'The Practice of Clinical Medicine as an Art and as a Science', *Medical Humanities*, **26**: 18–22.

Shepherd, M. (1990). 'Karl Jaspers: General Psychopathology', in *Conceptual Issues in Psychological Medicine*. London: Routledge, 276–281.

Slavney, P.R., McHugh, P.R. (1985). 'The Life-Story Method in Psychotherapy and Psychiatric Education: The Development of Confidence', *American Journal of Psychotherapy*, **39**: 57–67.

Spitzer, R.L., Endicott, J., Robins, E. (1975). *Research Diagnostic Criteria for a Selected Group of Functional Disorders*. New York, NY: Biometrics Research, New York Psychiatric Institute.

Spitzer, R.L., Endicott, J., Robins, E. (1978). 'Research Diagnostic Criteria: Rationale and Reliability', *Archives of General Psychiatry*, **35**: 773–782.

Stanghellini, G. (2009). 'The Meanings of Psychopathology', *Current Opinion in Psychiatry*, **22**: 559–564.

Strik, W. (2011). 'Clinical Handling and Understanding of Schizophrenia Should be Based on Pathophysiological Findings and Theories', *World Psychiatry*, **10**(1): 37–38.

Tyrer, P., Gunderson, J., Lyons, M., Tohen, M. (1997). 'Special Feature: Extent of Comorbidity Between Mental State and Personality Disorders', *Journal of Personality Disorders*, **11**(3): 242–259.

Van Praag, H. (1992). 'Reconquest of the Subjective. Against the Waning of Psychiatric Diagnosing', *British Journal of Psychiatry*, **160**: 266–271.

Wakefield, J.C. (2012). 'Are You as Smart as a 4th grader? Why the Prototype-Similarity Approach to Diagnosis is a Step Backward for a Scientific Psychiatry', *World Psychiatry*, **11**(1): 27–28.

Westen, D. (2012). 'Prototype Diagnosis of Psychiatric Syndromes', *World Psychiatry*, **11**(1): 16–21.

Wiggins, O.P., Schwartz, M.A., Spitzer, M.A. (1992). 'Phenomenological/Descriptive Psychiatry: The Methods of Edmund Husserl and Karl Jaspers', in M.A. Spitzer, F.A. Uehlein, M.A. Schwartz, C. Mundt (eds), *Phenomenological Language and Schizophrenia*. New York, NY: Springer, 46–69.

Woodruff, R.A., Goodwin, D.W., Guze, S.B. (1974). *Psychiatric Diagnosis*. New York, NY: Oxford University Press.

Zilboorg, G. (1967). *A History of Medical Psychology*. New York, NY: W.W. Norton & Company.

Chapter 14

On psychosis: Karl Jaspers and beyond

Josef Parnas

Introduction

Karl Jaspers' (1913/1963/1997) successive revisions of *General Psychopathology* provided a uniquely systematic and comprehensive conceptual and descriptive foundation of psychopathology. Jaspers' work is not without shortcomings, even if judged within its own historical context. Nonetheless, *General Psychopathology* was truly transformative in its emphasis of the particular nature (ontology) of the 'psychiatric object' (symptoms and signs), an ontology quite unlike that of extant spatiotemporal physical objects or things. Therefore, *General Psychopathology* insisted on an epistemology tailored to the nature of subjectivity, which required specific methods for the exploration and description of the latter. Another important task of psychopathology, said Jaspers, was to adopt a critical, reflective attitude towards psychiatric concepts and common assumptions. A thorough analysis could here prevent undue simplifications, distortions, and reifications. Moreover, a critical analysis of concepts and assumptions often disclosed their hidden, but unjustified metaphysical commitments.

Unfortunately, the impact of Jaspers on mainstream Anglophone psychiatry was minimal. Jaspers' work was certainly not consulted during the 'operational' remake of psychiatric nosology.

Unfortunately, the absence of 'Jaspersian' critical intellectual impulse is quite perceptible in the contemporary scene (Andreasen 2007). Many descriptive concepts are so much taken for granted that we use them as technical indicators of really existing kinds: e.g. DUP (duration of untreated psychosis), 'converting to psychosis' (i.e. entering 'psychosis', category by crossing a psychometric threshold). This problem is even more pronounced with the terms stemming from cognitive science, which are currently flooding the psychiatric idiom (e.g. 'mentalizing', 'meta-representation', 'monitoring', etc. (Skodlar et al. 2012)). Such terms become rapidly assimilated into the descriptive vocabulary of psychopathology, despite being phenomenologically and conceptually undigested, and despite the fact that originally they often referred to hypothetical sub-personal processes and were inapplicable for the phenomenal realm. When such reifications settle down as habit, any initial concerns of validity (if ever articulated) sink into oblivion.

The concept of psychosis, which has a central status in psychiatric description and classification and is used by psychiatrists on a daily basis, may be a subject to similar concerns.

The purpose of this chapter is to explore theoretical, clinical, and phenomenological aspects of the concept of 'psychosis'. There are timely reasons for such a critical appraisal.

Despite more than 30 years of intensive research in the framework of 'operational psychiatry', 'a gaping disconnect exists between the brilliant discoveries informing genetics and neuroscience and their almost complete failure to elucidate the causes (and guide the treatment) of mental illness' (Frances and Widiger 2012: 112). This statement echoes Jaspers' assessment of 'the poverty of the so far recognized relationships between events in the brain and abnormal psychic events' (Jaspers, 1963: 577). Despite this lack of progress, or because of it, we are now in the process of revising the diagnostic psychiatric systems, i.e. we are on the way to future editions of the *Diagnostic and Statistical Manual of Mental Disorders* (DSM) and International Classification of Diseases (ICD). One plausible reason for the 'gaping disconnect' is a longstanding and systematic neglect of conceptual and phenomenological issues underpinning empirical research, i.e. the issues, which were considered by Jaspers as foundational for the science of psychiatry. Psychiatric research necessarily begins with distinctions in the phenomenal realm, e.g. symptoms, signs, syndromes, or altered patterns of existence ('the psychiatric object' (Marková and Berrios 2009)). When invalid or distorted, such distinctions cannot avoid jeopardizing or impeding scientific developments. Therefore, following Jaspers, we need an epistemological approach that is adapted to the ontological particularities of the 'psychiatric object', rather than an approach dictated by theoretical prejudice or (apparent) easiness of application.

A brief history

A recent historical contribution (Burgy 2008) is mute on a central, but difficult and elusive question: what is psychosis?

Originally, the term 'psychosis' referred to psychological manifestations of brain (neural) disease, whereas 'neurosis' was the neural disease itself (Burgy 2008). These meanings were radically altered in the beginning of the twentieth century. 'Psychosis', after having emancipated itself from the very inclusive, nineteenth-century term 'dementia', came to designate a serious psychological disorder with hypothetical biological roots (Schneider 1950) and a 'global personality change', resistant to empathic understanding (Jaspers 1963/1997). A layman refers to psychosis as 'madness' (insanity, craziness, *folie*). 'For lay persons madness means senseless ravings, affectless confusion, delusion, incongruous affects, a "crazy" personality, and [lay persons] think this all the more the more sensible and orientated the individual remains' (Jaspers 1963/1997: 577–578). The expression 'affectless confusion' and the last part of the sentence is significant: the more we take the person to be emotionally composed and unimpaired in his basic intellective faculties, the more obviously his 'craziness' (irrationality) articulates itself as 'crazy'. In other words, should, for example, an epileptic source of the 'senseless raving' become apparent, the layman would be likely to consider the person as being somatically 'ill' rather than 'mad'.

If we assume that folk psychological understanding helps found the psychiatric terms, then it seems that psychosis is a predicate that we ascribe to someone who has seriously transgressed the intersubjective bounds of rationality or the shared 'we-perspective' on the world (Tomasello and Rakoczy 2006). A common way to define this transgression is to equate it with the presence of delusion(s) (delusionality). This equation is unsatisfactory for several reasons that will be addressed later. Most importantly, delusion does not exhaust all characteristics of 'madness', as a layman understands it. Delusion is but one of the 'psychotic symptoms' specified in the current diagnostic systems (DSM-IV and ICD-10). In other words, we need to expand the notion of (ir-) rationality beyond what may be articulated in a propositional belief format (delusions).

Nosological connotations of the concept of psychosis

Historically, psychosis was never considered on a purely descriptive-phenomenological level, disconnected from hypothetical, nosological-pathogenetic considerations. Rather, all definitions of psychosis were and are embedded in extra-clinical (extra-descriptive) references.

Both Kurt Schneider (1950) and Karl Jaspers (1963/1997) assumed neurobiological causes of psychosis (e.g. Jaspers' notion of an underlying 'process'). On the descriptive level both authors referred to a 'global personality change'. This term seems today to refer to the 'structure of subjectivity' rather than to 'personality' as it is currently understood. Unfortunately, Jaspers failed to define more closely the nature of that change. As is well known, he considered 'un-understandability' (elusiveness to empathic understanding) as an index of the underlying biological process. Schizophrenia, with its alterations of the sense of 'mineness' of experience (e.g. passivity phenomena), was Jaspers' prime example: 'Only negatively or metaphorically can we visualize this essentially changed psychic life in which these [...] experiences play a part' (Jaspers 1963/1997: 578).

Yet, Jaspers' assumption that un-understandability must imply 'organic' causes is 'non sequitur'. Claiming an organic background of un-understandability is not an analytic truth. Second, understandability is a matter of degree (see later in the section on delusions). Moreover, from a neuroscientific perspective, all mental phenomena are, in a sense, 'organically' caused, i.e. correlated with neurophysiological processes. The dichotomy between 'organic' and 'functional' disorders becomes increasingly blurred, and seems to be a function of technological sophistication. Biological research findings are being published on all studied psychiatric disorders.

The nosological issues were never a primary focus of continental phenomenology. However, to the extent that the distinction psychosis versus neurosis was being discussed, phenomenology pointed to the structural changes of subjectivity (alterations of the basic ontological frameworks of being-in-the-world, e.g. spatiality, temporality, self-awareness) as the hallmark of psychosis (Basso 2012; Tatossian 1979). Yet, within the framework of psychiatric operationalism, a phenomenological investigation of the 'structures of subjectivity' would be considered as being a form of 'theoretical' enterprise, outside the realm of pure, 'atheoretical' description. This is so because the operational approach considers psychiatric symptoms and signs as directly observable, well-delimited, mutually independent, thing-like entities, accessible and graspable in the third-person format (Nordgaard et al. 2012a). Going beyond this objectivist-operational frame is typically considered as engaging in a non-empirical, speculative endeavour.

Classic psychoanalysis considered psychosis to be a regression to pre-Oedipal developmental stages with the activation of the corresponding low-level 'primitive' defence mechanisms (Fenichel 1945). Today, psychoanalysis understands 'psychosis' and 'psychosis-proneness' as a specific pattern of psychological organization (Kernberg 1975). However, in the operational view, the notions of 'regression' or 'psychological organization' may be construed as referring to nosological constructs rather than to observable, descriptive realm.

The ICD-8 and ICD-9 (preceding the arrival of ICD-10 in 1992) (World Health Organization 1992) grouped the psychoses into a triad reflecting their assumed aetiologies: (1) endogenous/heritable (schizophrenia, manic-depressive illness), (2) organic/exogenous/toxic, and (3) psychogenic (reactive) psychoses. This latter kind was by definition 'understandable' as a consequence of a psychosocial trauma. The general descriptor of psychosis in the ICD-8/9 systems was 'deficient reality testing' (addressed in detail in the section entitled 'Reality, sense of reality, reality judgement, and reality-testing').

Contemporary diagnostic systems and the clinical application of the concept of psychosis

Although the current diagnostic systems claim an 'atheoretical', descriptive stance, the mainstream view, in continuity with Jaspers–Schneider, is that psychotic disorders are mainly 'biological' in nature, i.e. 'brain disorders' or 'diseases'.

In the DSM-IV (American Psychiatric Association 2000) the term psychotic refers to the presence of certain symptoms. The specific constellations of these symptoms vary across the diagnostic categories. In Schizophrenia, Schizophreniform Disorder, Schizoaffective Disorder, and Brief Psychotic Disorder, the term psychotic refers to delusions, any prominent hallucinations, disorganized speech, or disorganized or catatonic behaviour (a flamboyant subgroup of catatonic symptoms). In Psychotic Disorder Due to a General Medical Condition and in Substance-Induced Psychotic Disorder, psychotic refers to delusions or only those hallucinations that are not accompanied by insight. Finally, in Delusional Disorder and Shared Psychotic Disorder, psychotic is equivalent to being delusional. In the DSM-IV there is no use of the term 'psychosis' as a substantive.

The definition of psychosis in the ICD-10 (World Health Organization 1992) uses the same symptomatic indices (hallucinations, delusions, incoherence, gross disorganization, catatonic features). ICD-10 mentions the general concept of psychosis, but the definition is limited to a reference to a failure of 'reality testing' (which is another expression for lack of 'insight', because having insight into being ill reflects an aspect of reality testing). In brief, psychosis is descriptively undefined or under-defined in the diagnostic manuals.

In the 'prodromal' (At-Risk-Mental-State, AMRS) research, psychosis is defined through a prespecified psychometric threshold:

> We have chosen to operationalize a definition of psychosis based on the presence of clear-cut threshold level psychotic symptoms (delusions, hallucinations, and formal thought disorder,[1] scored above a psychometric threshold) occurring several times per week for at least 1 week in a help-seeking population … This definition of … psychosis is of course somewhat arbitrary, but it does at least have clear treatment implications and applies equally well to substance related symptoms, symptoms that have a mood component—either depression or mania—and schizophrenia spectrum disorders. (Yung et al. 2003: 21–22)

The AMRS approach represents a quantitative, dimensional assessment of psychopathology, followed by an arbitrary, but practically useful, carving out of the target category. Such an approach, however, relies on a series of epistemological assumptions on the nature

[1] It refers to maximal formal thought disorder: incoherence and neologisms.

of psychiatric object as comprising atomic, thing-like psychiatric symptoms and signs (Nordgaard et al. 2012a).

In the current daily European clinical practice the notion of psychosis is descriptively founded on the notion of deficient 'reality testing', attested by the presence of the psychotic symptoms (as stipulated in the ICD-10).

Finally, it is important to recall that legal and ethical concerns also permeate the notion of psychosis. This is to say that legal consequences do not merely follow from the concept of psychosis. Rather, the very existence of a category called 'psychosis' (madness) is linked to ethical, social, and political considerations. Madness implies a loss or lack of personal autonomy, responsibility, and accountability. A crime, committed (in Europe) in a psychotic state, is typically not sanctioned by the standard punitive measures, because a psychotic offender cannot be considered to have acted as an autonomous, free-willed individual.

Reality, sense of reality, reality judgement, and reality-testing

To say that psychosis involves 'lack of insight' or 'deficient reality testing' is merely a tautology and certainly does not help to define what psychosis is. 'Reality', used as a predicate, is often contrasted with the 'world of psychosis'. Psychosis is here conceived of as a standing outside of the realm of the real, in some sort of imaginary world. The real is typically defined as that which exists independently of our conscious acts (e.g. fantasy or imagination), with emphasis on the material world and objectivity and on the role of intersubjective agreement. However, the concept of reality is not defined nor discussed in the current diagnostic manuals or major textbooks.

For phenomenology reality is a reality of a 'lived world', i.e. a world imbued with meaning, relevance, and objectivity, all (co-)constituted by our (inter-)subjectivity, with symbolic-communicative, social, and cultural dimensions (Parnas and Sass 2008). This shared lived world is not just a container of individual objects or things. Rather, it functions as an encompassing background dimension, a horizon, or a condition of the objects' manifestation. Phenomenologically speaking, reality does not first present itself as a raw, naked, physical reality, revealed by elementary sense data and which we subsequently dress with layers of meaning, assisted by the aid of concepts and reflection. Rather, all perception happens from within our standard lived world, with its prior familiarity and trust that Husserl (1982) called 'Urdoxa' and Merleau-Ponty (2012), 'perceptual faith'.

> The belonging to the world is not a matter of having a belief-like intentional state with the content 'the world exists,' Rather, it involves ... having *a sense of reality*, by which I mean a grasp of the distinction between 'real,' 'present' and other *possibilities*, without which one could not encounter anything as 'there' or, more generally as 'real.' We generally take for granted that others share this same *modal space* with us and that they are able to encounter things in the same was as we do. (Ratcliffe 2012: 479–480)

This original belonging to the world, a *sense of reality* is a sense of embodied (self-)presence in the midst of a shared world (*Dasein*). The root of this sense is not primarily cognitive but affective in nature. 'Felt reality' is not the product of a dispassionate disclosing of the world. As Husserl (1982) mentions, our cognitive grasping of objects relies on a sense of being affected by, and belonging to, the world through inconspicuous affective-existential tonalities (Ratcliffe 2008), which make up the pre-reflective horizon of experience and frame our everyday commerce with objects, situations, and Others. These feelings constitute the very context in which cognition and reflection takes place (Damasio 1999, 2003). Their overall structure is 'touch-like' (Ratcliffe 2008). Like in touch, a self-presence and experience of otherness are inextricably interwoven in the same unitary experiential structure. These experiences are ways in which the world appears.

Very much in the same spirit, Jaspers (1963/1997) emphasized that we should distinguish between *primary* awareness of reality (*sense of reality*), which is an immediate (directly given and implicit) certainty of reality and a reality created through a *reflective* reality judgement. Conceptual reality carries conviction only if a kind of presence is experienced (Jaspers 1963/1997). Pierre Janet (1926) proposed a similar distinction between '*la fonction du réel*' and '*la notion du réel*'.

The sense of reality and unreflected presence in the intersubjective world is not based on a hypothetical 'reality testing' (defined in cognitive science as an ability to distinguish imagination from perception) or 'reality monitoring' (ability to distinguish external and internal stimuli). Both testing and monitoring (considered at a phenomenal level and not merely postulated as sub-personal neural processes) would imply incessant online comparisons of what we are experiencing with some representational models or criteria. We would continuously compare our perceptions and fantasies with each other, and with a reality model. But when I imagine myself sitting on the terrace of a Parisian café, my self-awareness of my imagining (my awareness of me, now being engaged in an act of imagining) is precisely that which constitutes my experience as a case of imagining. I need no reflective scrutiny to 'know' whether I am imagining or perceiving. In fact, even to say that 'I know that I perceive or imagine' borders on incoherence, because we do not have here an epistemic relation at all; we are simply dealing with a self-affection of intentionality of perception or imagination (Henry 1973).

It is possible (and perhaps likely) that processes like reality testing and monitoring do take place on a sub-personal (neural) level, but this is not reflected on the experiential level. On the other hand, as Jaspers points out, we do have a possibility of a reflective judgement about reality (as when I am assessing how much repair the roof of my summerhouse may need). Such explicit relation to reality is not a feeling or a pre-verbal experience, but a cognitive, conceptual attitude. It contains reflection, a changing of one's perspectives, and it involves judgements about reality. In this attitude we may mobilize additional cognitive resources (as when stretching our arms out upon entering a dark room, in order to compensate with movement and touch for the lack of visibility).

Yet, the important point to recognize is that we are not dealing here with a restricted, modular function of 'reality testing' or 'insight' but rather with general, complex, and multifaceted cognitive, reflective abilities. Such abilities may be diminished in psychosis but this decrease cannot be insulated from the psychotic process itself. An ability to improve on one's rational faculties is not independent of one's prior, pre-existing irrational predicament. In other words, both the concepts of 'insight' and of 'testing' seem to presuppose a distinction or separateness between the (intact) self and the phenomena of psychosis. But we 'are' psychotic rather than 'having' psychosis.

In summary, a modular process of 'reality testing' does not articulate itself as a phenomenal experience or function. For this reason, 'reality testing' should not be used as a psychiatric, phenomenological 'descriptor'. To say that a patient suffers from deficient reality testing or lacks an insight in his illness is just another way of saying that he is psychotic. Instead, we should say that the patient's (reflective) reality judgement (critical, socially-anchored, reflection) is radically compromised, while keeping in mind that we are not referring to any modular, specific function.

It is important to add that the distinction between experience and judgement is not absolute. Their relation is perhaps best conceived of as a dimensional transition between two gestaltic-prototypical opposites. For example, feelings and moods connect us 'understandingly' with the world (Heidegger 1953/1996). 'Understanding' (*Verstehen*), says Heidegger, is not just a specific or contingent faculty of cognition, but rather an 'Existential', i.e. 'a mode or structure of being-in-the-world'. Affectivity implies tacit disclosing of the world (i.e. it is a tacit cognitive achievement). A phenomenological notion of 'experience', as a translation of the German term '*Erlebnis*' (in French, *vecu*), refers to a pathic, passive living through a specific (self-)affection (e.g. a sensation of pain, a mood, a feeling of joy, but also a qualitative, pathic [self-affecting] aspect of an act of thinking about one's future). Experience is permeated by a dimension of qualia, i.e. of 'what it is like' to have that experience. A judgement, on the other hand, is considered as a cognitive act, a belief, or a propositional attitude about a certain state of affairs in the world. A judgement *posits* its object as being in a certain way (the so-called 'thetic' component, Husserl 1982). Experience may be associated with varying degrees of thetic positing: e.g. in seeing a tree in front of us, we implicitly posit the tree as actually existing *there*, in front of us. Conversely, all judgements display an experiential, affective dimension. There is a difference in 'what it is like' to *believe* that something, to *doubt* that something, or to *hope* that something (Zahavi 2005; *vide supra* on the self-affection of intentionality (Henry 1973)).

Rationality and irrationality

A layman's view of psychosis (madness) tells us that the person's rationality, i.e. her judgement, grasp, or understanding of reality, of the world, including herself, is markedly dislocated from what is contextually and socially adequate, acceptable and valid. The patient thus appears to exist outside the bounds of rationality in *a* certain radical way. Whether this radicality can be 'operationally' defined and whether we are dealing here with a dimensional transition or a categorical discontinuity will be addressed later. Here, we can add that the typical, constitutive, and interrelated aspects of radical irrationality comprise perspectival rigidity (inability to adopt the Other's perspective), communicative breakdown and existential solitude.

We briefly need to dwell on the issue of rationality. Traditionally, since Descartes' call for 'clear and distinct ideas', rationality is understood as 'theoretical rationality', i.e. a reasoning capacity dependent on serial, discursive-propositional steps, guided by inferential logic. The outcome of this process is typically propositionally structured as in a sentence 'I believe that we are heading towards recession'. To consider another person as an ideally rational being involves (most clearly in the analytic philosophical tradition) the following prerequisites: (1) we understand the person's reasons for acting in a given way (action is consistent with its intent); (2) we ascribe to her a rationality of mental states, i.e. her beliefs and desires comprise a consistent and coherent set or network; (3) her reasoning follows the rules of logic and of probability calculus; (4) she tends to optimize her knowledge and possesses transparent preferences/inclinations.

However, such an ideally rational human being, perhaps unsurprisingly, is not a very frequent finding of empirical population studies. Rather, it seems that humans tend to reason heuristically, violate the rules of logic, ignore probability calculus, and become easily biased by affective factors (Gigerenzer 2007).

Along these lines, cognitive science distinguishes between at least two types of rationality (Shafir and LeBoeuf 2002). One is 'theoretical'- serial, reflective, following logic, and proximate to the ideal type depicted by analytic philosophy. The other type is 'pragmatic', rapid, holistic, involving an affective dimension, and is context-sensitive. Future research will undoubtedly uncover an even greater heterogeneity of rationality.

Phenomenology was always familiar with these two types of rationality (variously designated): one, reflective, logical, and inferential, and the other, 'practical rationality'. This other type of reasoning 'is not a logic of the logicians but the logic of the world' (Tatossian 1979), a 'common sense' (understood here as '*sensus communis*' of Antiquity). It is a pre-reflective, pre-linguistic and pre-conceptual sense of affective salience, affordance, proportion, adequacy and relevance. It is an attunement, enabling one to negotiate one's way in a world that is not pre-defined and static, but dynamic and constantly changing, and moulded by the subject's own actions (Parnas and Bovet 1991; Parnas et al. 2002). It is an understanding of the world in the tacit mode of '*Zuhandenheit*' (Heidegger 1996), implicit in acting, especially in social, interpersonal relations. '*Background Capacities*' of the analytic tradition (Searle 1992) and '*habitus*' of the social anthropology (Bourdieu 1990) are overlapping designations of 'common sense'. The notions of 'common sense' and 'sense of reality' are, of course, intimately interconnected. Both imply a primary and basic constitution of meaning-horizon, which articulates itself out of our embodied self-presence in a shared world. Both are pre-reflective, passive processes (involving 'passive syntheses'(Husserl 1982)) that provide the foundation for the more explicit, active, and thematic intentionalities, including a reflective judgement. It is likely that the psycho-developmental notion of 'basic trust' is closely related to phenomenology's 'common sense' and 'sense of reality'.

Irrationality, the hallmark of psychosis, may be 'theoretical', propositionally structured in discursive thought contents, and presented as what we call delusions, reporting of hallucinations, or delusional explanations of abnormal experiences.

However, psychosis may also manifest itself as an irrationality of the pragmatic-affective kind, i.e. in a dislocation from intersubjectivity, which reveals itself through affectivity, expressivity and action (e.g. catatonia, hebephrenic behavioural style). This variant of psychotic irrationality may be called 'non-propositional', thereby indicating a significant distinction from delusionality, the latter being expressed in propositional statements ('I believe that … ').

We will look more closely at an example of 'non-propositional', expressive irrationality: catatonic posturing and catatonic stupor. Why do we take these phenomena as being indicative of the presence of psychosis? Typically, in such cases we do not have access to a self-report from the patient that could allow us to classify him as being delusional. Only in retrospect, the patient may, or may not, recall what went through his mind, and sometimes we learn something about, e.g. his catastrophic or cosmic experiences and the associated, plainly delusional contents (e.g. that a single movement might have led to a world-cataclysm). In the majority of cases we remain ignorant of the patient's experience and thought. What then, in a confrontation with such patients, justifies the label of 'psychosis'? First, there is a fundamental break of communication, and thus of intersubjectivity.

Second, the patient's distorted expression is, from a phenomenological perspective, not an autonomous 'external' feature but a gestalt-like manifestation of a certain whole, jointly constituted by the patient's expression and inner world. What justifies the label of 'psychosis' is the fact that in the catatonic expressivity we perceive an enacted understanding of the world that appears to be radically different from our own (i.e. we sense a radical dislocation from intersubjectivity).

Another variant of the 'non-propositional irrationality' may manifest itself through strange action episodes, the so-called 'crazy action' ('*Unsinnige Handlung*' (Conrad, 1958); '*dèlire en acte*' (Minkowski, 1927)), e.g. sudden aimless trips, strange impulsive acts, often so trivial that they elude the clinician's attention. From a theoretical point of view, action is perhaps an even more significant manifestation of (ir-)rationality than what can be expressed through language (i.e. delusional statements). As Pierre Janet (1926) noted, action is the ultimate confirmation of belief. Conrad offers an example of a behaviour that, in this particular case, turned out to be a forerunner of the onset of schizophrenia:

> H.K., 24, sergeant, was in a 'dreadful' state of tension since the beginning of the attack on France [in 1940], in which he participated. An exceptional soldier, much beloved by his superiors, full of ideals, but 'deeply' affected by several matters ... The dizziness of a victorious advance, punctuated with critical engagements with the enemy, was mixed up with feelings of deception in relation to his comrades, who could not resist the temptation of plundering; a behavior which he most deeply despised [...] When his troops' advance stopped in the vicinity of Paris, he took his service vehicle and, breaking the strict and explicit orders, drove with some privates under his command to Paris, in order to 'draw their attention on the cultural values of the enemy.' He was condemned to six weeks of prison. The psychosis broke out some months later. (Conrad, 1958: 35)

Here, the gross transgression of the discipline, completely incongruent with the sergeant's former exemplary conduct, appeared in its motivation—'to approximate his soldiers to the culture of the enemy'—as completely 'mad' in the eyes of his superiors[2] (Bovet and Parnas 1993).

What is characteristic in the sergeant's acting is a peculiar dislocation from common sense, justifying the designation of 'autistic activity' (Minkowski 1927). It is not so much the problem of logic and theoretical rationality, but rather an expression of a loss of attunement to the tacit, pre-reflective, pre-conceptual, socially shared and contextually adequate 'logic of the world' (common sense). His action reveals an understanding of the world that is seriously displaced from intersubjectivity (common sense). Taken in isolation, it would not suffice for the label of psychosis. Yet, this example is clinically very significant because, despite its apparent banality, it points to a lack of 'common sense', a trait feature of the schizophrenia spectrum disorders, often preceding the onset of a fully articulated psychosis (Parnas et al. 2002, 2011), and which, in a clinical situation, should awaken the psychiatrist's attention to a possibility of severe psychopathology.

Irrationality of action may sometimes be most clearly visible in a striking incongruence between the motivational/experiential content and the resulting activity: X, one of my patients, diagnosed with schizotypal disorder (who later developed a frank

2 What is a 'crazy action' is evidently culture-bound. In a contemporary Western army, the sergeant's act would not be considered as 'mad'.

schizophrenia), was tormented by pseudo-obsessive ruminations. He was overwhelmed by the thoughts that he perhaps might have once murdered a baby.[3] He spent his days walking through the city, searching inside the trash containers for a corpse of a baby. These ruminations were not clearly delusional. The patient considered them as 'obsessions' and was very well aware that he never murdered anyone. His 'obsessions' lacked the truly obsessive quality, because they did not evoke any immediate impulse of 'internal resistance' (ICD-10); thus, they were partly ego-syntonic. However, he was unable to resist the compulsive urge to search in the city trash containers, despite the fact that he had no rational reason to expect finding a corpse exactly in those containers. In most cases of such 'crazy actions', the patients' (post hoc) explanations are evasive, vague, or strangely illogical—and only with difficulty can be 'translated' into a propositional (delusional) belief-format.

Another example of the 'non-propositional irrationality' is a pervasive depressive condition with a profound sense of existential transformation, a sense of inability to reach out to the future, of 'not being able to ... ' and pervasive guilt feelings. Although all such features may not be quite translatable into a clearly articulated delusional format, they testify nonetheless (analogously to the catatonic expressivity) to a radically altered world-understanding.

Still other 'non-propositional' variants of irrationality comprise severe formal thought disorder (incoherence, neologisms), amnesia, disorientation, and global disorders of attention. They all affect cognition, behaviour, and communication (and hence rationality) to a degree where clinicians feel that the psychosis label is appropriate.

Delusion

Delusion is a paradigmatic index of psychosis. It is today a very broad concept, referring to 'false, erroneous beliefs', i.e. thoughts and convictions, articulated as propositional statements, e.g. 'I believe that the CIA contaminates the drinking water in order to make all males living here sexually impotent'.

Defining psychosis through the presence of delusion does not solve the issue of the definition of the former. The problem moves from defining irrationality of psychosis to defining the nature of delusion. Here, the problem even becomes amplified. First, a delusion defies any simple definition. Second, the DSM-IV and ICD-10 criteria are empirically (factually) incorrect. The common criteria (falsity, conviction, and incorrigibility) are usually ascribed to Jaspers. Yet, Jaspers (1963/1997) explicitly did not consider this triad as defining what delusion was (rather, it was a non-reducible change of the structure of subjectivity). He even described these features as 'external indicators' (*aussere Merkmale*), suggesting the presence of delusion, but not defining it. The DSM-IV-TR goes somewhat further, beyond the triad of falsity, conviction and incorrigibility:

> A false personal belief based on incorrect inference about external reality and firmly sustained in spite of what almost everyone else believes and in spite of what constitutes incontrovertible proof or evidence to the contrary. (American Psychiatric Association 2000: 765)

---

[3] Such rumination appear sometimes to be linked to an inability to distinguish between different modes of intentionality; here perhaps between a remembered fantasy and a factual memory.

In fact, all components of this definition have been questioned (e.g. Bovet and Parnas 1995; Sass 1994; Spitzer 1990). A delusion need not be (and sometimes is not) empirically false (e.g. delusions of jealousy may be empirically true); it may not be personal but involve other people or impersonal world affairs; it is not always about external reality (which is itself operationally undefined), for it may involve body or mind as themes; it needs not to be, and frequently is not, based on inferential reasoning; nor does it need to be believed with full conviction to be clinically significant.[4] The 'reality' of the DSM definition oscillates between the 'objective', mind-independent (in-itself) realist version and a normative, consensual-social convention. These two realities need not to coincide.

Although all delusional patients are psychotic, not all psychotic patients are delusional in the DSM/ICD operational sense of entertaining 'false beliefs'. It rarely happens that we assess (or find it feasible or sensible to assess) empirical truth or falsity of a potentially delusional claim. Rather, as clinicians, we focus on the content's probability, plausibility, and its way of presentation. In the patient's claims and their presentation, we may sense that it is not merely a question of falsity/truth of a single claim that matters. Something more global may be at stake, e.g. something that transpires through the patient's way of arguing. This gestalt-like whole comprises a fabric of branching, interconnected beliefs, attitudes, background assumptions, which ultimately inhere in the overall structure of consciousness and experiencing. It is these various contextual aspects, surrounding the focal propositional content, that help the clinician to classify a given statement as an instance of delusion. This role of contextual aspects is illustrated by a modified, reconstructed example from Heinimaa (2002):

> The example takes place in Helsinki, Finland. A man seeks a psychiatric emergency and complains of anxiety and insomnia, because he knows that Russia is going to invade Finland tomorrow. It all happens at the heydays of Russian-Western relations. You, a young doctor on duty, would be liable to consider the statement as delusional (you would be more cautious in your judgment if all this happened few days after the 2008 Russian invasion of Georgia). However, if the patient turns out to be the chief of Finland's Intelligence Service, you would suspend your initial hunch and proceed with a very thorough psychiatric assessment. It turns out that the patient is justifying his conviction by a personal experience from the previous evening. Then, he attended a cocktail party at the Russian Embassy and there he got a very unpleasant feeling that the party had a kind of arranged, fabricated atmosphere. All people stared at him. Upon this information, you would suspect a psychotic condition preceded by a delusional mood. Finally, if the patient tells you that *Russia has already invaded Finland three years ago* but no one has yet noticed it, you would be liable (assuming that the patient is not sarcastic or joking) to think that the patient's 'concept of invasion' (and its more encompassing framework) does not match yours, perhaps pointing to a degree of irrationality justifying the diagnosis of psychosis.

No simple definition of a propositional content is immune to changing contexts and normative factors. It goes without saying that the problem with defining of delusion weakens and destabilizes the validity of the entire group of 'psychosis-near phenomena' listed in the DSM/ICD such as self-reference, overvalued idea, paranoid ideation, and magical thinking.

---

[4] Clinically, this is a very difficult feature to assess, because patients often do not reveal their innermost convictions and often conceal their delusional ideation.

Is delusion a belief?

In cognitive and philosophical literature, the concept of belief is usually taken for granted, considered as univocally referring to a propositional attitude in which we assume something to be true. Anthropological and linguistic research emphasizes, however, an intrinsic vagueness of the term belief, which appears to cover a wide variety of mental states (Needham 1972). Thus, a more specific (and perhaps more serious) problem that confronts the definition of delusion as a 'false belief' is the question whether delusion can be considered as an instance of belief or reality-assertion at all (e.g. 'the CIA poisons the water in order to ... '). As is well known, Jaspers distinguished between the 'true, or primary' delusions and 'delusion-like ideas' (secondary delusions). Thus, it is Jaspers' delusion-like ideas, rather than true delusions, that correspond to what the DSM and ICD manuals designate today as delusions, i.e. false, erroneous judgements of some state of affairs.

Primary delusion involves a characteristic 'mode of experience'—in which the content of any experience, e.g. occurrent perception, thought, or recollection—articulates or reveals a delusional significance in a direct, un-mediated way. '*Unmittelbar*' is the word used in the German edition of Jaspers, i.e. not only temporally instantaneous, but also entailing another sense, i.e. in 'a direct way, non-mediated by reflection or inference'. The delusional meaning, for example, of a percept, articulates itself in the perceived content like a revelation, formally similar to a strong aesthetic experience:

> A patient walking up the staircase to his psychiatrist's office, noticed through a window, a canvas with intense blue color, among some furniture stabled in the yard. Seeing the painting with its blue color, the patient became aware of being insane [an example of empirically true delusion]. (Blankenburg 1965: 289)

This *primary* articulation of delusional meaning is, according to Jaspers, not empathically understandable, partly because it is not mediated through the inferential reflections that the psychiatrist can emulate in his own mind. Primary delusion is not an inferential or empirical error, a mistaken view of reality. 'To say simply that a delusion is a mistaken idea which is firmly held by the patient and which cannot be corrected gives only a superficial and incorrect answer to the problem', wrote Jaspers. It is 'primary' in the (patho-)genetic, rather than temporal sense. It points to a shattering of the basic forms of experience and hence a transformation of the patient's total awareness of reality (Jaspers 1963/1997; Schneider 1959). What is changed is not an *opinion* about reality but the very structure of the global perspective on the world: the patient's existential-ontological framework (Bovet and Parnas 1995; Parnas 2004). Primary delusion cannot be considered as a 'knowledge statement about empirical matters' (i.e. beliefs) but more as a quasi-metaphorical statement (Blondel 1914; Parnas 2004; Spitzer 1990), expressing (pathic) alterations 'in the structure of experience', which affect the very 'sense of reality', i.e. the sense of embodied self-presence to the shared world (i.e. the existential feelings (Ratcliffe 2008)). The ontological framework of experience is modified with an emergence of altered articulations of space, time, causality and self-identity. 'The significance is of a special kind; it always carries a great import, is urgent and personal, *a sign or message from another world*' (Schneider 1959: 104). For the patient, his delusional 'evidence' stems primarily from a non-conceptual 'felt' experience; the latter being a touchstone of a private, unique and absolute sense of certitude (Müller-Suur 1950, 1954, 1962). This certitude, even if 'thematically' vague in the nascent stages of delusional experience is nonetheless overwhelming from the very start. The '*sense of uncertainty*' of delusional mood is itself '*absolutely certain*' (Müller-Suur 1950). The schizophrenic certainty articulates itself passively as an illuminating self-affection or sensation, whereas the 'paranoiac' delusional certainty is 'achieved', i.e. it is hard-earned, through observation and reflection over time (Müller-Suur 1950, 1954). Primary delusion cannot be challenged by some more fundamental dataset. The patients typically do not seek social validation, are indifferent to empirical proofs and only rarely act upon their delusions (Parnas 2004). The sense of certainty (i.e. originary delusional experience) often persists, even after the patient is said to have remitted from a frankly delusional condition.

For the secondary/primary distinction of Jaspers, we have proposed another, more descriptive terms: 'empirical' (secondary) versus 'autistic solipsistic' (primary) delusions[5] (Parnas 2004). Empirical delusions display a propositional belief-structure, concern our shared mundane framework, and involve an incorrect *judgement of reality* but the *sense of reality* remains mainly intact. These delusions typically deal with worldly affairs in which the patient is engaged and where he seeks the evidence supporting his claims. A statement 'I know that I am persecuted by my boss' is an epistemic statement with a structure similar to that of a statement 'I know that Berlin is the capital of Germany'.

'Autistic-solipsistic' (primary) delusions are of self-experiential origin (with *altered sense of reality*) and reflect a fundamentally altered existential-ontological structure of subjectivity (Parnas 2004). The cardinal point here is to realize that in the 'autistic-solipsistic' delusions, reasoning processes 'do not just follow from experience but are embedded in it. They emerge from the chiasm of experience and judgement'. The nature of reasoning processes (judgements) is not independent of the changes in the structure of experience. The sense of reality, 'presupposed in entertaining beliefs', may be changed or lost: 'With an altered *sense of reality*, patients cannot take things to be the case in the usual way, as the sense of "is" and "is not" has changed' (Ratcliffe 2008: 194). We thus disagree with Jaspers on the issue of incomprehensibility of schizophrenia (Parnas and Sass 2008). We may grasp (at least to a certain degree) the nature of the patient's experience upon adopting a phenomenological stance, in which we suspend our common sense assumption of sharing with the patient the same 'modal space'. Through this kind of 'radical empathy' (Ratcliffe 2012), we attempt to make manifest what is most frequently overlooked, namely the altered structures of the patient's lived world, with other forms of spatiality, temporality, and selfhood etc. For the patient, his delusional evidence stems primarily from the pre-reflectively lived anomalous experience, a source of a private and unique conviction, which cannot be grasped within a 'defective reality-testing' model (Sass 1994). We may encounter here 'a double book-keeping' (i.e. a peculiar co-existence of rationality and irrationality[6]). First-person accounts of such states suggest that the patient often feels a unique and superior access to (another) reality, ahead of, and more 'sophisticated' than what is currently accepted as valid in the socially prevailing world-view (Saks 2007, 2009).

[5] Such rumination appear sometimes to be linked to an inability to distinguish between different modes of intentionality; here perhaps between a remembered fantasy and a factual memory.

[6] An example, given by Bleuler (1950) is of a university professor, who after his discharge as 'cured', dedicated a treatise to his mistress, signed 'Lord of the Universe'.

Hallucination and psychosis

Since Esquirol, hallucination has been defined as 'perception without an object'. This definition survived basically unchanged to become incorporated in the contemporary diagnostic systems. Analogously to the issue of delusion, the notion of hallucination was problematized in 1855 at a debate of the Societé Médico-Psychologique in Paris. Three questions, some still resonating in our time, were discussed (Berrios 2006): (1) can hallucination be considered as a 'normal' experience? (2) Is there a seamless continuum between sensation, image, and hallucination? (3) Is the nature of hallucinations similar to that of dreams and ecstatic trance states?

In general, hallucination has been, and still is, considered mechanistically, as an abnormal signal from dysfunctional brain module(s) (a view of hallucination proposed quite early by Tamburini (1876) as a form of *epilepsie sensorielle*, quoted in Ey 1973: 915). Hallucinations are claimed to occur in a substantial proportion of normal people and across a wide variety of psychiatric (including non-psychosis) diagnoses (Larøi et al. 2012). These latter claims are perhaps in part explained by methodological deficiencies in many recent studies (Stanghellini et al. 2012). Moreover, the view of hallucination as an abnormal *species of perception* has been regularly questioned (Ey 1973; Merleau-Ponty 2012).

In relation to psychosis, our concern comprises two 'interrelated issues': first, does it make sense to consider hallucination as a unitary experiential phenomenon, and, second, does hallucination always signify a psychotic loss of rationality (and if so, in what way)?

It seems that the answer to both questions is negative. For example, in the visual hallucinations of a full-blown delirium tremens, the hallucinatory object is experientially given as a fully transcendent entity, characterized by 'corporeality' (*Leibhaftigkeit*), and integrated in the patient's perceptual field. The patient therefore reacts as he would react to a perception. He is psychotic because his entire lived reality is altered. He has lost both a normal 'sense' and 'judgement' of reality. However, his hallucination remains a temporally circumscribed abnormal event, and is considered as such after recovery. Another type of organic hallucination is 'eidolia', often with an intense and lively, transcendent pictorial character. However, the patient remains aware of its imaginary nature: '[l'eidolie] fascine la conscience du sujet sans l'engager dans le jugement de réalité' (Ey 1973: 334). 'The pictures, however lively, remain mere *images* for the patient, pointing nowhere beyond themselves and without belonging to the perceived reality' (Ey 1973: 334). The patient is not suffering from psychosis because 'il est à la foi conscient de la présence de ce qui est percu et de son absence de réalité' (Ey 1973: 340). He remains in the intersubjective perceptual world, with intact sense *and* judgement of reality. Moreover, 'the [morbid] experience is not a part of the historical continuity of his personality nor is it at the center of his lived situation' (Ey 1973: 339).

In the auditory-verbal hallucinations of schizophrenia, the subject is only rarely confronted with a hallucinatory object that appears as phenomenologically entirely transcendent (external) or 'objective'. Nor is the experiencing of the hallucinatory object always best captured by the sensory, i.e. acoustic-auditive terms.

At the origin of hallucination there is a progressive objectivation of the subject himself who thereby becomes his own object. Hallucination articulates itself from an original pathic affection, gradually reversed and articulated as *another presence* (e.g. the transition from a loss of thought-ipseity over audible thoughts to auditory hallucinations). The sense of this new alterity has typically no spatial or temporal structures characteristic of perceptual modality. There is a sense of oppressing proximity ('the dark space' (Minkowski 1936)) and lack of a thick temporal contour. The affection happens abruptly and its proximity precludes any evasion to a protective distance. In short, hallucination happens *within the intimacy of subjectivity itself*. Hallucination is 'lived as a radical, unique inversion of the subjective and the objective ... which happens in the private intimacy of consciousness' (Ey 1973: 69). As an essentially *pathic event* (Straus 1935; Gennart 2011), the original affection is undeniably real and true (as affection) from the first person perspective. We, as psychiatrists, rephrase this experience into the third-person terms, calling it 'hallucination'. The patient often expresses the experience of 'another presence' in the available sensory vocabulary even though his actual experience often lacks perceptual qualities (e.g. 'soundless voices' (Bleuler 1911)). Most often, the patient distinguishes his perceptions from hallucinations and typically does not expect the psychiatrist to be able to hear his 'voices'. Merleau-Ponty (2012) says that what protects a normal man from hallucinations is an intact structure of the lived space. We can rephrase it by saying that a normal man is protected from hallucinations by his 'sense of reality', i.e. by living pre-reflectively immersed in the shared perceptual world (in the shared modal space). Analogously to the origin of autistic-solipsistic (primary) delusions, auditory hallucinations in schizophrenia reflect a profound 'experiential alteration' that may found another ontological framework and stance (e.g. a claim of a unique access to the deeper layers of reality). To the extent that the patient is able to keep his mundane and private frameworks adequately separated, he is in a successful position of 'double book-keeping'. When enacting or overwhelmed by his hallucinatory experience, the patient's sense and judgement of reality become sufficiently impaired as to qualify his condition as an instance of psychosis. In this perspective, hallucination and delusion, as well as passivity phenomena, appear to be much more closely related (Ey 1973; Gennart 2011) than what is commonly represented in the psychiatric literature. In the individual patient, these phenomena often substitute or complement each other.

Unitary and neurotoxic psychosis

For some years there has been a vigorous revival of the notion of 'Unitary Psychosis', merging the schizophrenic and affective spectrums into one disorder. A major source of this revival is to be suspected in the ongoing massive simplification of psychopathology (e.g. a psychopathological description limited to 'positive' and 'negative' symptoms). The corresponding checklists and scales are insensitive to qualitative, experiential, and gestaltic differences (a heterogeneity illustrated by the above exposition of psychotic phenomena). Such descriptive simplification bolsters the notion of Unitary Psychosis because it facilitates the empirical findings of 'dimensionality' of symptomatic distributions with absent 'points of rarity'. In addition, a demonstration of few, shared genetic markers and some similarities in neurocognitive profiles in schizophrenia and bipolar illness are taken to validate the unitary idea. Yet it is a conceptual error to assume that if x is a part of both y and z, it is also responsible for the distinctive articulations of y and z. Lawrie et al. (2010) rightly noted that the unitary proposal is both vaguely conceptualized and empirically unfounded. We can add that the distinction between schizophrenia and bipolar illness should be ideally linked to the considerations on the prototypical 'whatness' of these disorders (residing in the alterations of the structure of subjectivity (Parnas 2011, 2012)), rather than to rely on the quantitative checklist-scores. Consider these two contrastively constructed cases:

1. Bipolar disorder. 40-year-old married man, owner of a successful business, energetic, efficient, sociable, with a history of two severe manic episodes with hyperactivity, sleeplessness, flight of ideas, and grandiose projects of competing Google out of business. One of the episodes necessitated involuntary admission. Prophylactic lithium treatment.
2. Schizophrenia. 40 years old, living alone, unemployed bachelor, who always had a sense of being confined to the interiority of his mind, with a diminished sense of self-presence and a sense of lacking immersion in the world, feeling profoundly different from, and unable to reach out to others, socially isolated, spending most of his time visiting para-psychological websites. Three past hospitalizations with a paranoid-hallucinatory psychotic condition. On continuous antipsychotic medication.

Does it make sense to claim that these two patients suffer from the same disorder because there is some genetic vulnerability overlap? No, this scenario emphasizes the fact that the ontology of the psychiatric object (the patient's experience, expression and existence) should play a foundational role in any sensical psychiatric classification.

The hypothesis of neuro-toxicity of 'untreated psychosis' has been intensely investigated for the last 15 years (McGlashan 2006; Yung et al. 2003). This idea was originally motivated by the findings of a cognitive decline in some patients over the course of psychotic illness. The hypothesis generated a worldwide research interest in delaying the onset and shortening the duration of a full-blown psychosis. We will not discuss here the empirical merits of the neurotoxicity hypothesis or its adaptability in the face of negative findings.

Rather, we will assess its dominant conceptual articulation. The original claim is that untreated positive psychotic symptoms, i.e. delusions and hallucinations, exert toxic effects on the underlying neural substrate, leading to neurodegenerative changes, which in turn are responsible for cognitive and functional decline. However, such formulation is incoherent if viewed on the philosophical premises of neurobiological research. Mainstream neuroscience assumes an ontological monism (identity theory) of a physicalist type. On this view, hallucinations and delusions are identical with malfunctioning neural substrate. In other words, psychosis does not 'really' exist as a meaningful and causally relevant phenomenological entity, but simply is the malfunctioning substrate. In a less radical formulation, psychosis is a causally inert epiphenomenon of neurobiological processes. Therefore, in order for the neurotoxicity hypothesis to be meaningful in its original formulation, it must presuppose some sort of (minimal) dualism or strong emergentism, in which the mental domain, 'qua its mental nature', exerts downwards-causal effects. Otherwise, neurotoxicity simply means that psychosis *is* a neurodegenerative process, which perhaps may be arrested or diminished by direct biological effects of antipsychotic drugs. On the other hand, potential beneficial effects of psychosocial interventions would appear to be more enigmatic in this perspective.

Category, dimension, experience, judgement

All clinicians are familiar with 'threshold cases', where it may seem arbitrary, or even impossible, to classify a patient in binary terms, either as psychotic or as non-psychotic. In the empirical, quantitative research, we almost by necessity obtain dimensionally distributed data, and it seems that dimensional models of psychopathological data appear to be more reliable and more valid than the corresponding categorical approaches (Markon et al. 2011).

Many patients, especially those with schizotypal or spectrum disorders, display reality judgements or report anomalous experiences that we qualify as 'sub-threshold' or 'psychosis-near' (Parnas and Sass 2011; Parnas et al. 2005). It is important to note that an 'experience as such', no matter how unusual, by itself can never justify the label of 'psychosis'. Whatever affection I happen to live in my first-person perspective, it has undoubtedly a reality- and truth-status 'as my experience'. The schizophrenia spectrum patients live a variety of anomalous self-experiences (self-disorders), with varying degrees of felt concreteness (Parnas and Sass 2011), yet often without any clear concomitant dislocation from the shared social framework (intersubjectivity). A thorough analysis of how different articulations of anomalous experience may relate to the concept of psychosis is beyond the scope of this essay. Suffice to say here is that in order to address such issues we need more sophisticated descriptive and conceptual tools than merely the scores on scales of positive symptoms and 'operational' definitions of those symptoms.

In general, as illustrated earlier, anomalous experience becomes an index of psychosis only if it translates itself into judgements or behaviours that testify to a radically irrational understanding of the world.

Conclusions

Psychosis is a multi-dimensional notion designating a condition of being afflicted by a 'radical irrationality' or a radical 'displacement from intersubjectivity', the latter broadly understood as a social matrix of the 'we-perspective'. This irrationality manifests itself either through 'propositional' thought contents and their linguistic propositional expressions (delusions), or it is 'implicit' in the alterations of other anthropological dimensions, such as action, expression, affectivity, and existential patterns.

The nature and degree of 'radical irrationality' cannot be specified in advance, without regard for contextual and normative factors. In other words, the concept of psychosis resists a simple, unequivocal 'operational' definition, a fact that always led to compensatory attempts of invoking hypothetical causal mechanisms. However, we are today still without biological- or other extra-clinical markers to demarcate the concept of psychosis (a situation very aptly illustrated by the recent diagnostic debate on the mental state of a Norwegian mass killer, Anders Behring Breivik). Heinimaa has observed that only 'a person' (rather than a 'symptom') may be psychotic (Heinimaa 2000). A 'person' is a primitive (non-reducible) term (Strawson 1959), referring to a unique human being, with her particular personality, dispositions, and biography. The concepts of person and context rule out the possibility of a simple operationalization of the notion of psychosis.

The concept of psychosis, although useful, perhaps even indispensable from clinical-descriptive, therapeutic, ethical, and legal psychiatric perspectives, has probably a limited utility in research. This is partly due to the problems of description and definition addressed earlier, but also due to the fact that major mental disorders manifest themselves as *spectra* or quasi-continua, comprising psychotic and non-psychotic conditions. Thus, the schizophrenia spectrum disorders, e.g. schizophrenia and schizotypy, may share aetiological mechanisms (Parnas et al. 2005) that need not reflect or coincide with instances of 'radical irrationality' within such spectrum. The widely recognized lack of progress in psychiatric research has generated much criticism of the classificatory diagnostic approach, with proposals to focus elsewhere: either on *domains* of psychopathology (e.g. depression, reality distortion) (Carpenter 2007) or on behavioural constructs with known neural bases (in the Research Domain Criteria, e.g. negative and positive valence systems, arousal/regulatory systems) (Cuthbert and Insel 2010). The phenomenological approach to psychopathology suggests a somewhat different diagnosis and cure for psychiatry's own current malaise. A key problem is that our very conception of our object of study has been vastly oversimplified, and that this ontological oversimplification has been accompanied by reliance on methodologies (e.g. the structured interview) that are unable to capture the subtle forms of experience and expression that constitute the essential 'psychiatric object' (Nordgaard et al. 2012a, 2012b)

How are we to proceed as psychopathologists, according to Jaspers? In his view it is vital to obtain as correct and detailed an understanding of the patient's experiential life as possible. This includes not merely an exploration of 'what' the patient experiences but also 'how' he experiences, his way of experiencing. This latter task demands an effort to address the 'structures of subjectivity', perhaps the most crucial aspect of phenomenological investigation. Jaspers urges us to elicit and attend to the patients' self-descriptions, while paying close attention to their expressive behaviour and whatever results various psychological tests can deliver. This combination of methods can be difficult to carry out and is fallible. There is, however, no alternative, short of giving up entirely on the very project of psychiatry itself-because, as Jaspers put it, 'a psychopathology which simply confines itself to what can be directly perceived through the senses becomes inevitably a psychopathology without a psyche' (1997: 20).

References

American Psychiatric Association. (2000). *Diagnostic and Statistical Manual of Mental Disorders, Fourth Edition, Text Revision*. Washington, DC: American Psychiatric Association.

Andreasen, N.C. (2007). 'DSM and the Death of Phenomenology in America: an example of unintended consequences', *Schizophrenia Bulletin*, **33**: 108–112.

Basso, E. (2012). 'From the Problem of the Nature of Psychosis to the Phenomenological Reform of Psychiatry. Historical and Epistemological Remarks on Ludwig Binswanger's Psychiatric Project', *Medicine Studies*, 3(4): 415–452.

Berrios, G. (2006). *The History of Mental Symptoms*. Cambridge: Cambridge University Press.

Blankenburg, W. (1965). 'Zur Differentialphänomenologie der Wahrnehmung. Eine Studie über abnormes Bedeutungserleben', *Nervenarzt*, **36**: 285–298.

Bleuler, E. (1911). 'Dementia Praecox oder Gruppe der Schizophrenien', in G. Aschaffenburg (ed), *Handbuch der Psychiatrie*. Spezieller Teil, 4. Abteilung, 1. Häfte. Leipzig: Deuticke. Reprinted in Zinkin, J., Lewis, N.D.C. (trans.) (1950). *Dementia Praecox or the Group of Schizophrenias*. New York, NY: International University Press.

Blondel, C. (1914). *La conscience morbide. Essay de psychopathologie générale*. Paris: Felix Alcan.

Bourdieu, P. (1990). *The Logic of Practice* (R. Nice, trans.). London: Polity Press.

Burgy, M. (2008). 'The Concept of Psychosis: Historical and Phenomenological Aspects', *Schizophrenia Bulletin*, **34**: 1200–1210.

Carpenter, W. (2007). 'Deconstructing and Reconstructing Illness Syndromes Associated with Psychosis', *World Psychiatry*, **6**: 92–93.

Conrad, K. (1958). *Die beginnende Schizophrenie. Versuch einer Gestaltanalyse des Wahns*. Stuttgart: Thieme

Cuthbert, B.N., Insel, T.R. (2010). 'Toward new approaches to psychotic disorders: the NIMH Research Domain Criteria project', *Schizophrenia Bulletin*, **36**: 1061–1062.

Damasio, A. (1999). 'How the Brain Creates the Mind', *Scientific American*, **281**: 112–117.

Damasio, A. (2003). 'Feelings of Emotion and the Self', *Annals of the New York Academy of Sciences*, **1001**: 253–261.

Ey, H. (1973). *Traité des Hallucinations*, Vols I and II. Paris: Masson.

Fenichel, O. (1945). *The Psychoanalytic Theory of Neurosis*. New York, NY: W.W. Norton & Company, Inc.

Frances, A.J., Widiger, T. (2012). 'Psychiatric Diagnosis: Lessons from the DSM-IV Past and the DSM-5 Future', *Annual Review of Clinical Psychology*, **8**: 109–130.

Gennart, M. (2011). *Corporéité et présence. Jalons pour une approche du corps dans la psychose*. Argenteuil: Le Cercle Hermeneutique.

Gigerenzer, G. (2007). *Gut Feelings: The Intelligence of the Unconscious*. New York, NY: Viking Press.

Heidegger, M. (1996). *Being and Time* (J. Stambaugh, trans.). Albany, NY: State University of New York Press. (Original work published in 1953.)

Heinimaa, M. (2000). 'On the Grammar of Psychosis', *Medicine, Health Care and Philosophy*, 3: 39–46.

Heinimaa, M. (2002). 'Incomprehensibility: the Role of the Concept in DSM-IV Definition of Schizophrenic Delusions', *Medicine, Health Care and Philosophy*, **5**: 291–295.

Henry, M. (1973). *The Essence of Manifestation* (G. Etzkorn, trans.). The Hague: Martinus Nijhoff.

Husserl, E. (1982). *Ideas Pertaining to a Pure Phenomenology and to a Phenomenological Philosophy. First book* (E. Kersten, trans.). The Hague: Kluwer.

Janet, P. (1926). *De l'angoisse à l'extase*. Paris: Felix Alcan.

Jaspers, K. (1913). *Allgemeine Psychopathologie* (1st edn). Berlin: Springer.

Jaspers, K. (1963). *General Psychopathology* (7th edn) (J. Hoenig, M.W. Hamilton, trans.). Chicago, IL: University of Chicago Press.

Jaspers, K. (1997). *General Psychopathology* (7th edn) (J. Hoenig, M.W. Hamilton, trans.). Baltimore, MD: Johns Hopkins University Press.

Kernberg, O.F. (1975). *Borderline Conditions and Pathological Narcissism*. New York, NY: Jason Aroson.

Larøi, F., Sommer, I.E., Blom, J.D., Fernyhough, C., Ffytche, D.H., Hugdahl, K., *et al.* (2012). 'The Characteristic Features of Auditory Verbal Hallucinations in Clinical and Nonclinical Groups: State-of-the-Art Overview and Future Directions', *Schizophrenia Bulletin*, **38**: 724–733.

Lawrie, M.S., Hall, J., McIntosh, A.M., Owens, D.G.C. (2010). 'The continuum of psychosis: scientifically unproven and clinically impractical', *British Journal Psychiatry*, **197**: 423–425.

Markon, K.E., Chmielewski, M., Miller, C.J. (2011). 'The Reliability and Validity of Descrete and Continuous Measures of Psychopathology: A quantitative review', *Psychological Review*, **137**: 856–879.

Marková, I.S., Berrios, G.E. (2009). 'Epistemology of mental symptoms', *Psychopathology*, **42**: 343–349.

McGlashan, T.H. (2006). 'Is active psychosis neurotoxic?', *Schizophrenia Bulletin*, **32**(4): 609–613.

Merleau-Ponty, M. (1945/2012). *Phenomenology of Perception* (D.A. Langes, trans.). London: Routledge.

Minkowski, E. (1936). *Vers une cosmologie. Fragments philosophiques*. Paris: Aubier-Montaigne.

Minkowski, E. (1927). *La schizophrénie. Psychopathologie des schizoïdes et des schizophrenes*. Paris: Payot.

Müller-Suur, H. (1950). 'Das Gewissheitsbewusstsein beim schizophrenen und beim paranoischen Wahnerleben', *Fortschritte der Neurologie Psychiatrie und ihrer Grenzgebiete*, **18**: 44–51.

Müller-Suur, H. (1954). 'Die Wirksamkeit allgemeiner Sinnhorizonte im schizophrenen Wahnerleben', *Fortschritte der Neurologie Psychiatrie und ihrer Grenzgebiete*, **22**: 38–44.

Müller-Suur, H. (1962). 'Das Schizophrene als Ereignis', in H. Kranz (ed), *Psychopathologie Heute*. Stuttgart: Thieme, 81–93.

Needham, R. (1972). *Belief, Language, and Experience*. Chicago, IL: The University Chicago Press.

Nordgaard, J., Sass, L.A., Parnas, J. (2012a). 'The Psychiatric Interview: Validity, Structure and Subjectivity', *European Archives of Psychiatry and Clinical Neuroscience*, first published online September 2012 (doi: 10.1007/s00406-012-0366-z).

Nordgaard, J., Sæbye, D., Parnas, J. (2012b). 'Assessing the validity of a structured psychiatric diagnostic interview in a first-admission hospital sample', *World Psychiatry*, **11**: 181–185.

Parnas, J., Bovet, P. (1993). 'Schizophrenic delusions: a phenomenological approach', Schizophr Bull, **19**(3):579-97.

Parnas, J. (2004). 'Belief and pathology of self-awareness: A phenomenological contribution to the classification of delusions', *Journal Consciousness Studies*, 11: 148–161.

Parnas, J. (2011). 'A disappearing heritage: The clinical core of schizophrenia', *Schizophrenia Bulletin*, 7(6): 1121–1130.

Parnas, J. (2012). 'The Core Gestalt of Schizophrenia', *World Psychiatry*, 11(2): 67–69.

Parnas, J., Bovet, P. (1991). 'Autism in Schizophrenia Revisited', *Comprehensive Psychiatry*, **32**: 7–21.

Parnas, J., Bovet, P., Licht, D. (2005). 'Cluster A Personality Disorders: A Review (followed by peer commentaries)', in M. Maj, H. Aksiskal, J.E. Mezzich, A. Okasha (eds), *Personality Disorders*. WPA Series: Evidence and Experience in Psychiatry. Chichester: John Wiley & Sons, 1–74.

Parnas, J., Bovet, P., Zahavi, D. (2002). 'Schizophrenic Autism: Clinical Phenomenology and Pathogenetic Implications', *World Psychiatry*, 1: 131–136.

Parnas, J., Sass, L.A. (2008). 'Varieties of "Phenomenology": On Description, Understanding, and Explanation in Psychiatry', in K. Kendler, J. Parnas (eds), *Philosophical Issues in Psychiatry: Explanation, Phenomenology, and Nosology*. Baltimore, MD: Johns Hopkins University Press, 239–277.

Parnas, J., Sass, L.A. (2011). 'The Structure of Self-consciousness in Schizophrenia', in S. Gallagher (ed), *The Oxford Handbook of the Self*. Oxford: Oxford University Press, 521–546.

Ratcliffe, M. (2008). *Feelings of Being: Phenomenology, Psychiatry and the Sense of Reality*. Oxford: Oxford University Press.

Ratcliffe, M. (2012). 'Phenomenology as a Form of Empathy', *Inquiry: An Interdisciplinary Journal of Philosophy*, **55**(5): 473–495.

Saks, E. (2007). *The Center Cannot Hold. A Memoir of my Schizophrenia*. London: Virago.

Saks, E. (2009). 'Some Thoughts on Denial of Mental Illness', *American Journal Psychiatry*, **166**: 972–973.

Sass, L. (1994). *The paradoxes of delusion*. Ithaca, NY: Cornell University Press.

Schneider, K. (1950). *Klinische Psychopathologie* (3th enlarged edn of the contributions to psychiatry). Stuttgart: Thieme. Reprinted in Hamilton, M.W., Anderson, E.W. (trans.) (1959). *Clinical Psychopathology*. New York, NY: Grune and Stratton.

Searle, J. (1992). *The Rediscovery of the Mind*. Cambridge, MA: The MIT Press.

Shafir, E., LeBoeuf, R.A. (2002). 'Rationality', *Annual Review of Psychology*, **53**: 491–517.

Skodlar, B., Henriksen, M.G., Sass, L.A., Nelson, B., Parnas, J. (2012). 'Cognitive-Behavioral Therapy for Schizophrenia—A Critical Evaluation of its Theoretical Framework from a

Clinical-Phenomenological Perspective', *Psychopathology*, first published online October 2012 (doi: 10.1159/000342536).

Spitzer, M. (1990). 'On Defining Delusions', *Comprehensive Psychiatry*, **31**: 377–397.

Stanghellini, G., Langer, A.I., Ambrosini, A., Cangas, A.J. (2012). 'Quality of Hallucinatory Experience: Difference Between Clinical and Non-Clinical Samples', *World Psychiatry*, **11**: 110–113.

Straus, E. (1935). *Vom Sinn der Sinne. Ein Beitrag zur Grundlegung der Psychologie*. Berlin: Springer.

Strawson, P. (1959). *Individuals*. London: Menthuen.

Tamburini, A. (1876). *Contribuzione alle fisiologia e patologia del linguaggio*. Reggio Emilia.

Tatossian, A. (1979). *Phénoménologie des psychoses*. Paris: Masson.

Tomasello, M., Rakoczy, H. (2006). 'What Makes Human Cognition Unique? From Individual to Share to Collective Intentionality', *Mind and Language*, **18**: 121–147.

World Health Organization. (1992). *The ICD-10. Classification of Mental and Behavioural Disorders. Clinical descriptions and diagnostic guidelines*. Geneva: World Health Organization.

Yung, A.R., Phillips, L.J., Yuen, H.P., Francey, S.M., McFarlane, C.A., Hallgren, M., *et al.* (2003). 'Psychosis Prediction: 12-Month Follow Up of a High-Risk ("Prodromal") Group', *Schizophrenia Research*, **60**: 21–32.

Zahavi, D. (2005). *Subjectivity and Selfhood: Investigating the First-Person Perspective*. Cambridge, MA: MIT Press.

Chapter 15

Delusional atmosphere and the sense of unreality

Matthew Ratcliffe

Introduction

Recent approaches to delusions in philosophy and the cognitive sciences generally construe them as propositional attitudes that arise due to a combination of anomalous perceptual contents and cognitive disturbances. For example, Stone and Young (1997) claim that certain delusional beliefs are explanations of affectless and thus strange perceptual experiences, which are arrived at and maintained due to reasoning biases. Davies et al. (2001) offer a slightly different explanation, according to which the delusional content is integral to perception. The belief is then generated in the same way as most other beliefs, via the unquestioning acceptance of perceptual content as veridical. So, in their view, the problem stems not from faulty reasoning but from a failure to veto certain anomalous perceptual contents. An alternative approach is proposed by Campbell (2001), who suggests that the delusional belief causes the associated perception, rather than vice versa. However, what his 'rationalist' account continues to share with perception-first or 'empiricist' accounts is a commitment to explaining delusions in terms of causal relationships between perceptual and belief contents. The emphasis of most recent discussions is upon monothematic, circumscribed delusions, with the Capgras delusion (the belief that a familiar has been replaced by an impostor) receiving most attention, followed by the Cotard delusion (the belief that one is dead or no longer exists). However, there is a tendency to think of delusions more generally in terms of propositional attitudes and associated perceptual contents.

What might Jaspers have said about these various models of delusion formation? This remark from his *General Psychopathology* gives us an indication: 'It is a pity to waste time on torturous, meaningless argument or on imaginary models, however much they clamour for attention' (Jaspers 1963/1997: 22). I suspect this might well have been his reaction (although my own view is that such an appraisal is too harsh). He would have been similarly downbeat about orthodox conceptions of delusion in psychiatry, which are epitomized by the oft-quoted *Diagnostic and Statistical Manual of Mental Disorders* (DSM) definition to the effect that delusions are mistaken beliefs arising from faulty inferences (DSM-IV-TR; American Psychiatric Association 2004: 821). As Jaspers puts it:

> To say simply that a delusion is a mistaken idea which is firmly held by the patient and which cannot be corrected gives only a superficial and incorrect answer to the problem. Definition will not dispose of the matter. (Jaspers 1963/1997: 93)

What is the problem? For one thing, Jaspers emphasizes the need to adopt a kind of empathetic attitude in order to appreciate psychopathological phenomena. It would, in his view, be a mistake to rely exclusively upon a detached, impersonal, objective standpoint towards the delusional person or her delusions: 'The process is not only one of simple observation, like reading off a measurement, but the exercise of a self involving vision in which the psyche itself is glimpsed' (Jaspers 1963/1997: 21). For Jaspers, the best sources we have for this kind of empathetic/phenomenological understanding are patient descriptions offered in the context of interaction, where there is the possibility of clarification through dialogue. Adoption of this empathetic approach does not require the rejection of objective accounts of delusions; the two are complementary. Indeed, as we will see, Jaspers concedes that empathetic understanding (*Verstehen*) ultimately fails when it comes to certain kinds of delusion, leaving us with only an impersonal, medical construal to go on. But this does not imply that empathy is unnecessary in such cases, as we only discover the limits of empathy by adopting an empathetic approach in the first place.[1]

However, Jaspers' principal complaint is that, once we adopt a phenomenological approach, we come to appreciate that conceiving of delusions principally in terms of beliefs is not so much incorrect as beside the point; there is a failure to engage with what is most fundamental to them. Various authors have since challenged the view that delusions are beliefs. For example, Berrios (1991) goes so far as to suggest that they are empty speech acts, and Currie and Jureidini (2001) propose that they are not beliefs but 'mistaken imaginings'. Others, who continue to maintain that delusions are beliefs, have stressed the need for more permissive or nuanced conceptions of belief (Bayne and Pacherie 2005; Bortolotti 2005). Jaspers has a different concern though, and would regard the question of whether or not delusions are beliefs as something of a distraction too. What is missing, he suggests, is an adequate understanding of the nature and role of perceptual changes that are largely responsible for the alleged 'beliefs'. There is a tendency to think of these in terms of perceptual contents of one kind or another (although there is disagreement regarding the kinds of properties that perceptual content incorporates). However, Jaspers draws attention to another aspect of perceptual experience—the elusive 'atmosphere' that pervades it. He suggests that delusions originate in an all-enveloping change to the 'form' of experience ('form' being the manner in which things are encountered by us, as 'perceived', 'judged', 'felt', and so on), rather than localized, anomalous perceptual contents (Jaspers 1963/1997: 58–59). Specific delusional contents are symptomatic of this more general shift in 'mood' or 'atmosphere'. Thus, to make particular perceptual and/or belief contents one's exclusive focus is to abstract them from a phenomenological context outside of which they cannot be properly grasped and to neglect the core, underlying phenomenon. If this is right, we need not conclude that content-based approaches to delusion in philosophy, cognitive neuropsychology, and elsewhere are completely misguided. Nevertheless, given that they are founded upon an inadequate conception (or no conception at all) of an aspect of experience that is central to delusion, they surely require both revision and a change of emphasis.

[1] Phenomenology is not to be identified with empathy, as it is also pursued in the first person. However, in the second-person case, Jaspers regards empathetic understanding as synonymous with phenomenological understanding. I thus treat the two as interchangeable for current purposes.

In what follows, I begin by outlining Jaspers' account of 'delusional atmosphere' or 'delusional mood', focusing upon the 'sense of unreality' that is central to it. Then I critically discuss his well-known claim that certain 'primary delusions' or 'delusions proper' cannot be understood phenomenologically. I reject that view and instead sketch how we might build upon Jaspers' insights by developing a clearer, more detailed phenomenological analysis of delusional atmosphere, thus further illuminating how certain delusional beliefs arise. However, I concede that this task poses a particular challenge for empathy, and suggest that a distinctive kind of empathy is required in order to overcome it. I call this 'radical empathy'. I conclude by considering how we might relate a phenomenological approach along these lines to non-phenomenological research on delusions, and tentatively suggest that recent neurobiological work on 'predictive coding' might offer a complementary way of explaining them. I do not claim (or seek) to naturalize the phenomenology through neurobiology, but I at least maintain that there is potential for fruitful commerce between the two.

Delusional atmosphere

Jaspers distinguishes what he calls 'delusion proper' from 'delusion-like ideas'. The latter, he says, emerge in understandable ways from experience, whereas the former originate in what he describes as a '*transformation in our total awareness of reality*' (Jaspers 1963/1997: 95).[2] According to Jaspers, the delusional belief (the focus of most accounts of delusions proper) is a 'secondary' judgement that arises in the context of a more 'primary' delusional experience; it is a content-specific symptom of a non-specific shift in the person's relationship with the world. He refers to the experience as 'delusional atmosphere' or 'delusional mood', and describes it as follows:

> Patients feel uncanny and that there is something suspicious afoot. Everything gets a new meaning. The environment is somehow different—not to a gross degree—perception is unaltered in itself but there is some change which envelops everything with a subtle, pervasive and strangely uncertain light. A living-room which formerly was felt as neutral or friendly now becomes dominated by some indefinable atmosphere. Something seems in the air which the patient cannot account for, a distrustful, uncomfortable, uncanny tension invades him. (Jaspers 1963/1997: 98)

His claim is not simply that a delusional atmosphere causes delusional beliefs to arise. Rather, primary delusions only become intelligible possibilities in the context of a shift in the overall structure of experience. By analogy, a checkmate situation would not be intelligible outside of a chess game. Thus, in order to understand the delusion, one has to understand the experience in which it is embedded. The problem, according to Jaspers, is that empathetic understanding reaches its limit somewhere along the way.

Delusional atmosphere involves some sort of perceptual change. However, it is not a change in one or more circumscribed perceptual contents, and its precise nature is difficult to convey. As Jaspers says, things are 'somehow' different, in a way that is 'indefinable'. In fact, it is seemingly paradoxical, insofar as 'perception is unaltered'. If one somehow

2 Radden (2011: xv) suggests that 'delusions' are a 'heterogeneous assemblage' and that accounts such as Jaspers', which involve a 'bulwark of central cases', are therefore problematic. I agree with that view and will suggest that what Jaspers calls 'delusional atmosphere' is itself heterogeneous in character.

managed to compile a complete inventory of perceived properties before and after the relevant experiential change, everything would be much the same; red things would still be red, squares would still be square, and so on. What has changed then? Central to delusional atmosphere is an aspect of experience that is seldom acknowledged, let alone described—what we might call the 'sense of reality': 'the experience within which delusion takes place is that of experiencing and thinking that something is real' (Jaspers 1963/1997: 93). Having a sense of reality is not a matter of taking however many things to be real. Instead, it comprises a sense of what it is to be real or unreal. One might suggest that this amounts to no more than taking various propositions to be true or untrue, in other words to having beliefs. However, Jaspers recognizes that a sense of reality is not exclusive to attitudes of belief; it is also integral to perceptual experience. When we perceive something, our perception incorporates not just a sense of 'what it is' but also a sense 'that it is'. It appears as 'there', 'present', 'part of the same world as the perceiver'. Delusion proper, he maintains, originates in an alteration of this ordinarily taken-for-granted sense of things as 'there', where nothing presents itself in that way anymore.

A sense of perceptual presence does not add up to a sense of reality; we can have a belief about what is the case without the relevant state of affairs being perceptually present at the time. However, Jaspers claims that the kind of conviction required for belief is parasitic upon a more fundamental experience of reality. If the experienced world were drained of the sense that things 'are', one's judgements and assertions regarding what is the case would lack conviction. We can, Jaspers says, think up as many definitions of 'reality' as we want, but our thoughts about reality will never add up to a grasp of reality. What is needed is 'something more that this purely logical concept of reality; there is also *the reality we experience*' (Jaspers 1963/1997: 93). If we follow this line of thought, the position we end up with is more elaborate than the view that perceptual experience incorporates a changeable sense of things as 'real', upon which belief depends. There is more to a sense of reality than taking things to be perceptually present and having beliefs. A sense of what it is to be 'not there' depends upon a sense of what it is to be 'there'. More generally, a sense of what it is to be 'not real' depends upon a sense of what it is to be 'real'. So other kinds of intentional state, such as imagining, remembering, anticipating, doubting, and so forth (all of which incorporate a sense of these distinctions) equally depend upon the experienced sense of reality. When that sense of reality is altered, their form is altered along with it (Ratcliffe 2008, 2012). Delusional atmosphere is thus an all-encompassing change in the shape of experience and thought.

One might be tempted to simply dismiss Jaspers' view that perceptual experience incorporates a sense of reality, on the basis that it doesn't reveal itself to first-person phenomenological reflection. Jaspers would acknowledge that most of us are oblivious to the sense of reality most of the time. It is so constant, so engrained, that it is overlooked and only reveals itself when it wavers. So it is not something that we first come to understand and only later apply to psychopathology. Rather, the relevant phenomenological achievement is made salient to us in a second-person way, through permutations of the sense of reality reported by patients. It should be added that delusional atmosphere is not the only form of 'unreality' experience, as illustrated by various first-person accounts of 'derealization' (Jaspers 1963/1997: 63). However, it is not entirely clear from Jaspers' discussion how delusional atmosphere differs from other forms of unreality experience: is the difference one of intensity or are there also qualitative differences? Even so, he at least makes clear that certain delusional beliefs are symptomatic of some kind of shift in the structure of experience and, with it, the sense of reality. And this is why an emphasis upon specific belief contents is misplaced; such contents need be understood as originating in the context of a non-localized change in form. Indeed, Jaspers goes so far as to say that the content of the belief may well be largely 'accidental' in some instances (Jaspers 1963/1997: 99).

What kinds of delusion are accommodated by Jaspers' approach? Presumably, it applies to various delusions that occur in schizophrenia, some of which are elaborate and polythematic. But does it apply equally to the circumscribed, monothematic delusions that have been a focus of recent attention in philosophy and elsewhere? One problem is that delusions such as the Capgras and Cotard delusions are individuated by their contents. These contents are surely not epiphenomenal, given the frequency of their occurrence. However, Jaspers' account emphasizes form and treats content as superficial at best. Thus, even if delusional atmosphere is necessary for the formation of monothematic delusions, it is surely not sufficient, as some additional factor is needed to account for the specificity of the belief. Nevertheless, it is arguable that delusional atmosphere has some role to play here. It has been noted that monothematic delusions are not just associated with specific changes in perceptual content. In addition, there is often a change in the perceptual feel of everything. For example, as well as maintaining that an alleged impostor looks somehow different, a Capgras patient might complain of a more pervasive perceptual change, where 'everything looks strange' and things 'look painted or not natural' (Ellis and Young 1990: 240).[3]

Something else that monothematic delusions share with other kinds of delusion is a resistance to change. As Jaspers observes, the delusional person will maintain the belief 'in the face of all other experiences to the contrary and against all argument' (Jaspers 1963/1997: 104). He indicates that this too can be accounted for in terms of delusional atmosphere. Beliefs usually originate against the backdrop of a shared, social world. The sense of belonging to a public world, in which one occupies a contingent perspective, is integral to the sense of reality. Furthermore, an associated receptiveness to social norms and to the influence of other people plays a vital role in the formation and regulation of beliefs. It is this public world to which the status 'incorrigible' ordinarily attaches. But, with the onset of delusional atmosphere, 'socially accepted reality totters, people become adrift', and reality 'becomes reduced to an immediate and shifting present' (Jaspers 1963/1997: 104). So delusional atmosphere involves at least partial loss of a consensus reality, and thus erosion of a distinction between what is 'part of the public world' and what is 'imagined by me'. Following this loss, a sense of stubborn conviction that attaches to many normal beliefs might remain, but it is no longer anchored to a public world, to a realm where beliefs can be questioned, debated, revised and abandoned. Delusional beliefs are thus formed without the constraining influence of that world, and are also insulated from interpersonal negotiation. The position Jaspers gestures towards here bears some resemblance to Wittgenstein's view that our beliefs rest upon a bedrock of 'hinge' propositions that are accepted as certain, which Campbell has appealed to in order to argue that some delusions are 'hinge' or 'framework' propositions (Campbell 2001; Wittgenstein 1975). The similarities are even more evident if it is accepted that what

3 See Ratcliffe (2008: chapters 5 and 6) for an account of how changes in the overall form of experience might dispose one towards specific belief contents, such as 'I am dead' or 'My spouse has been replaced by a robot'.

Wittgenstein calls a hinge 'proposition' is not really a proposition at all, but something habitual and non-conceptual in nature (Rhodes and Gipps 2008).[4]

Delusions and unintelligibility

So far, I have outlined Jaspers' view that delusional beliefs are embedded in a global change in the structure of experience, and emphasized that a sense of unreality is central to it. But how can 'delusional atmosphere' (and thus the nature of those delusional beliefs that arise within it) be further understood? Many have remarked that it is extremely difficult to describe. As Jaspers says, 'description always proceeds by metaphor'. Indeed, he goes so far as to say that 'it is impossible to express the experiences directly' (Jaspers 1963/1997: 62). He is surely right that people struggle to communicate such experiences. To quote Sass (1992: 46), 'even the most articulate schizophrenics are usually reduced to helplessly repeating the same, horribly inadequate phrase: everything is strange, or everything is somehow different'. However, that people have difficulty expressing something does not imply that its expression is impossible. Furthermore, even if the experience is not, or even cannot, be understood in the first person, it might be possible for a phenomenologically sensitive interpreter to shed further light upon it. Jaspers instead maintains that the 'primary experiences' underlying delusions proper are beyond the reach of phenomenological understanding:

> If we try to get some closer understanding of these primary experiences of delusion, we soon find we cannot really appreciate these quite alien modes of experience. They remain largely incomprehensible, unreal and beyond our understanding. (Jaspers 1963/1997: 98)[5]

However, he does not make sufficiently clear where the limits lie. There cannot be a total embargo on phenomenological understanding here, as Jaspers himself offers a description of delusional atmosphere that incorporates some degree of empathetic insight. Furthermore, he indicates that the transition from atmosphere to belief is something we can make sense of. Delusional atmosphere incorporates a pervasive and unpleasant feeling of uncertainty. Those afflicted with it search for some 'fixed point', any fixed point, to which they can 'cling', and the delusional belief is the outcome of that search. Jaspers adds that this is akin to something we all do on occasion: 'Whenever we find ourselves depressed, fearful or at a loss, the sudden clear consciousness of something, whether true or false, immediately has a soothing effect' (Jaspers 1963/1997: 98). Even so, he insists that primary delusions can only be grasped non-phenomenologically, in terms of a disease process:

> Delusions proper are the vague crystallisations of blurred delusional experiences and diffuse, perplexing self-references which cannot be sufficiently understood in terms of the personality

---

[4] Also complementary is Sass's analysis, according to which certain delusional utterances originate in forms of experience that involve loss of a public reality and thus a quasi-solipsistic predicament (e.g. Sass 1994). It is also helpful, in my view, to consider the role sometimes played by a loss of 'trust', where trust is construed as a habitual background to experience and thought, rather than in terms of propositional attitudes (Bernstein 2011). An all-pervasive breakdown of trust in oneself, the surrounding world and, principally, other people would amount to loss of a public reality that ordinarily operates as a backdrop to the formation and maintenance of beliefs. It would thus be a profound shift in how one finds oneself in the world (Earnshaw 2011).

[5] 'Understanding' (*Verstehen*) is synonymous here with empathetic/phenomenological appreciation.

or the situation; they are much more the symptoms of a disease process that can be identified by the presence of other symptoms as well. (Jaspers 1963/1997: 107)

So it is not the transition from the experience to the belief that resists characterization but the experience itself. And, insofar as we cannot understand delusions empathetically without understanding the core experiences that underlie them, delusions cannot be empathized with. However, Jaspers' account suffers from a lack of clarity over what it is to 'emerge comprehensively from other psychic events' (Jaspers 1963/1997: 106–107). Just what are the limits of phenomenological comprehension? Surely, it is not restricted to the domain of rational or non-rational inferences from perceived or misperceived states of affairs, given that Jaspers himself stresses—on apparently phenomenological grounds—the limitations of thinking about delusions in such a way. And what is the nature of the alleged limit; is it something specific to human psychology or are there grounds for making a stronger claim to the effect that no empathizing consciousness of any kind could ever comprehend the relevant phenomenon?[6]

Regardless of where Jaspers might draw the line, I want to suggest that further phenomenological understanding of delusional atmosphere is possible. Nevertheless, it should also be acknowledged that the kinds of experiential transformation Jaspers addresses are somehow qualitatively different from and much harder to empathize with than more mundane phenomenological differences between people. As Rhodes and Gipps (2008: 299) observe, there is a 'vertiginous feeling' that we have; we are confronted with something that 'puts a strain on the foundations of our comprehension of the world'. Why is this? The problem is not specific to delusional atmosphere. It applies to any experiential change that involves a shift not just in mental state contents but in a way of 'finding oneself in the world' that such contents presuppose. Although the relevant aspect of experience is seldom recognized, it is a consistent theme in the phenomenological tradition.[7] For instance, Husserl (e.g. 1973, 1989) addresses a sense of the world's existence that is presupposed by our various experiences and thoughts. That both parties share the same 'world', in this sense of the term, is something that empathetic understanding ordinarily overlooks; the possibility of difference at that level is not even entertained. Instead, the world is taken for granted as a shared backdrop, as something that *we* belong to. For Husserl and others, this presupposed phenomenological achievement does not take the form of a belief with the content 'the world exists'; it is comprised of a bodily, non-conceptual, habitual sense of practical dwelling, which, in the usual case, is taken as certain (Ratcliffe (2013)). This 'world' is also a central theme in phenomenological psychopathology. Many anomalous experiences are claimed to involve changes in how we find ourselves in the world (and thus in the form of all experience and thought), rather than more superficial phenomenological changes that occur against an intact backdrop of belonging.[8] It is this difference, I suggest, that accounts

6 See Henriksen (2011) for a recent discussion of incomprehensibility in schizophrenia.

7 Most of the work I am thinking of appeared after the publication of the first edition of Jaspers' *General Psychopathology* in 1913. So I am not suggesting that Jaspers should have taken it into account. Rather, I am exploring how his insights might be further clarified and elaborated in the light of subsequent thought.

8 For some recent statements, see, for example, Sass (2003), Stanghellini (2004), Rhodes and Gipps (2008), and Fuchs (2013).

for why delusional atmosphere is both qualitatively different from and also more difficult to understand than more familiar kinds of experience. Outside of the phenomenological tradition, the relevant aspect of experience is seldom acknowledged, let alone characterized, and so alterations in its structure are both hard to comprehend and easy to misinterpret in terms of more specific perceptual or thought contents.

However, changes in the form of experience are, in my view, not quite as exotic as Jaspers' account might suggest. The sense of 'finding oneself in the world' shifts in a range of different and often subtle ways, not just in psychiatric illness but throughout the course of everyday life. Many of these shifts also incorporate alterations in the sense of reality (as one would expect if phenomenologists such as Husserl are right to maintain that a sense of the world's existence is inextricable from a sense of practical belonging). I have referred to the many variants of our sense of reality and belonging as 'existential feelings', examples of which include the following:

> People sometimes talk of feeling alive, dead, distant, detached, dislodged, estranged, isolated, otherworldly, indifferent to everything, overwhelmed, suffocated, cut off, lost, disconnected, out of sorts, not oneself, out of touch with things, out of it, not quite with it, separate, in harmony with things, at peace with things or part of things. There are references to feelings of unreality, heightened existence, surreality, familiarity, unfamiliarity, strangeness, isolation, emptiness, belonging, being at home in the world, being at one with things, significance, insignificance, and the list goes on. People also sometimes report that 'things just don't feel right,' 'I'm not with it today,' 'I just feel a bit removed from it all at the moment,' 'I feel out of it' or 'it feels strange'. (Ratcliffe 2008: 68)

More elaborate descriptions of existential feelings often feature in literature, and they are also a common theme in first-person accounts of psychiatric illness. Delusional atmosphere, I suggest, is a kind of existential feeling or, more likely, several subtly different kinds. If we accept that less extreme changes in the form of experience are fairly widespread, such phenomena are perhaps not so far removed from everyday experience as they might seem. Of course, supplying a name, and adding that something may not be so unfamiliar after all, does not amount to a better understanding of what the relevant experiences consist of or how they differ from each other. However, I will now suggest that we can further refine our understanding of delusional atmosphere by turning to the phenomenology of possibility.

The phenomenology of possibility

Existential feelings in general are difficult to describe (even if it is accepted that some of them are fairly commonplace). As discussed, one problem is that they involve shifts in a sense of reality and belonging that is seldom an explicit object of reflection or discussion. A further problem is that everything can appear much the same as before and yet profoundly different, as illustrated by Jaspers' description of delusional atmosphere. I have suggested elsewhere that the nature of this difference can be understood once we acknowledge the phenomenological role of possibility (e.g. Ratcliffe 2008, 2012). An important theme in Husserl's work (e.g. 1973, 1989), later developed in a largely complementary way by Merleau-Ponty (1962), is the 'horizonal' structure of experience. In brief, when we see an entity, such as a cup, Husserl maintains that we not only see what actually appears to us at the time. We perceive an object of a certain type, rather than a two-dimensional image that is subsequently inferred to be the appearance of such an object. Husserl proposes that this phenomenological achievement is to be accounted for in terms of possibilities. The object appears *as* something that I might walk around in order to reveal a hidden side, and also as something that is accessible to some or all of the other senses. In addition, it appears as something that is actually or potentially available to other people. These various kinds of possibility together form a structured system, which Husserl calls the entity's 'horizon'.

Elaborating on Husserl's approach (in ways that I think he would have endorsed), I want to maintain that experience incorporates practical as well as perceptual possibilities, for oneself as well as for others, some of which take the form of potential activities and others potential happenings. These possibilities present themselves as *significant* in various different ways. Something might appear as 'useable' in some context of practical activity or perhaps, more specifically, as 'something to be grasped right now'. A potential activity might appear urgent, non-urgent, difficult, effortless, pleasant, unpleasant, relevant to some future goal or ongoing project, and so on. Experience incorporates many other kinds of significant possibility too, including possibilities that involve other people in various ways. According to Husserl, the various possibilities that the world offers are inextricable from our bodily phenomenology. Bodily constraints, capacities, and dispositions are implicated in whether or not something is perceivable and equally, I suggest, in whether and how it might be practically significant. It is 'through' our bodies that we experience the various kinds of possibility offered by the world. Jaspers likewise maintains that perception of the world is inextricable from our bodily phenomenology. The body, he says, is a 'background for consciousness' (Jaspers 1963/1997: 88).[9]

If something along roughly these lines is accepted, we can begin to further interpret phenomena such as delusional atmosphere. Of course, a change in the possibilities that one experiences could amount only to a localized difference in the content of perception. A cup would look different if it no longer appeared as 'something to be picked up or seen from another angle', but this would not involve an all-enveloping transformation of the form of experience. However, I suggest that shifts in existential feeling, including delusional atmosphere, can be understood in terms of changes in the kinds of possibility that experience incorporates. Suppose that nothing presented itself as practically significant in any way, that one inhabited a realm from which that kind of possibility, rather than just some of its instances, was altogether absent. This would surely amount to a profound transformation of the sense of reality and belonging. Nothing would appear quite 'there', given that an appreciation of being able to act upon one's environment in ways that have significant consequences is integral to a sense of being part of the world. There is plenty of testimony to suggest that experiential changes like this can indeed happen. Changes in the sense of reality can take many other forms too. Some involve the diminution or absence of 'possibilities for others', the result being erosion of the distinction between one's own perspective and a shared public world. And there are various other kinds of alteration in the shape of interpersonal possibilities. For example, people might cease to offer possibilities such as support and communion, and instead appear only in the guise of threat (Ratcliffe 2008).

It is important to add that the horizonal structure of experience is dynamic. As Husserl (e.g. 1973) emphasizes, one anticipates the realization of possibilities. When they are realized,

[9] See, for example, Stanghellini (2008, 2009) for a more recent and complementary approach to the body in the context of phenomenological psychopathology.

further possibilities present themselves, and the process proceeds in a structured fashion. Anticipation, Husserl suggests, ordinarily takes the form of habitual certainty. As one walks across the road, it is taken as given that one's foot will again find itself upon a hard, flat surface. As one opens the kitchen door in the context of routine activity, one presupposes that the room will appear much as it always does. Against this backdrop of certainty, there are localized experiences of doubt and uncertainty. Hence significant possibilities are not always experienced as 'merely possible'; they can also appear in the guise of different forms of anticipation as certain, uncertain, or doubtful, with certainty being the default mode. And what is anticipated may or may not be realized, the resultant experience involving fulfilment of expectation or surprise. Different kinds of significance can be attached to both anticipated and actualized possibilities. For example, anticipated novelty can take the form of excitement or dread, and a surprise can be nice or nasty. Certain changes in existential feeling can be understood in terms of global changes to this anticipation-fulfilment structure. For example, everything might present itself as contingent, changeable, unpredictable, in a way that could amount to a feeling of insecurity, of being lost, adrift. Alternatively, everything might present itself as surprising. Here, anticipation does not take the form of doubt or uncertainty. Instead, everything appears somehow contrary to what was anticipated. Again, this could take different forms. Everything might appear mysterious, intriguing and new. Alternatively, things might look odd in a disturbing, menacing way. We can thus begin to appreciate how everything might look 'the same but different'. Actual properties of entities, such as colour and shape, may be unchanged. But the kinds of possibility that frame one's experience and thought have changed and nothing presents itself as offering quite what it used to.

Such an approach further illustrates why an appreciation of existential feeling and, more specifically, delusional atmosphere demands a distinctive form of empathy. When we empathize with people in more mundane contexts, we tend to take for granted that both parties inhabit a common modal space. In other words, we assume that others have access to the same kinds of possibility that we do, regardless of how much their various experience and thought contents may differ from our own. What is required in order to empathize with different forms of world experience is a kind of empathy that acknowledges the presupposed world as a phenomenological achievement and also recognizes its variability. One needs to suspend the assumption of a shared modal space in order to contemplate changes in the kinds of possibility that experience incorporates. So, rather than maintaining that delusions proper are incomprehensible, it is arguable that phenomenological understanding can progress further—to some extent at least—through a kind of 'radical empathy' (Ratcliffe 2011, 2012).[10] Others have similarly pointed out that empathy can proceed further once the shared world we habitually take as certain is recognized as a fragile phenomenological accomplishment. For example, Henriksen (2011) describes the empathetic project of attempting to 'reconstruct the altered framework in schizophrenia' and understand its effect upon a person's experiences and thoughts. Rhodes and Gipps (2008: 299) adopt a similar approach, in maintaining that we can 'pursue the imaginative exercise of temporarily suspending those certainties that

[10] In order to empathize in this way, one need not have an explicit, articulate grasp of what one is doing. By implication, one need not construe it in terms of possibility. Indeed, I do not wish to maintain that it can only be articulated in those terms. This is just my own preferred way of conveying it.

constitute the bedrock of our reason itself, certainties that are implicitly challenged by the delusional belief'.[11]

One might respond on behalf of Jaspers that this kind of empathy is simply impossible, but Jaspers does not consider its possibility. So it is tempting to simply assert that the onus of proof is upon the proponent of incomprehensibility. However, a positive case can also be made for it by pointing to all those instances where alterations in the form of experience *have been* described, in phenomenological psychopathology and elsewhere (Ratcliffe 2008, in press). For instance, Sass (1992, 1994, Chapter 7, this volume) and others have offered elaborate accounts of forms of experience that nurture the development of delusions, thus illuminating what Jaspers claimed to be incomprehensible.[12] Even if one were to dismiss a specific phenomenological account as false or at least questionable, such accounts still serve to illustrate that this kind of enquiry is possible.

What, then, does 'delusional atmosphere' involve? My aim here has been to sketch an approach for further understanding it, rather than to offer a comprehensive characterization. However, I will briefly mention three features that appear central to some or all instances of delusional atmosphere. First of all, as mentioned by Jaspers and developed in considerable detail by Sass (e.g. 1994), there can be a change in one's sense of inhabiting a shared, public world, which involves loss of certain kinds of interpersonal possibility from experience. The line between 'my experience' and 'how the world is' becomes blurred, the result being a quasi-solipsistic predicament. Second, as Sass also observes, there is practical disengagement and passivity. The world no longer solicits practical activity in the usual way, and one's relationship with it becomes oddly voyeuristic. Yet objects are not entirely devoid of significance. Although they do not invite activity, they seem strange, somehow fascinating, perhaps horrifying. So there remains a kind of perceptual curiosity. Lopez-Ibor (1982) offers an account of this, according to which there is a diminished sense of agency and, with it, a loss of practical solicitation from the world. Instead of things appearing significant in relation to one's own agency, a seemingly autonomous significance emanates from them, and everything therefore looks strangely different.

A third aspect that is central to many descriptions (including Jaspers' own) is an all-enveloping sense of novelty or surprise.[13] This, I suggest, is plausibly accounted for in terms of a structural change in the interplay between anticipation and fulfilment. Perhaps expectation of some kind remains, but one lacks a sense of its fulfilment. Hence everything seems odd; there is a pervasive feeling of its being somehow contrary to how it should be.

---

[11] However, Rhodes and Gipps (2008) do not make sufficiently clear the distinction between the form and content of experience. In appealing to Wittgensteinian hinge propositions, their account could refer equally to deeply entrenched experiential contents and to the experiential form that I have characterized as a possibility space.

[12] As Sass and Parnas (2007: 65) remark, 'a phenomenological understanding of a disturbed overall mode of consciousness or lived-world may allow one to make sense out of seemingly bizarre actions and beliefs that might otherwise seem completely incomprehensible'.

[13] Sheets-Johnstone (2007) considers the phenomenological role of something like 'surprise' in many instances of schizophrenia. There is an interesting contrast here between the world of at least some schizophrenic people and the world of severe depression, as the latter involves no anticipation that anything could ever be relevantly different to one's current predicament and no sense of novelty either (Ratcliffe 2010).

Something like this would happen if, for example, one still anticipated perceiving things as practically significant but lacked the ability to experience anything in that way. Here, experience would lack possibilities of kind *p*, but retain a sense of *q*, where q is the possibility of *p*. In contrast, it could be that a certain form of anticipation is lacking, that one no longer anticipates possibilities of type *p* but remains capable of experiencing their fulfilment. An account along such lines would be consistent with Lopez-Ibor's view. For example, anticipated practical significance might be lacking, due to a diminished sense of being a locus of projects and agency. At the same time, things might still present themselves as significant. However, that significance would no longer be anchored to one's pursuits in any way and so everything would look strange, perhaps unpleasantly so. I am not sure that we need to choose between these two scenarios. It could be that 'delusional atmosphere' is heterogeneous, and accommodates a wide range of subtly different changes in the form of experience. And it is worth noting that Jaspers does not restrict the term 'atmosphere' to 'delusional atmosphere'. He acknowledges that there are other kinds of variation in this aspect of experience. For example, 'just as the perceptual world may be experienced as something strange or dead, so it can be experienced as something *entirely fresh* and of *overpowering beauty*' (Jaspers 1963/1997: 63). However, there is a fine line between the uncomfortable, uncanny strangeness that he emphasizes in the delusional case and a sense of the world as wonderfully mysterious, novel and profound, and it is arguable that both variants have 'delusional forms'. In any case, the issue is—I suggest—amenable to further phenomenological investigation. Hence, in summary, Jaspers' work provides us with a valuable starting point for a detailed, nuanced phenomenological study of changes in the overall form of experience, along with a treasure trove of first-person descriptions and insightful remarks. However, he gives up too early, having adopted a conception of empathy that is too restrictive.

Belief

An issue that I have not yet addressed is whether the delusional 'beliefs' that crystallize out of delusional atmosphere are indeed beliefs. Granted, Jaspers maintains that they are secondary and that that an overemphasis upon belief distracts from the primary phenomenon. Even so, the question can still be asked. In my view, the conclusion Jaspers' discussion points towards is that there cannot be a simple 'yes' or 'no' answer. It is not clear whether or not delusions are beliefs because it is not clear what the limits of the category 'belief' are. First of all, it is important to distinguish a sense of belonging to a world from specific belief contents. For example, if someone complains that he doubts the world's existence, that belief could take the form of assenting to the proposition 'it is possible that the world does not exist'. Alternatively, it could originate in a changed form of experience, where everything seems unreal to the extent that one's habitual, practical confidence in the world's existence can no longer be maintained (Jaspers 1963/1997: 93–94). As Jaspers says of severe derealization, 'patients have to handle things to make sure they are really still there, have to convince themselves of the existence of the ground by stamping on it' (Jaspers 1963/1997: 63).

So the first thing to be decided is whether 'belief' applies to contents that one accepts in the context of an already given world and also changes in the form of experience, or just the former. A further complication is that a change in the overall shape of experience not only disposes one towards certain beliefs; it also alters the form of belief. The sense of conviction that attitudes of 'belief' incorporate is variable in structure. In the context of a world that seems unreal, all of one's utterances lack the kind of conviction that is ordinarily associated with belief. And it is not clear whether these utterances express a different kind of belief or an attitude other than belief. One might restrict 'belief' to more everyday instances of conviction. But it is arguable that everyday beliefs also involve various different kinds of conviction. My belief that I will die, when it takes the form of a profound and dreadful revelation, is quite different from my belief that I had porridge for breakfast this morning, even though I might be equally convinced of both. Shifts in the sense of reality and belonging can affect the form (or forms) of belief in a range of ways. To quote Jaspers:

> Belief in reality can range through all degrees, from a mere play with possibilities via a double reality—the empirical and the delusional—to unequivocal attitudes in which the delusional content reigns as the sole and absolute reality. (Jaspers 1963/1997: 106)

Talk of a 'double reality' is not intended simply to suggest that there is a halfway house between entertaining possibilities and being certain of something, where one oscillates between believing that *p* and not believing that p. Instead, Jaspers is drawing attention to an altered form of experience where the person seems at the same time to believe that *p* and believe that *not p*. She inhabits a delusional reality where *p* is the case, but she keeps one foot in consensus reality where *p* is not the case. The phenomenology of this 'double bookkeeping' is further described by Sass (1994: 3):

> Many schizophrenic patients seem to experience their delusions and hallucinations as having a special quality or feel that sets these apart from their 'real' beliefs and perceptions, or from reality as experienced by the 'normal' person. Indeed, such patients often seem to have a surprising, and rather disconcerting, kind of insight into their own condition.

Jaspers also indicates that there are various other kinds of conviction. For example, certain compulsive beliefs involve believing that *p* while knowing *p* to be false; 'a *struggle* ensues between the conviction and knowing the opposite to be true' (Jaspers 1963/1997: 134–135). Hence believing something cannot simply be identified with taking it to be the case or knowing it to be true.[14] The issue of whether or not the term 'belief' should be restricted to attitudes that arise in the context of certain forms of experience but not others (and, if so, which ones and why) has not been systematically addressed, let alone resolved. It is therefore unclear whether or not the utterances and associated convictions that are symptomatic of experiential form *x* and those that are symptomatic of experiential form *y* should both count as beliefs. Thus, Jaspers' account not only suggests that the question of whether or not delusions are beliefs is secondary. It also points (in my view, at least) towards the conclusion that the question has been formulated in too simplistic a way. In so doing, it illustrates how engagement with psychopathology has the potential to both complicate and illuminate philosophers' conceptions of 'belief'.

Non-phenomenological understanding

Phenomenology is only one aspect of Jaspers' *General Psychopathology*, and he acknowledges that phenomenological understanding alone does not add up to a comprehensive appreciation of the relevant phenomena. Indeed, he states that the phenomenological attitude

[14] See Hunter (2011) for a detailed discussion of such 'alienated beliefs'.

is only 'one point of view among many and holds a subordinate position at that' (Jaspers 1963/1997: 48). The question thus arises as to whether and how we might relate his insights to current non-phenomenological work on delusions. A word of caution is needed here. Jaspers does not restrict a psychological understanding of meanings to the context of 'phenomenological understanding'. Hence it would be wrong to construe his contrast between 'phenomenological' and 'non-phenomenological' solely in terms of a contrast between 'phenomenological' and 'causal-mechanistic'.[15] However, my concern here is more specifically with the latter. I have already made clear why Jaspers parts company with 'perceptual content plus belief' models: they fail to acknowledge the nature of delusional atmosphere and its driving role, and any non-phenomenological approach premised upon such models would equally fail to do so. There is, however, at least one neurobiological approach that is consistent with much of what Jaspers says: the 'predictive coding' approach.[16] The basic idea is that cognition is centrally concerned with successful prediction. At a non-phenomenological or 'subpersonal' level, the brain is sensitive to mismatches between what is expected and what actually occurs. In the event of a mismatch, an error signal is generated, which triggers processes that work to reduce or eliminate future mismatches. It has been suggested that at least some delusions arise due to a global misalignment between predictions and error signals. As a result, everything presents itself as different from what was expected, despite the absence of genuine conflict between expected and actual perceived properties. The phenomenological correlate of this is the mundane looking salient, in ways that are consistent with the all-enveloping sense of strangeness that features in delusional atmosphere. It has been suggested that delusional beliefs arise out of a need to somehow account for what has happened, again complementing Jaspers' view. As Corlett et al. (2009: 1) put it:

> Prediction error theories of delusion formation suggest that under the influence of inappropriate prediction error signal, possibly as a consequence of dopamine dysregulation, events that are insignificant and merely coincident seem to demand attention, feel important and relate to each other in meaningful ways. Delusions ultimately arise as a means of explaining these odd experiences.

Corlett et al. maintain that a pervasive change in the appearance of things is associated with an unpleasant sense of uncertainty. There is a felt need to resolve that uncertainty by latching onto anything that might make sense of what has happened, thus re-establishing a degree of order and predictability: 'a delusion represents an explanatory mechanism, an attempt to impose order on a disordered perceptual and cognitive world' (Corlett et al. 2010: 348). Hence we have a non-phenomenological explanation that complements Jaspers' view of delusions as tension-relievers that crystallize out of delusional atmosphere: 'affectively charged uncertainty drives delusion formation, through establishment of predictive associations that, while maladaptive, represent attempts to render the world more predictable' (Corlett et al. 2010: 353). Of course, there is much more to be said. The relevant disturbance might involve expected events failing to occur, unexpected events occurring or both. Furthermore, a global failure of anticipation and a resultant sense of unexpectedness could take many different forms. Things might look strangely unfamiliar,

---

[15] See Sass (Chapter 7, this volume) for a good discussion of Jaspers on phenomenological and non-phenomenological understanding.

[16] Thanks to Andy Clark for pointing out to me the relevance of research on predictive coding.

somehow fascinating, utterly novel, threatening or horrifying. More fine-tuning and clarification is thus required at both the phenomenological and non-phenomenological levels. Nevertheless, the parallels between the two approaches at least point to the potential for mutual enrichment. For example, subtle phenomenological distinctions between variants of delusional atmosphere might help facilitate different versions of prediction error theory, while a non-phenomenological emphasis on prediction error might serve to corroborate phenomenological accounts that appeal to a global shift in the form of experience, involving changes in the anticipation-fulfilment relation.

References

American Psychiatric Association. (2004). *Diagnostic and Statistical Manual of Mental Disorders, Fourth Edition, Text Revision*. Washington, DC: American Psychiatric Association.

Bayne, T., Pacherie, E. (2005). 'In Defence of the Doxastic Conception of Delusions', *Mind & Language*, **20**: 163–188.

Bernstein, J. (2011). 'Trust: On the Real but Almost Always Unnoticed, Ever-changing Foundation of Ethical Life', *Metaphilosophy*, **42**: 395–416.

Berrios, G.E. (1991). 'Delusions as "Wrong Beliefs": A Conceptual History', *British Journal of Psychiatry*, **159**(14): 6–13.

Bortolotti, L. (2005). 'Delusions and the Background of Rationality', *Mind & Language*, **20**: 189–208.

Campbell, J. (2001). 'Rationality, Meaning, and the Analysis of Delusion', *Philosophy, Psychiatry, & Psychology*, **8**: 89–100.

Corlett, P.R., Krystal, J.H., Taylor, J.R., Fletcher, P.C. (2009). 'Why do Delusions Persist?', *Frontiers of Human Neuroscience*, **3(12)**: 1–9.

Corlett, P.R., Taylor, J.R., Wang, X.-J., Fletcher, P.C., Krystal, J.H. (2010). 'Toward a Neurobiology of Delusions', *Progress in Neurobiology*, **92**: 345–369.

Currie, G., Jureidini, J. (2001). 'Delusion, Rationality, Empathy: Commentary on Davies et al.', *Philosophy, Psychiatry, & Psychology*, **8**: 159–162.

Davies, M., Coltheart, M., Langdon, R., Breen, N. (2001). 'Monothematic Delusions: Towards a Two-Factor Account', *Philosophy, Psychiatry, & Psychology*, 8: 133–158.

Earnshaw, O. (2011). 'Recovering the Voice of Insanity: A Phenomenology of Delusions.' Unpublished PhD thesis, Durham University, UK.

Ellis, H.D., Young, A.W. (1990). 'Accounting for Delusional Misidentification', *British Journal of Psychiatry*, **157**: 239–248.

Fuchs, T. (2013). 'Temporality and Psychopathology', *Phenomenology and the Cognitive Sciences*, 12(1): 75–104.

Henriksen, M.G. (2011). 'On Incomprehensibility in Schizophrenia', *Phenomenology and the Cognitive Sciences*, first published online 11 January 2011 (doi: 10.1007/s11097–010–9194–7).

Hunter, D. (2011). 'Alienated Belief', *Dialectica*, **65**: 221–240.

Husserl, E. (1973). *Experience and Judgment* (J.S. Churchill, K. Ameriks, trans.). London: Routledge.

Husserl, E. (1989). *Ideas Pertaining to a Pure Phenomenology and to a Phenomenological Philosophy: Second Book* (R. Rojcewicz, A. Schuwer, trans.). Dordrecht: Kluwer.

Jaspers, K. (1963). *General Psychopathology* (7th edn) (J. Hoenig, M.W. Hamilton, trans.). Manchester: Manchester University Press.

Jaspers, K. (1997). *General Psychopathology* (7th edn) (J. Hoenig, M.W. Hamilton, trans.). Baltimore, MD: Johns Hopkins University Press.

Lopez-Ibor, J. (1982). 'Delusional Perception and Delusional Mood: A Phenomenological and Existential Analysis', in A.J.J. Koning, F.A. Jenner (eds), *Phenomenology and Psychiatry*. London: Academic Press, 135–152.

Merleau-Ponty, M. (1962). *Phenomenology of Perception* (C. Smith, trans.). London: Routledge.

Radden, J. (2011). *On Delusion*. London: Routledge.

Ratcliffe, M. (2008). *Feelings of Being: Phenomenology, Psychiatry and the Sense of Reality*. Oxford: Oxford University Press.

Ratcliffe, M. (2010). 'Depression, Guilt and Emotional Depth', *Inquiry*, **53**: 602–626.

Ratcliffe, M. (2011). 'Phenomenology is not a Servant of Science', *Philosophy, Psychiatry, & Psychology*, **18**: 33–36.

Ratcliffe, M. (2012). 'Phenomenology as a Form of Empathy', *Inquiry*, 55(5): 473–495.

Ratcliffe, M. (2013). 'Phenomenology, Naturalism and the Sense of Reality', Royal Institute of Philosophy Supplement **72**: 67–88.

Rhodes, J., Gipps, R.G.T. (2008). 'Delusion, Certainty and the Background', *Philosophy, Psychiatry, & Psychology*, **15**: 295–310.

Sass, L.A. (1992). *Madness and Modernism: Insanity in the Light of Modern Art, Literature, and Thought*. New York, NY: Basic Books.

Sass, L.A. (1994). *The Paradoxes of Delusion: Wittgenstein, Schreber, and the Schizophrenic Mind*. Ithaca, NY: Cornell University Press.

Sass, L.A. (2003). '"Negative Symptoms," Schizophrenia, and the Self', *International Journal of Psychology and Psychological Therapy*, **3**: 153–180.

Sass, L.A., Parnas, J. (2007). 'Explaining Schizophrenia: The Relevance of Phenomenology', in M. C. Chung, K.W.M. Fulford, G. Graham (eds), *Reconceiving Schizophrenia*. Oxford: Oxford University Press, 63–95.

Sheets-Johnstone, M. (2007). 'Schizophrenia and "the Comet's Tail of Nature": A Case Study in Phenomenology and Human Psycho-Pathology', *Philoctetes*, **1**: 5–26.

Stanghellini, G. (2004). *Disembodied Spirits and Deanimated Bodies: The Psychopathology of Common Sense*. Oxford: Oxford University Press.

Stanghellini, G. (2008). 'Schizophrenic Delusions, Embodiment and the Background', *Philosophy, Psychiatry, & Psychology*, **15**: 311–314.

Stanghellini, G. (2009). 'Embodiment and Schizophrenia', *World Psychiatry*, **8**: 56–59.

Stone, T., Young, A.W. (1997). 'Delusions and Brain Injury: The Philosophy and Psychology of Belief', *Mind & Language*, **12**: 327–364.

Wittgenstein, L. (1975). *On Certainty* (D. Paul, G.E.M Anscombe, trans.). Oxford: Blackwell.

Chapter 16

The self in schizophrenia: Jaspers, Schneider, and beyond

Thomas Fuchs

Introduction

The concept of self-disorders has always played a major role for the psychopathology of the psychoses. In his *General Psychopathology*, Jaspers distinguished what he called ego-consciousness (*Ich-Bewusstsein*) from object-consciousness and characterized it by the sense of activity, unity, identity, and ego-demarcation. On this basis, Kurt Schneider later coined the term '*Ich-Stoerungen*' (ego-disorders) for the experience of one's thoughts, actions, feelings, or bodily sensations being influenced or manipulated by others. However, neither the term 'self-disorder' nor 'ego-disorder' appears in the tenth revision of the International Classification of Diseases (ICD-10) or the fourth edition of the *Diagnostic and Statistical Manual of Mental Disorders* (DSM-IV), although these symptoms are attributed major importance for a valid diagnosis of schizophrenia. Instead, thought insertion, thought withdrawal, made actions or feelings are regarded as bizarre delusions, commonly referred to as delusions of influence, control, or passivity.[1]

It has often been criticized by continental psychopathologists that this conception of ego-disorders as delusions misses their core disturbance which consists not in a cognitive distortion of reality but in a more fundamental alteration of self-awareness and demarcation of self from the environment (Kraus 2010; Spitzer 1988). Only secondarily do these alterations of self-experience give rise to corresponding delusional convictions. The concept of ego-disorders therefore characterizes a group of core schizophrenic symptoms which may not be ranged on the same level as, for example, simple delusions of persecution.

Moreover, the term 'ego-disorder' may serve as a mediating term which connects the core syndrome of acute schizophrenia with a more basic symptom level, namely the level of prodromal or basic self-disorders which have been investigated by Huber (1983, 1995), Klosterkoetter (1988, 1992), and more recently by Parnas and his group (Parnas et al. 2005a, 2005b; Raballo et al. 2012). The study of the transition from prodromal to acute psychotic symptoms, for example, from alienated thoughts to thoughts aloud and full-blown thought insertions, is of particular importance for understanding the nature and the course of schizophrenia as leading from basic self-disturbances on a pre-reflexive level to disorders of

[1] There is no consistent English translation of 'Ich-Stoerung'. I use the term 'ego-disorder' instead of 'I-disorder' (Spitzer 1988) which seems a bit awkward in the English language. However, there is no reference implied to the psychoanalytic 'ego psychology' and its theory of psychosis (e.g. Federn 1953).

ego-demarcation. The term 'ego-disorder' seems better suited to express this transition. On the other hand, Jaspers and Schneider themselves have contributed to impeding the investigation of transitional phenomena, since they conceived of ego-disorders as all-or-nothing symptoms for the sake of clear-cut nosological distinctions.

In this chapter I will give a short historical introduction into the problem of self-disorders. Then I will analyse the connection of ego-disorders with more basic disorders of self-awareness. I will argue that full-blown delusions of alien control are based on a disturbance of the intentionality of thinking, feeling, and acting. This disturbance of intentionality, for its part, may be traced back to a lack of pre-reflexive self-awareness as it has been proposed by more recent phenomenological approaches to schizophrenia. Finally, I look at the intersubjective disturbances that arise as a consequence of self-disorders which, as I will argue, are always disorders of self-with-others at the same time.

A short history of self-disorders

The phenomena of self-alienation and self-disorders gained particular attention for the first time in German and French psychopathology around 1900. Stoerring (1900) and Pick (1909) had already emphasized the disturbance of the sense of activity or agency (*Aktivitaetsgefuehl*) in psychotic patients: 'They lack the sense of agency, the sense of striving in thinking and acting'. Oesterreich (1907) saw the core of self-consciousness in the affects and attributed the alienation of reality to a loss of self-affection. Dugas and Moutier (1911) introduced the notion of depersonalization to denote the disturbance of an integrative mental process which they thought 'personalizes' mental acts and endows them with a sense of mineness: 'Personalization is the act of a psychical synthesis, of appropriation or attribution of states to the self' (Dugas and Moutier 1911: 13). Later, Berze (1914: 130) attributed depersonalization to a 'dynamic insufficiency of single intentions': 'Since the ego may be regarded as a product of the fusion or integration of the ... single intentions, the weakness of the power of consciousness must manifest itself in a decrease of personality or ego-consciousness'.

Drawing on these approaches in the first edition of his *General Psychopathology* (1913), Jaspers characterized 'personal consciousness' (which he termed 'ego-consciousness' later on) by four formal features:

1. ego-consciousness in contrast to the external world and to others
2. sense of activity
3. sense of identity over time
4. sense of unity or of being one and the same person.

Among these features, the *sense of activity* was crucial for Jaspers, since through it perceptions, sensations, thoughts, feelings, and actions are 'personalized'. The experience of one's mental acts as not being one's own, as alien or automatic was termed 'depersonalization' by Jaspers.

Later editions of *General Psychopathology* were increasingly influenced by Kurt Schneider. Jaspers now put the sense of activity in the first place and further divided it into:

1. *Existenz-* or *Daseinsbewusstsein* (awareness of existence or of being-there), whose disturbance meant a self-alienation in different degrees.

2. *Vollzugsbewusstsein* (awareness of agency), whose disturbance was now equivalent to experiencing one's thoughts or actions as being made, controlled or withdrawn from outside.

In his *Clinical Psychopathology* which first appeared in 1950, Kurt Schneider, for his part, referred to Jaspers' criteria and stated, somewhat simplifying, that in clinical practice only the sense of activity may actually be disturbed (Schneider 1959). However, since the notion of activity could hardly be attributed to feelings and spontaneous thoughts, he substituted the sense of activity by the term 'mineness' (*Meinhaftigkeit*). Disturbances of mineness became now equivalent to the major schizophrenic self-disorders or experiences of alien control. In the last edition from 1967, Schneider subsumed thought insertion, thought withdrawal, thought broadcasting, and all phenomena of 'made' feelings, sensations, and actions under the term 'ego-disorders', characterizing them as an abnormal permeability of the boundary between ego and environment. By this, he implicitly referred to the first of Jaspers' original criteria, namely ego-consciousness in contrast to the external world and to others. This permeability became the hallmark of ego-disorders which in Schneider's system assumed the status of first-rank symptoms for the diagnosis of schizophrenia.

It cannot be denied that Jaspers' and Schneider's emphasis on the concept of ego-consciousness and its disorders marked a crucial progress in the psychopathology and nosology of schizophrenia. On the other hand, the concept also showed a number of remarkable flaws:

1. First, the term 'depersonalization' taken by Jaspers from Dugas and Moutier remained too unspecific. It took a long time until it was removed from the field of schizophrenic ego-disorders and finally came to denote a separate diagnostic entity, namely neurotic depersonalization disorder (ICD-10 F.48.1).
2. The notions of 'sense of existence' (*Daseinsbewusstsein*), 'sense of activity' (*Vollzugsbewusstsein*), 'mineness', and 'ego-demarcation' were neither clearly distinguished nor philosophically grounded terms. It remained inconclusive whether or not *Daseinsbewusstsein* only referred to feelings and bodily sensations and *Vollzugsbewusstsein* only to thoughts and actions, all the more since neither Jaspers nor Schneider came to grips with the question which mental acts and states should be regarded as activities and which not.
3. The possibility of transitional phenomena leading from basic disorders of *Daseinsbewusstsein* to disorders of *Vollzugsbewusstsein*, or from lower to higher levels of self-awareness disappeared, for the already mentioned reason of clear-cut nosological distinctions.

The level of basic self-awareness in schizophrenia had previously come into view, namely in the monograph of the Viennese psychiatrist Joseph Berze, referred to earlier (*Die primaere Insuffizienz der psychischen Aktivitaet*, 1914). He regarded the primary disorder in schizophrenia as a diminished state of awareness or mental activity which he called *hypophrenia*. Kronfeld (1922) and Minkowski (1927) also developed concepts of the schizophrenic core disturbance as a loss of basic mental activity, or of vital contact to reality. But it was not until the 1960s that Huber and his group reactivated these approaches by their concept of 'basic symptoms', later to be extended by Klosterkoetter's investigations of the transitions from basic to full-blown psychotic symptoms (Huber 1983, 1995; Huber et al. 1979;

Klosterkoetter 1988, 1992). However, these concepts still lacked a phenomenological background and rather consisted in a meticulous compilation of single and unrelated symptoms. It was only through the phenomenological approach put forward by Parnas and Louis Sass in the late 1990s that these basic symptoms were integrated to form a unified concept of schizophrenia as a *disorder of basic self-awareness or ipseity*, manifested in a combination of loss of self-affection and complementary hyper-reflexivity (Parnas and Sass 2001; Sass 2000; Sass and Parnas 2003). This approach also resulted in the development of the *Examination of Anomalous Self-Experience* (Parnas et al. 2005b), an in-depth phenomenological interview covering the pre-psychotic or prodromal stages that may extend over years before the manifest psychosis.

From self-disorders to ego-disorders

In these interviews, patients often describe a feeling of a pervasive inner void or lack of presence in the world. This may also be expressed in complaints about a certain opacity of consciousness (feeling like 'in a fog' or 'surrounded by invisible walls') or a general existential feeling of being alien to the world. The disturbance permeates the whole experiential field:

> It is as if I am not a part of this world; I have a strange ghostly feeling as if I was from another planet. I am almost non-existent. (Parnas et al. 2005b: 245)
>
> A feeling of total emptiness frequently overwhelms me, as if I ceased to exist. (Parnas et al. 2005b: 245)
>
> I constantly have to ask myself who I actually am. It is hard to explain … most of the time I have this very strange thing: I watch myself closely, like how am I doing now and where are the 'parts.' … It is not easy when you change from day to day. As if you were a totally different person all of a sudden. (de Haan and Fuchs 2010: 329)

The level of experience that is concerned in these patients is not that of the I or Ego. It is the more foundational level of pre-reflexive self-awareness which was not yet clearly defined by Jaspers and Schneider, and which may be conceived as follows: for each experience to occur it is necessary to assume a first-personal givenness of the experience. Tasting chocolate, feeling pain, running on the street, remembering one's last holidays—all this implies experiencing what it is like to taste, feel, run, remember etc. (Nagel 1974; Zahavi 2005). In order for something to come to awareness or to be experienced, there has to be a basic self-awareness or self-experience. Thus, the first-person perspective inhabits all modes of intentionality and imbues them with a sense of mineness. Self-awareness is inherent in any kind of experience, not as an objectified 'I' or Ego, but as a *tacit self-presence* that is the presupposition for reflexively identifying myself. Accordingly, Parnas and Sass have based their notion of basic self in particular on the work of the French phenomenologist Michel Henry who emphasized the affective basis of conscious life and termed it self-affection or *ipseity*—a fundamental sense of being alive and being present that permeates every perception, cognition, emotion or action (Henry 1973).

Now it seems that this basic or pre-reflexive sense of self or mineness may well be identified with Jaspers' *Existenz-* or *Daseinsgefuehl*—although neither he nor Schneider took a closer look at its possible alterations in schizophrenia. Disturbances of the *Aktivitaetsgefuehl* (sense of activity or agency) would then be equivalent to the full-blown psychotic passivity experiences or ego-disorders. In these, it is the higher level of *reflexive* self-consciousness that is concerned, because the patients explicitly attribute their alienated experiences to others. Whereas basic self-awareness characterizes subjectivity already on the earliest stages of life, reflexive self-consciousness only arises when children develop the capacity to take the perspective of others, which normally takes place in the second year of life (Fuchs 2012). With this, they also become able to *explicitly* distinguish themselves from others. What Schneider called the lack of ego-demarcation or permeability of ego-boundaries is therefore only possible on the level of reflexive self-consciousness (Fuchs 2010).[2] Now the crucial question is: what is the possible relationship between disturbances of mineness and disturbances of agency, or basic self-disorders and ego-disorders?

Before examining this question, a short digression might be in order for reasons of clarification. It has become usage in recent cognitive science to distinguish between the sense of 'ownership' and the 'sense of agency' (Gallagher 2000, 2004). Inserted thoughts or controlled actions are still owned by the subject insofar as they belong to his own mental life. However, they lack the sense of agency, that is, of being performed or enacted by the subject. To be sure, no schizophrenic patient claims that inserted thoughts occur in the mind of someone else, or that controlled actions occur in someone else's body; there is still a subjective experience of the thoughts or movements. Ownership must not be confused with mineness, however. What I own—such as my property, my car, my fortune—is precisely not what 'is me'. Obviously the sense of mineness is more basic than the sense of certain mental acts belonging to me. Therefore, disturbances of mineness and of agency may well be connected: thoughts or actions which lack the sense of mineness may also lose the sense of agency although I still 'own' them as belonging to my mental life. We thus arrive at the distinction of: (1) mineness or ipseity, (2) agency, and (3) ownership. The first is disturbed in basic self-disorders; the second in psychotic ego-disorders, whereas the third is preserved in most cases, except perhaps for nihilistic delusions where patients even deny the existence of their mental life itself. Now back to the question: are disturbances of mineness and disturbances of agency related, and if so, in what way?

A possible connection lies in the concept of 'intentionality' which we haven't taken into account so far (and which is only casually mentioned by Jaspers, let alone related to schizophrenia). Intentionality means the inherent directedness of consciousness towards its contents and objects. This directedness is mediated through single sensations, movements, perceptions or thoughts that are combined and synthesized to form meaningful patterns or *Gestalten*. When reading this sentence, for example, you are immediately directed to its meaning through the single letters or words that you are reading—you read the letters *as* the meaning you are directed to. One could also say that the letters and words as such withdraw from our attention and become *transparent* for the meaning they convey (Fuchs 2005; Polanyi 1967). This is also expressed by the notion of the 'intentional arc' coined by Merleau-Ponty (1962: xvii, 137, 243). Through the medium of integrated elements of sensation, movement, or thoughts, the subject is directed towards the meaning or goal of its conscious act (Figure 16.1).

[2] Drawing on Jaspers, Scharfetter (1995, 1999) has described five dimensions of ego-disorders in schizophrenia (disorders of ego-vitality, ego-activity, ego-consistency, ego-demarcation, and ego-identity). However, these dimensions do not clearly separate disorders on the pre-reflexive level (such as ego-vitality) from disorders on the reflexive level (such as ego-demarcation).

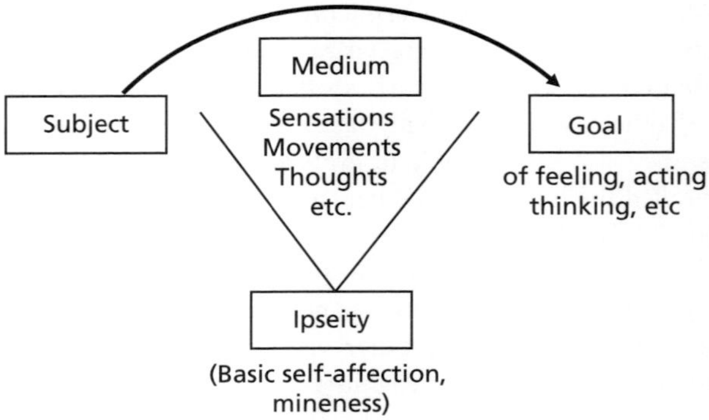

Figure 16.1 Intentional arc.

This mediation is bound to a more basic medium, namely to ipseity: the intentional arc is embedded in the basic self-affection of the subject. Ipseity is what 'animates' the single sensations, perceptions, movements or thoughts and endows them with a sense of mineness and meaningfulness. On the contrary, a lack of self-affection leads to an opacity of the medium. To take an everyday example: if we temporarily lose the sensation in our arm because of a nerve compression, the arm does not only feel numb and somehow alien, but the hand is no longer able to serve as a medium of touch too. Instead of conveying a sense of the touched surface, the movements of the hand will be awkward or clumsy, and it will appear as an alien, thing-like or material object—an obstacle instead of a medium. So we can say: *the mineness of the mediating elements is what makes them transparent, while a loss of mineness results in a growing opacity of the medium.*

Now we can apply this principle to schizophrenia: if a lack of ipseity or basic self-affection extends on the single bodily sensations, movements, perceptions, or thoughts, they will no longer serve as fluent media of intentionality but become resistant and opaque. The subject is experientially separated from the mediating processes which it normally embodies, and these processes will become disintegrated or fragmented, resulting in what may be called a 'disembodied mind' (Fuchs 2005; Stanghellini 2004). The relation of the subject to the world is then deprived of its immediacy, leading to a fundamental alienation. Sensations, perceptions, movements, or thoughts will increasingly appear as objects or obstacles that conceal the world instead of giving access to it. Consciousness will be like a window that has become blind.

However, we have to bear in mind that there might also be a reciprocal relationship: a disintegration of habitual patterns of perception, movement or thought may also lead to a sense of alienation and loss of mineness. To a certain degree, this kind of alienation is an everyday experience: if we repeat a familiar word several times slowly and aloud it may sound strange to us—the coupling of syllables and meaning is dissolved. In the same way, when focusing on a single part of the body, it often no longer functions as a component of integrated habits. If the musician concentrates on his single fingers, he will stumble in his run, as we also will when running down the stairs and thinking of the single steps. The explication of single elements by hyper-reflexive awareness thus disturbs the former familiarity and leads to an alienation and loss of mineness. This may also occur in schizophrenia, as a 'pathological explication' caused by the disintegration of habits or Gestalten (Fuchs 2012; Sass 2000).

Now we have all elements that we need to analyse the possible connection of basic self-disorders and ego-disorders in the course of schizophrenia. There are two stages that we can distinguish in principle:

1. alienation, resulting from a loss of mineness or ipseity
2. externalization, resulting from a loss of agency.

I will take a closer look at these stages, using the example of thought alienation and externalization which finally leads to the experience of thought insertion.

Alienation of thinking processes

Let us start with a historical example of schizophrenic self-alienation:

> If a thought passed quickly through his brain … he was forced to direct back his attention and scrutinize his mind in order to know exactly what he had been thinking. In one word, he is preoccupied by the continuity of his thinking. He fears that he may stop thinking for a while, that there might have been 'a time when my imagination had been arrested.' … He wakes up one night and asks himself: 'Am I thinking? Since there is nothing that can prove that I am thinking, I cannot know whether I exist.' In this manner he annihilated the famous aphorism of Descartes. (Hesnard 1909: 180)

In vain, this patient tries to banish his existential fear of losing himself by constantly observing his own thoughts. His attempt towards self-assurance fails because retrospection and reflection never reach the source of thoughts which should imbue them with a sense of mineness. If the intentional act is no longer embedded in basic self-affection, it remains unrealized and has to be repeated emptily, resulting in hyper-reflexivity (Sass 1992, 2000). On the other hand, the alienation of the thinking process may also arise from a primary disintegration, as is the case in formal thought disorder:

> 'While speaking, I suddenly lose the thread and don't know what I was going to say.'—'Sometimes there are strange thoughts in me that come out of the blue.' 'I have to pick out thoughts and put them together. I can't control the actual thoughts I want.… I think something but I say it different.… (Last time) I could not get the words that were correct to make up a sentence and I knew I was not saying the right thing'. (Chapman 1966: 236)

In these and similar reports of schizophrenic patients we can notice a 'lack of tension' in the intentional arc which normally guides the thoughts, keeps them on the track, as it were, and prevents unfitting thoughts or words from intruding. The train of thoughts suddenly breaks off, interfering thoughts may arise and interrupt the intended course of thinking. Huber spoke of a '*loss of the conductivity of thinking*' (*Verlust der Leitbarkeit der Denkvorgaenge* (Huber et al. 1979: 122)) which also implies an increasing awareness of the single elements of thinking instead of its overall meaning and goal.

Objectification of thoughts

On the next level, these fragmented or intruding thoughts gain increasingly object-like character, as shown in the following cases:

> Each time I think a thought I get a counterthought on the other side of my brain. (Parnas et al. 2005b: 242)
>
> Thoughts always pass down obliquely into the very same spot. (Parnas et al. 2005b: 242)

> Sometimes my thoughts are audible in my head as if I would speak them. (thoughts aloud). (Author's own patient)

With the medium of thoughts being alienated, they lose their transparency for intentional content. Lacking the implicit sense of mineness, the thoughts are no longer 'inhabited' by the self. Instead, they are like material objects localized somewhere in the head, or they become audible and the patient listens to his own thinking. Nevertheless, there is no complete alienation of the thoughts, because they are still integrated in the intentional field and experienced as one's own; in other words, their agency is preserved.

Loss of agency and externalization of thoughts

The next and crucial stage is reached when the dissolution of the intentional arc of thinking is advanced to the point where the fragmented and intruding thoughts appear to be imposed on the patient from the outside:

> I could no longer think the way I wanted to ... It was as if one could no longer think oneself, as if one were hindered from thinking. I had the impression that all what I think were no longer my own ideas at all ... as if I wouldn't be the one who is thinking. I began to wonder whether I am still myself or an exchanged person. (Klosterkoetter 1988: 111, author's own trans.)

What this patient experiences is not only loss of conductivity, but a passivity and disempowerment of her thinking process as a whole. This loss of agency is equivalent to the stage of externalization: the thoughts are no longer experienced as self-generated, but as made or inserted from outside. This is precisely the stage which can be termed '*Ich-Stoerung*' or 'ego-disorder', implying a dissolution of the boundary between self and others.

There have been a lot of debates on how this externalization could be explained. Some Anglo-American authors such as Maher (1988) have relied on rational concepts, assuming that the patients try to explain their irregular experiences in a way which suggests itself: a thought that I did not generate myself must have come to me from outside. However, apart from the fact that this conclusion seems not at all natural or logical, Maher's assumption is not consistent with the phenomenon of inserted thoughts either. In the earlier case example the patient obviously retains a last reservation toward her own experience: She uses an 'as-if' clause two times, thus expressing that 'it cannot be as it seems'. She still knows that her thoughts cannot possibly be someone else's. The externalization is thus not based on an inference or a mere delusion, but is *a peculiar quality of the thoughts themselves.* Jaspers already emphasized that the inserted thought 'occurs *with the immediate awareness* that not the patient but a foreign power thinks it' (Jaspers 1968: 102, italics by the author).

In Frith's neurocognitive theory of schizophrenia, the externalization is explained by a putative self-monitoring mechanism which compares a prior intention to think with the actual thought itself (Frith 1992). This is assumed in analogy to the efference copy mechanism in motor action—the copy prepares the sensory system for the change in the perceptual field resulting from the body's action. Following Feinberg (1978), Frith assumes a similar comparator mechanism for thinking too. If there is a dysfunction of this self-monitoring mechanism, a thought will arise without anticipation and therefore be experienced as coming from outside. However, apart from this efference copy being only a hypothetical assumption in the case of thoughts, it is even not clear what an 'intention to think a thought' could mean. When I intend to think something, I am already thinking it (see Gallagher 2004 for a critique). Moreover, many unbidden thoughts appear in our mind without being deliberately evoked, and yet we do not attribute them to someone else.

Elsewhere I have given a different explanation (Fuchs 2007, 2013) which is based on the temporal disintegration of the intentional arc and shall be outlined briefly. According to Husserl's concept of inner time consciousness, the synthetic temporal processes of presentation, protention, and retention also create a basic continuity of self-awareness that is thus inherent in the intentional arc. With growing fragmentation of these synthetic processes, the diminishment of ipseity may reach the point of creating intermittent gaps in the basic continuity of self-awareness. As a result, the fragments of the intentional arc will not only be experienced as meaningless objects or obstacles but as completely foreign to oneself, as being inserted or, if further externalized, as auditory hallucinations or voices. The discontinuity of self-awareness thus eliminates the sense of agency, leaving the broken pieces of the intentional arc as radically alien experiences. This discontinuity may be regarded as a final result of the diminishment of ipseity which is already found in prodromal states of schizophrenia.

Delusion of thought insertion

At the last stage, the reservation of the 'as-if' is finally given up, and the patients are firmly convicted that others are able to actually influence their thoughts.

> Everybody is able to transmit thoughts onto him. Sometimes he tries to defend himself … but then they try to wipe out his own thoughts by pressure. His own and alien thoughts are intermingled … This 'speech in the head' (*Kopfsprache*) is constantly present and emanates from his comrades. (Conrad 1992: 96)

Here the ego-disorder has definitely turned into a delusion of thought insertion or thought control. What is concerned now is not only the basic, pre-reflexive self but the reflective self or 'I' that is constituted by taking the other's perspective while at the same time distinguishing self and other as different persons. Delusions of control imply a disturbance of both these aspects of intersubjectivity: on the one hand, the patient is unable to take the other's perspective, that means, to transcend his own point of view and to call his delusional conviction into doubt. On the other hand, he is also unable to clearly distinguish between himself and others. This loss of ego-boundaries also shows itself in what Bleuler (1911) called 'transitivism':

> When I look at somebody my own personality is in danger. I am undergoing a transformation and my self is beginning to disappear. (Chapman 1966)
>
> A young man was frequently confused in a conversation, being unable to distinguish between himself and his interlocutor. He tended to lose the sense of whose thoughts originated in whom, and felt 'as if' the interlocutor somehow 'invaded' him, an experience that shattered his identity and was intensely anxiety-provoking. (Parnas 2003: 232)
>
> The others' gazes get penetrating, and it is as if there was a consciousness of my person emerging around me … they can read in me like in a book. Then I don't know who I am any more. (Fuchs 2000: 172)

Such reports show that 'being conscious of another consciousness' may threaten schizophrenic patients with a loss of their self. How could this be explained? In current neurocognitive accounts, the sense of self is regarded as being generated by inferential self-monitoring processes. Corresponding explanations of symptoms such as transitivism, thought insertion or passivity experiences rely on the concept of 'shared representations', i.e. overlapping neuronal representations for the execution of an action and for the observation of the same action in others (Decety and Sommerville 2003). A hypothetical failure of the action attribution system (neuronal 'who' system (Georgieff and Jeannerod 1998)) then leads to self-other confusion and delusional misattribution.

However, such modular explanations miss the basic disturbance of self-awareness that precedes the acute psychotic symptoms often by years. From a phenomenological perspective, the self-other distinction is automatically constituted in every experience as an aspect of non-reflective self-awareness (Parnas 2003). If the primary sense of self or ipseity is disturbed, then taking the other's perspective will become precarious, for it implies the threat of a loss of one's self on the personal or reflexive level as well. Thus, we arrive at the following result: in ego-disorders, the basic schizophrenic self-disorder reaches the point of a fundamental disturbance of subjectivity and intersubjectivity, marked by a loss of the boundaries between self and others. Delusions of alien influence or control are thus not primary cognitive distortions or meta-representational faults but rather the final result of a loss of self on the pre-reflexive level. No matter how these particular disturbances of self–other demarcation are finally termed, there is no question that their absence in international classifications results in a severe drawback for a differentiated psychopathology of schizophrenia.

Conclusion

Jaspers' concept of self-awareness, its dimensions, and disorders may be regarded as a milestone for the psychopathology of the psychoses. In particular, it laid the ground for Schneider's elaboration of the concept of ego-disorders in schizophrenia. On the other hand, in the approach of the Heidelberg school, the aim of drawing clear-cut nosological distinctions prevailed over more fine-grained analyses of transitional phenomena. For this and other reasons, the pre-reflexive self and its disorders in schizophrenia were largely left out of accounts. Nevertheless, Jaspers' term *Daseinsbewusstsein* may be regarded as prefiguring current phenomenological concepts of schizophrenia as a disturbance of basic self-awareness, that is, as a diminished self-affection or ipseity. This can be found in its pure form particularly in the prodromal stages of schizophrenia, leading to a growing sense of alienation and separation from the world and others. While the patients are still aware of their personal self and of course are able to reflect on themselves, this (hyper-)reflexion always comes too late and cannot substitute for the lack of basic self-affection.

The relation of these basic disturbances to ego-disorders on a higher level may be based on the concept of intentionality. The intentional arc of conscious life is realized through the mediating or tacit function of sensations, perceptions, movements, or thoughts which, being combined and synthesized, become transparent for the subject's over-arching intentions or goals. This transparency, however, depends on the basic medium of self-affection or mineness. A loss of mineness results in an alienation and growing opacity of the mediating elements which appear in the field of awareness as thing-like obstacles. Inserted thoughts or verbal hallucinations are the remnants of the broken intentional arc which the patient encounters in his own experience. The fragmentation of the intentional arc in combination with a loss of temporal self-coherence finally leads to ego-disturbances involving a loss of boundaries of self and other. They may be regarded as the experiential core of delusions of influence and alien control.

As we can see, understanding the transition from basic self-disorders to full-blown delusions of alien control presupposes the concepts of intentionality, intersubjectivity, and ego-disorders. Regarding the latter as merely bizarre delusions is equivalent to a surrender of any sophisticated psychopathology.

References

Berze, J. (1914). *Die primaere Insuffizienz der psychischen Aktivitaet: Ihr Wesen, ihre Erscheinungen und ihre Bedeutung als Grundstoerung der Dementia praecox und der Hypophrenien ueberhaupt*. Leipzig: Deuticke.

Bleuler, E. (1911). *Dementia praecox oder Gruppe der Schizophrenien*. Leipzig: Deuticke.

Chapman, J. (1966). 'The early symptoms of schizophrenia', *British Journal of Psychiatry*, **112**: 225–251.

Conrad, K. (1992). *Die beginnende Schizophrenie. Versuch einer Gestaltanalyse des Wahns* (6th edn). Stuttgart: Thieme.

Decety, J., Sommerville, J.A. (2003). 'Shared representations between self and other: a social cognitive neuroscience view', *Trends in Cognitive Science*, **7**: 527–533.

de Haan, S., Fuchs, T. (2010). 'The Ghost in the Machine: Disembodiment in Schizophrenia. Two Case studies', *Psychopathology*, **43**: 327–333.

Dugas, L., Moutier, F. (1911). *La depersonnalisation*. Paris: Felix Alcan.

Federn, P. (1953). *Ego psychology and the Psychoses*. London: Imago Publishing.

Feinberg, I. (1978). 'Efference Copy and Corollary Discharge. Implications for Thinking and its Disorders', *Schizophrenia Bulletin*, **4**: 636–640.

Frith, C.D. (1992). *The Cognitive Neuropsychology of Schizophrenia*. Hillsdale, NJ: Erlbaum.

Fuchs, T. (2000). *Psychopathologie von Leib und Raum. Phänomenologisch-empirische Untersuchungen zu depressiven und paranoiden Erkrankungen*. Darmstadt: Steinkopff.

Fuchs, T. (2005). 'Corporealized and Disembodied Minds. A Phenomenological View of the Body in Melancholia and Schizophrenia', *Philosophy, Psychiatry, & Psychology*, **12**: 95–107.

Fuchs, T. (2007). 'The Temporal Structure of Intentionality and its Disturbance in Schizophrenia', *Psychopathology*, **40**: 229–235.

Fuchs, T. (2010). 'Phenomenology and Psychopathology', in S. Gallagher, D. Schmicking (eds), *Handbook of Phenomenology and the Cognitive Sciences*. Dordrecht: Springer, 547–573.

Fuchs, T. (2011). 'The Psychopathology of Hyperreflexivity', *Journal of Speculative Philosophy*, **24**: 239–255.

Fuchs, T. (2012). 'The Phenomenology and Development of Social Perspectives', *Phenomenology and the Cognitive Sciences*, first published online July 2012 (doi: 10.1007/s11097-012-9267-x).

Fuchs, T. (2013). 'Temporality and Psychopathology', *Phenomenology and the Cognitive Sciences*, 12(1): 75–104.

Gallagher, S. (2000). 'Philosophical Conceptions of the Self: Implications for Cognitive Science', *Trends in Cognitive Science*, **4**: 14–21.

Gallagher, S. (2004). 'Neurocognitive Models of Schizophrenia: A Neuro-Phenomenological Critique', *Psychopathology*, **37**: 8–19.

Georgieff, N., Jeannerod, M. (1998). 'Beyond Consciousness of External Events: A Who System for Consciousness of Action and Self-Consciousness', *Consciousness and Cognition*, **7**: 465–477.

Henry, M. (1973). *The Essence of Manifestation*. The Hague: Nijhoff.

Hesnard, A.L.M. (1909). *Les Troubles de la Personnalité dans les états d'asthenie Psychiques*. Paris: Alcan.

Huber, G. (1995). 'Prodrome der Schizophrenie', *Fortschritte der Neurologie und Psychiatrie*, **63**: 131–138.

Huber, G. (1983). 'Das Konzept substratnaher Basissymptome und seine Bedeutung fuer Theorie und Therapie schizophrener Erkrankungen', *Nervenarzt*, **54**: 23–32.

Huber, G., Gross, G., Schuettler, R. (1979). *Schizophrenie. Eine verlaufs- und sozialpsychiatrische Langzeitstudie*. Berlin: Springer.

Jaspers, K. (1968). *General Psychopathology* (7th edn) (J. Hoenig, M.W. Hamilton, trans.). Chicago, IL: University of Chicago Press.

Klosterkoetter, J. (1988). *Basissymptome und Endphaenomene der Schizophrenie*. Berlin: Springer.

Klosterkoetter, J. (1992). 'The Meaning of Basic Symptoms for the Genesis of the Schizophrenic Nuclear Syndrome', *Psychiatry and Clinical Neurosciences*, **46**: 609–630.

Kraus, S. (2010). 'Existential a prioris and the phenomenology of schizophrenia', *Dialogues in Philosophy, Mental and Neuro Sciences*, **3**: 1–7.

Kronfeld, A. (1922). 'Ueber schizophrene Veraenderungen des Bewusstseins der Aktivitaet', *Zeitschrift fuer die gesamte Neurologie und Psychiatrie*, **74**: 15–68.

Maher, B.A. (1988). 'Anomalous Experience and Delusional Thinking: The Logic of Explanations', in T.F. Oltmanns, B.A. Maher (eds), *Delusional Beliefs*. New York, NY: Wiley, 15–33.

Merleau-Ponty, M. (1962). *Phenomenology of Perception* (C. Smith, trans.). London: Routledge and Kegan Paul.

Minkowski, E. (1927). *La Schizophrenie*. Paris: Payot.

Nagel, T. (1974). 'What is it Like to be a Bat?', *The Philosophical Review*, **83**: 435–450.

Oesterreich, K. (1907). 'Die Entfremdung der Wahrnehmungswelt und die Depersonalisation in der Psychasthenie: ein Beitrag zur Gefuehlspsychologie', *Journal für Psychologie und Neurologie*, **9**: 15–53.

Parnas, J. (2003). 'Self and schizophrenia: a phenomenological perspective', in T. Kircher, A. David (eds), *The Self in Neuroscience and Psychiatry*. Cambridge University Press, 217–241.

Parnas, J., Handest, P. (2003). 'Phenomenology of Anomalous Self-Experience in Early Schizophrenia', *Comprehensive Psychiatry*, **44**: 121–134.

Parnas, J., Handest, P., Jansson, L., Saebye, D. (2005a). 'Anomalous Subjective Experience among First-Admitted Schizophrenia Spectrum Patients: Empirical Investigation', *Psychopathology*, 38: 259–267.

Parnas, J., Møller, P., Kircher, T., Thalbitzer, J., Jansson, L., Handest, P., *et al.* (2005b). 'EASE: Examination of Anomalous Self-Experience', *Psychopathology*, **38**: 236–258.

Parnas, J., Sass, L.A. (2001). 'Solipsism, Self, and Schizophrenic Delusions', *Philosophy, Psychiatry, & Psychology*, 8: 101–120.

Pick, A. (1909). 'Zur Pathologie des Ich-Bewusstseins', *Archiv fuer Psychiatrie und Nervenkrankheiten*, **38**: 22–23.

Polanyi, M. (1967). *The Tacit Dimension*. Garden City, NY: Anchor Books.

Raballo, A., Sæbye, D., Parnas, J. (2012). 'Looking at the Schizophrenia Spectrum Through the Prism of Self-disorders: An Empirical Study', *Schizophrenia Bulletin*, **37**: 344–351.

Sass, L.A. (1992). *Madness and Modernism. Insanity in the Light of Modern Art, Literature, and Thought*. New York, NY: Basic Books.

Sass, L.A. (2000). 'Schizophrenia, Self-Experience, and So-Called Negative Symptoms', in D. Zahavi (ed), *Exploring the Self: Philosophical and Psychopathological Perspectives on Self-Experience* Amsterdam: John Benjamins, 149–182.

Sass, L.A., Parnas, J. (2003). 'Schizophrenia, consciousness, and the self', *Schizophrenia Bulletin*, **29**: 427–444.

Scharfetter, C. (1995). 'The ego/self experience of schizophrenic patients', *Schweizer Archiv für Neurologie und Psychiatrie*, **146**: 200–206.

Scharfetter, C. (1999). Schizophrenic ego disorders—argument for body including therapy', *Schweizer Archiv für Neurologie und Psychiatrie*, **150**: 1–15.

Schneider, K. (1959). *Clinical Psychopathology* (M. W. Hamilton, trans.). Oxford: Grune & Stratton.

Spitzer, M. (1988). 'Ich-Stoerungen: In search of a theory', in M. Spitzer, F.A. Uehlein, G. Oepen (eds), *Psychopathology and Philosophy*. Berlin: Springer, 167–183.

Stanghellini, G. (2004). *Disembodied Spirits and Deanimated Bodies: The Psychopathology of Common Sense*. Oxford: Oxford University Press.

Stoerring, G. (1900). *Vorlesungen ueber Psychopathologie in ihrer Bedeutung fuer die normale Psychologie*. Leipzig: Engelmann.

Zahavi, D. (2005). *Subjectivity and Selfhood: Investigating the First-Person Perspective*. Cambridge, MA: MIT Press.

Chapter 17

Understanding mood disorders: Karl Jaspers' biological existentialism

S. Nassir Ghaemi

For Karl Jaspers, character was indeed destiny; he strongly believed that one could not separate a philosophy from the philosopher. One's personal character was reflected in one's philosophy. Hence before we ask what Jaspers the psychiatrist and philosopher thought about mood disorders, we should ask what Jaspers the man experienced (an aspect of Jaspers not systematically discussed in most previous biographical or historical works).

Beginning with his family, Jaspers' brother Enno seems likely to have had bipolar illness. As Jaspers' biographer puts it: Enno was 'boisterous', 'enjoyed extravagant living', 'fun-loving', 'energetic', 'reckless … squandering his pocket money', and had an 'unnatural optimism about new projects' (Kirkbright 2004). Karl was the opposite in all these respects, and the two brothers conflicted personally. Eventually, Enno 'had a spiral of bad luck, imprudent money deals, the loss of several jobs, and three broken engagements' ending in 'two bankruptcies and a likely cocaine addiction' (Kirkbright 2004). Jaspers wrote of Enno in a letter: 'He cannot do anything with himself and is seized by a greed for entertainment, activity and adventure that are only to be satisfied with financial means that are considerable. All childishness, good nature and lack of formality is, as I must see Enno, shot through with ceaseless egocentric striving for money for consumption' (Kirkbright 2004: 104–105). This is a good description of mania. Enno himself wrote as follows: 'I feel myself in mind and body so fit and capable of achieving as I have never done in recent years. And this feeling of strength at least gives me confidence' (Kirkbright 2004: 105). Kirkbright attributed Enno's 'mood swings' to cocaine, but his manic symptoms long predated his cocaine use. By the late 1920s, as his financial circumstances worsened, Enno sunk into a deep depression, and, despite Jaspers' financial support and efforts to get him psychiatric help, committed suicide in 1931.To the end, Enno and Karl conflicted about money. Jaspers' parents seemed reconciled, writing to Karl: 'Our dear Enno, yesterday evening at 10 o'clock, was gently laid to rest, without a fight, at his own will' (Kirkbright 2004: 106) Enno left a suicide note for Karl:

> Dear Kally! … So I am at an end. At the moment, I am making use of that powder [poison] that I once mentioned to you I have in my possession. The 'family' will later reconsider its position, look seriously and be genuinely shattered, and will admit that all 'guilt' is on my side … And in the end the old farmer's instinct that covets gold can only discover: the man is dead; the ducats are saved. Fare well. Your Enno. (Kirkbright 2004: 106)

Karl did not attend the funeral; his wife Gertrud did.

This family history raises the question whether Jaspers himself suffered from a mood illness. I have found no evidence in biographical documentation of manic symptoms for Jaspers, unlike his brother, but there is plenty of evidence of depressive symptoms. Most writers have followed Jaspers himself in ascribing these depressive states to his chronic pulmonary illness (probably idiopathic pulmonary fibrosis). But, if Enno Jaspers indeed had bipolar illness, the strong genetic nature of this condition would increase the probability that Jaspers was likely predisposed to depressive symptoms himself.

Jaspers certainly interpreted his own depression existentially, rather than pathologically. It is likely that many of Jaspers' insights—such as about limit-situations, death, loss—grew out of his depressive experience, as suggested by psychological studies that show that people with depression have enhanced realism and increased empathy compared to non-depressed persons (Ghaemi 2011). In fact, the cornerstone of Jaspers' psychiatry—the concept of empathy—may have grown out of Jaspers' own personal experience with depression.

As explained later, I do not see a reason for a dichotomy between positive and negative aspects of depression, or between existential and pathological perspectives on depression. The two parts go hand in hand. Depression can be a disease, and yet existentially insightful; it can be harmful and beneficial at the same time. Jaspers' life may be another example of this truth.

A strong suggestion that Jaspers' depression was at least partly pathological has to do with his suicidality. Jaspers was not opposed to the idea of suicide, contrasting 'free death' (*Freitod*) as opposed to 'self-murder' (*Selbstmord*) (Kirkbright 2004: 169). It is well-known that in the Nazi era, Jaspers had a suicide pact with his Jewish wife Gertrud. This has tended to be seen as an honourable if difficult last-resort decision made only in the event of the Gestapo visit that would have inevitably led to Gertrud's extermination. Hence Jaspers had stockpiled plenty of medication, mainly barbiturates, if needed, in Heidelberg.

But this suicide pact went beyond Nazism. Gertrud, who had lifelong recurrent depression, had planned to kill herself if Jaspers' pulmonary illness should have led to his death in the Nazi era (Kirkbright 2004: 329). Further, in Basel, 20 years after the end of Nazism, Jaspers was still prepared for and preoccupied with suicide. In old age in 1966, Jaspers was explicit in private with Hannah Arendt, going into great technical detail:

> A 'respectable means of committing suicide' has been a problem for us [Karl and Gertrud] since the Nazi period and remains one … The drugs always have to be reasonably fresh; they spoil with time. The Nazis, always in the forefront in technical matters, used capsules containing cyanide along with some other ingredients that prevented the dreadful burning in the throat and esophagus and speeded up absorption though the stomach.… We had morphine, but not in heavy enough concentrations that one injection would have sufficed. I found at the time that even good physicians … were short on practical advice—They had Veronal [a barbiturate], which is relatively stable. You have to take a lot of it. But with tea that poses no great problem. Then you become unconscious, profoundly so, and you die of pneumonia in a few days if the stomach is not pumped out. With very large doses (several tubes) the process can be speeded up. My brother committed suicide with heroin, which, if you have connections, you can acquire in the illegal drug trade … The 'free world' is not free because it prohibits suicide. (Arendt and Jaspers 1992: 652–653)

Another time, he called the suicide of a poet-friend of Arendt's 'an act of the greatest self-mastery' (Arendt and Jaspers 1992: 617). The editors of this correspondence (one of whom was Jaspers' last assistant Hans Saner) commented in a footnote that after the death of Karl and Gertrud, 'six capsules of potassium cyanide, large amounts of morphine, and several packages of Veronal were found in their house' (Arendt and Jaspers 1992: 796). This was Switzerland in the 1960s, not Germany in the 1930s. Jaspers commitment to suicide was existential, and probably biological too, not merely circumstantial.

Besides Enno, Jaspers was faced with depression or manic-depression in two other close persons in his life, his wife Gertrud, and his hero Max Weber, who I'll discuss at the end of this chapter.

In his personal letters to his student and friend Hannah Arendt, Jaspers was matter of fact about Gertrud's depression:

> The touch of depression that Gertrud was experiencing when you were here has disappeared again completely. She has regained her natural equilibrium and does not blame herself for anything. She has experienced these swings back and forth her whole life long, a consequence of her genetic inheritance, which, measured against the effects it could have had, has manifested itself in a mild way, but it has been bad enough. But the good, healthy times always come back. (Arendt and Jaspers 1992: 566–567)

Here is Jaspers the husband, writing like a pure Kraepelinian psychiatrist (as explained later) about the recurrent depression Kraepelin defined as a manic-depressive condition. Like Kraepelin, Jaspers diagnosed, prognosed, and did not intervene, since nature cured more effectively than physicians could.

Taking history seriously

Now from Jaspers the man to Jaspers the philosopher, and later Jaspers the psychiatrist.

Jaspers engaged in philosophizing, a verb, not philosophy, a noun. His thinking was about asking questions and engaging in critique respectfully, not for the sake of verbal debate but to seek to know the truth. He once said that he wanted his remarks to be taken as questions (Jaspers 1951).

In that spirit, I believe the most salient feature of psychiatry today is eclecticism (Ghaemi 2003). People believe everything and nothing. All is permitted, but there are no laws. Science is routinely disparaged by critics, while it is also wielded as a weapon to enforce conformity. In the past, when dogmatism rather than eclecticism ruled, one could aim one's critique at orthodox psychoanalysis or biological reductionism. Though those worn out phrases are repeated, few mainstream powers in current psychiatry overtly advance those ideologies. The 'biopsychosocial' model is a catchphrase often used to allow one to do whatever one wants (Ghaemi 2009). Drugs are given without systematic reasons; and with the third edition of the *Diagnostic and Statistical Manual of Mental Disorders* (DSM-III) onwards, decisions regarding diagnostic definitions are increasingly made without regard to scientific evidence but with a primary focus on what is 'pragmatically' useful, in the opinions of the decision-makers.

This eclecticism has a philosophical basis in something else, a larger cultural phenomenon which has existed for about a century, a washing away of old values—both of the medieval religious past, but also of the rationalist Enlightenment past, a veering towards conceptual relativism where power supplants truth, where the death of God is followed by the death of science. Postmodernism is a phrase that captures this cultural change (though like other general phrases—socialism, communism, capitalism—it is a generic term that can have many detailed meanings) (Kaplan 1993).

Many critics of psychiatry today see the advances in neuroscience and the rise in use of medications as reason for sharp criticism based, philosophically, on postmodernism, and clinically, on eclecticism. They sometimes erroneously even use Karl Jaspers as a thinker in support of their opinions. In fact, Jaspers was a 'biological existentialist', and his support of science and biology are part of his overall philosophy. They are especially important in seeking to understand how his ideas can be applied to mood disorders.

Jaspers was quite explicit that we need to take truth seriously, including biological and scientific truths:

> We have heard the outcry: Science destroys faith. Critics doubt the eternal truth which shines forth in modern science. They deny and attack philosophical enlightenment, they turn against liberalism, attack tolerance as heartless indifference. In short, they reject the power to attain knowledge, in freedom, and advocate philosophical suicide. There can be no integrity or human dignity without a true scientific attitude. Where science is lost man falls into the twilight of vague edifying sentiments, of fanatical decisions arrived at in self-willed blindness. (Jaspers 1951: 4–7)

Unfortunately, Jaspers' direct warning was realized in the experience of psychiatry in the last half century, as discussed later.

The cultural context

In the discipline of the history of psychiatry, the mainstream view is that the ideas of the past must be left in the past (Berrios and Porter 1999). They are not relevant to the present, and certainly not the future. Every idea is apposite to its age, we are told, in truly Hegelian fashion. Everything that is real is right, it seems; how nice that we can never be wrong. And yet we are never fully right either, because our heirs tomorrow will have new ideas, different from ours, and their ideas are right too. This historical relativism may be fine for literary criticism, where much postmodernism has taken root, but when it branches out to psychiatry, as its hero Foucault so explicitly did (Foucault 1988), and thence to medicine and science, some of us think we should hesitate (Kaplan 1993).

Some of us think that since patients die, there appear to be diseases. These are real entities, not historically relative ones, although our understanding of them obviously changes over time (Shorter 1997). Since medications appear to kill patients, they are real entities, not figments of capitalist imagination. (If real, they may even save lives.) Some might argue that mental disorders may exist, and people can suffer and even commit suicide because of them, but still those mental disorders are value-laden in how we define them (Sadler 2002). My response would be that there are values involved in understanding any biological disease; consider the values involved in our views in the past on AIDS, or tuberculosis, or syphilis, or Addison's disease. Neurosyphilis in particular causes symptoms that are indistinguishable from mania or depression. Does this mean that neurosyphilis is some special 'value-laden mental disorder' which conflicts with the fact that it is a biological disease? Values do not refute the spirochete.

We are faced with a major cultural dilemma: the past is dead, and the future unborn. Or stated in Nietzsche's terms, God is dead, and there is nothing to replace him. Postmodernists revel in God's passing, and they want to make sure that no one, and nothing, dares replace him. The main pretender is science, so science becomes the enemy (Dennett 1999/2000). In psychiatry, this translates to a harsh rejection, or deep suspicion, of biology, whether research in genes and the brain or treatment with drugs (Bracken and Thomas 2001).

Jaspers criticized overly biological approaches in psychiatry, but he fully supported biological psychiatry within limits. He was a biological existentialist, not a nihilist postmodernist. That was the key difference between him and Heidegger (Olson 1994). Heidegger was quite critical and sceptical of modern science, as is well known (Videla 1994), and Foucault highly esteemed Heidegger as one of the modern world's greatest philosophers (Rayner 2007).

Here I will try to show how Jaspers' ideas help us understand mood disorders today, daring to think that the past can inform the present, and, using Jaspers' own method in history of philosophy, to take the ideas of this past thinker seriously on their own, not as historically relative constructions of times long gone.

Method-based psychiatry

Now we come to Jaspers the psychiatrist and mood disorders. The central idea of *General Psychopathology* is, I think, method-based psychiatry, or, as Jaspers puts it, 'methodological consciousness'. He used the two basic methods of *Erklären* and *Verstehen* to divide up all of psychiatry, to throw light on the phenomena of psychiatry, including diagnosis and treatment. Each method was valid within its limits, and needed to be used and respected. Neither method alone was scientifically valid. He would approach mood disorders in this 'method-based' way, with the specific methods used depending on what was scientifically most valid. Thus, for the biological disease of manic-depression—which today we call bipolar disorder and severe recurrent unipolar depression (Goodwin and Jamison 2007)—the Jaspersian approach would be consistent with a fully biological method, treatment with mood stabilizing medications like lithium, and biological research into causes and pathophysiology. For the mostly environmental condition of neurotic depression (as we'll see), which is combined with a biological component of the personality trait of neuroticisim, a Jaspersian approach would be mostly existential, seeking to help someone understand and cope with living.

These two diagnoses—manic-depression and neurotic depression—cover the vast majority of presentations of mood disorders. A purely anti-biology approach would not do justice to either Jaspers' philosophy or his psychiatry. Yet the existential, empathic work that Jaspers introduced in *General Psychopathology* also is obviously central to his way of thinking. Too often, however, Jaspers' phenomenology gets emphasized to the exclusion of his method-based philosophy. Phenomenology is then used to attack biology, and becomes yet another justification for cynicism about science, which Jaspers so vigorously opposed, whether in the hands of Nazism or post-Second World War postmodernism: 'The rejection of Enlightenment is treason against man' (Jaspers 1951).

Current nosology of mood disorders

Jaspers' ideas are relevant to the nosology of mood disorders today. The mainstream view on mood disorders today is derived from a combination of the views of Emil Kraepelin and his opponents, like Karl Leonhard (a follower of Kraepelin's opponent, Carl Wernicke) (Leonhard 1979). Kraepelin made the classic distinction between chronic psychosis (dementia praecox, later schizophrenia) and recurrent mood illness with psychosis (manic-depressive insanity). Later researchers extended Kraepelin's nosology to include non-psychotic mood episodes, hence manic-depressive illness (MDI). Wernicke, following his teacher Karl Kleist, mistrusted Kraepelin's broad MDI concept, and later Leonhard used new genetic research methods to argue that MDI comprised two definably different (based on course and genetics) subtypes: unipolar depression and bipolar disorder (Ungvari 1993).

In 1980, DSM-III combined the Kraepelinian separation of schizophrenia from mood illnesses with the Leonhardian separation of mood illnesses into the two unipolar and bipolar groupings. Thus DSM-III is not simply neo-Kraepelinian, as many state (Klerman 1986), but *also neo-Leonhardian*, an idea not present in prior histories of psychiatry. It is only partially, not completely, neo-Kraepelinian.

The impetus to DSM-III was, in good measure, scientific (Klerman et al. 1984). Prior to 1980, Kraepelin's views had been dethroned by neo-Freudian nosologic nihilism (diagnosis didn't matter; most everything was treatable with psychoanalysis of some variety) (Menninger 1963) and challenged by Leonhardian genetic and epidemiology research (Leonhard 1968). No one knew what to believe. DSM-III justly rejected neo-Freudian dogmatism, and combined the Kraepelinian and Leonhardian views. This was helpful, as many say, at least in terms of giving psychiatry a common language with some empirical basis: reliability. It was hoped that reliability would be a way station to validity (Klerman et al. 1984), but cultural postmodernism intervened, infecting the psychiatric profession with increasing vigour in the 1980s and onwards, so that the fourth revision of DSM in 1994 involved the primacy of a purely 'pragmatic' approach to nosological change: if the leaders of DSM-IV thought a change would help the profession, they would make it; if not, not (Frances 2010; Phillips et al. 2012). It was as simple as that. The leaders disliked lithium and neuroleptics presumably because they cause more side effects than the new generations of antidepressants (Frances 2010). This resulted in an expansion of the unipolar depression concept to the bloated 'major depressive disorder' (MDD) concept of today (Ghaemi et al. 2012), where almost any depressive symptom gets labeled with MDD and treated with one of a dozen modern antidepressants.

When pragmatism becomes extreme, as in the work of Rorty (1991), then it merges into an extreme postmodernism. There are no objective truths or realities, because truth and reality is only dependent on subjective grounds: what works for us. This is a critique William James (2011) faced repeatedly, and he responded with an anti-postmodernist reply. He admitted that objective truths and realities existed, but he claimed an epistemological pragmatism: we could only know those objective truths through their impact on how they worked in our personal experiences. This is a claim closer to Jaspers than to Heidegger and Rorty and Foucault and the DSM-IV leadership.

Many have justly criticized this epidemic of MDD and antidepressants, but for the wrong reasons, in my view. With the postmodernist mindset that there is no truth and life is all about a struggle for power, critics have looked for an enemy and found it in the pharmaceutical industry, or academics who get paid by that industry, or both. Such conspiracy theories though perhaps partially true, do not do justice to another possibility: MDD might be overdiagnosed and overtreated but not every psychiatric illness is necessarily overdiagnosed and overtreated. Specifically bipolar disorder might still be underdiagnosed and mistreated pharmacologically (Smith and Ghaemi 2010).

Into this welter of confusion and debate, we might justly ask what insights might be found in the thinking of that one thinker who so many psychiatrists today have ignored, and whose ideas definitely were ignored by the makers of DSM-III and their DSM-IV followers: Karl Jaspers.

Jaspers and Kraepelin

It is important to appreciate that when the young Karl Jaspers became a psychiatric resident at the University of Heidelberg in 1908, he entered a department that until just five years earlier had been run by the great nosologist himself: Kraepelin had been chairman at Heidelberg for a dozen years (1891–1903), the period of his most creative productivity in nosological revisions of his textbook (Baldessarini 2002; Kirkbright 2004). The department, under Franz Nissl, was completely Kraepelinian through and through.

So, as a senior resident three years after his arrival, Jaspers wrote his *General Psychopathology* in the shadow of Kraepelin. He struggled with making sense of psychiatry, as expounded by Kraepelin, in the light of Jaspers' own insights about phenomenology and science, the latter especially being influenced by Jaspers' philosophical mentor, Max Weber (Jaspers 1957/1986).

Weber's theory about 'ideal types' was central to Jaspers' critique of Kraepelin (Schwartz and Wiggins 1987), as was the phenomenological method as involving the clinical use of empathy (Havens 1967). A third important feature of Jaspers' nosology was the central philosophical theory, derived from Dilthey via Weber, of the distinction between *Erklären* (causal explanation) and *Verstehen* (meaningful understanding) (Ghaemi 2009; Wiggins and Schwartz 1991). In what follows, I'll trace how these ideas led to Jaspers' nosology, and later, how these ideas may apply to current thinking about mood illnesses.

Jaspers on nosology

Jaspers explains his views on nosology in part IV of *General Psychopathology* ('Conception of psychic life as a whole', in chapter XII, 'The synthesis of disease entities—Nosology': 564–616). He directly addresses the perspective of the empirical/biological school, led in his age by Kraepelin, criticizing the concept that psychiatric illnesses could be reduced to diseases of the brain, but supporting Kraepelin's clinical empirical approach:

> There has been *no fulfillment* of the hope that clinical observation of psychic phenomena, of the life-history and of the outcome might yield *characteristic groupings* which would *subsequently be confirmed in the cerebral findings*, and thus pave the way for the brain-anatomists.... The original question: are there only *stages and variants* of one unitary psychosis or is there *a series of disease-entities* which we can delineate, now finds its answer: *there are neither*. The latter view is right in so far that the idea of disease-entities has become a fruitful orientation for the investigations of special psychiatry. The former view is right in so far that no actual disease-entities exist in scientific psychiatry. (Jaspers 1959/1997: 568–570)

I would disagree with the blanket statement that there are no actual diseases in psychiatry, yet still appreciate that Jaspers was correct for his time: as of 1911, or 1942, there were no proven diseases in psychiatry (neurosyphilis—a huge exception—excluded?).

Raised in the hub of Kraepelin's world, Jaspers wanted to argue against reducing psychiatry to nothing but diagnosis:

> In the psychiatric assessment of a case ... except in the case of well-known cerebral changes, diagnosis is the least relevant factor. If it is made the main issue, it will prejudge what ideally should emerge from the investigation. What matters is the process of analysis. The chaos of phenomena should not be blotted out with some diagnostic label but bring illumination through the way it is systematically ordered and related. Psychiatric diagnosis is too often a sterile running round in circles so that only a few phenomena are brought into the orbit of conscious knowledge. (Jaspers 1959/1997: 20)

This doesn't mean diagnosis is completely irrelevant; later, in part IV, Jaspers explains why a classification scheme is important in psychiatry:

> We have detailed knowledge of particular phenomena, of causal connections and meaningful connections, etc., but complex disease entities remain an endless, inextricable web. The individual configurations of disease are not like plants which we can classify in a herbarium. Rather it is just what is a 'plant'—an illness—that is most uncertain. *What* do we diagnose? ... Diagnosis is expected to characterize in a comprehensive manner the whole morbid occurrence which has assailed the person and which stands as a well-defined entity among others.... But however we devise (a diagnostic schema) we realize that it cannot work; that we can only make temporary and arbitrary classifications; that there are a number of different possibilities which account for the fact that different workers construct entirely different schemata; and that classification is always contradictory in theory and never quire squares with the facts. Why then do we keep on making this vain attempt? In the first place we want to see properly what this idea of disease-entity has *achieved* in respect of the *over-all picture* of existing psychic disorders, and particularly where we have failed because it is the basic and radical failure which makes us aware of the actual state of our knowledge. In the second place every *presentation of special psychiatry* requires some classification of psychosis at its base. Without some such schema it cannot order its material. In the third place we need a classification in order *to make statistical investigations* of a large case material. (Jaspers 1959/1997: 604)

Jaspers goes on to explain his philosophy of nosology:

> An ideal schema would have to satisfy the following requirements: It must be such that any given case would have only one place within it and every case should have a place. The whole plan must have a compelling objectivity so that different observers can classify cases in the same way.... We abandon the idea of disease-entity and once more have to bear in mind continually the various points of view (as to causes, psychological structure, anatomical findings, course of illness and outcome) and in face of the facts we have to draw the line where none exists. Such classification therefore has only a provisional value. It is a fiction which will discharge its function if it proves to be the most apt for the time. There is no "natural" schema which would accommodate every case. (Jaspers 1959/1997: 605)

This approach is not entirely uncongenial to the postmodernist pragmatism of DSM-IV: it is atheoretical as to aetiology; 'fictions' are propounded explicitly and without apology. The difference, as we'll see, is that Jaspers' approach does not close the door on biological disease; it only seeks to admit that when such a disease-approach is not justified, it shouldn't be taken.

DSM-Jaspers

When looking at his actual clinical constructs, Jaspers proposes a nosology quite similar to the big shift in 1980 to DSM-III and the ninth revision of the International Classification of Diseases (ICD-9). He proposes dividing psychiatric conditions into three main groups (Jaspers 1959/1997): Group I, 'Known somatic illnesses with psychic disturbances' (such as cerebral tumours, meningitis), coincides with DSM's 'Axis III' which describes psychiatric conditions secondary to known medical illnesses. Group II, 'The three major psychoses' ('genuine epilepsy', schizophrenia, and manic-depressive illness), would correspond with the major mood and psychotic disorders on DSM's 'Axis I' of primary psychiatric conditions (with epilepsy moved to Axis III since a cerebral basis has long-been established for it). Group III is the 'Personality disorders', which corresponds to DSM's 'Axis II' also defined as personality disorders. Heuristically, with the caveats given previously, Jaspers goes on to accept Kraepelin's definition of the distinction between schizophrenia and manic-depressive illness based on the outcome criterion as the main factor, i.e. invariably poor outcome with schizophrenia and frequent recovery with manic-depressive illness. A key observation is that *Jaspers' Group II is pure Kraepelin, unaltered and unchanged.*

The distinction is that Jaspers saw Kraepelin's diagnoses not as proven diseases, but as only current approximations to possible diseases. In the appendix to *General Psychopathology*, written in the later revisions, Jaspers reviews the matter (Jaspers 1959/1997: 825–859):

> Kraepelin was responsible for one of the most fruitful lines of research, the investigation of the whole life-history of the patient. He … laid the foundations for psycho-pharmacology.… But Kraepelin's basic conceptual world remained a somatic one which in the company of the majority of doctors he held as the only important one for medicine, not only as a matter of preference but in an absolute sense. The psychological discussions in his Textbook are brilliant in parts and he succeeded with them as it were unwittingly. He himself regards them as temporary stopgaps until experiment, microscope and test-tube permitted objective investigation. (Jaspers 1959/1997: 852–853)

It is worth emphasizing that Jaspers writes of Kraepelin as 'laying the foundations for psychopharmacology', a curious fact given that Kraepelin was so often identified with 'therapeutic nihilism'. Decades before DSM-III, Jaspers saw that Kraepelin's nosology would match up well with a medication-oriented approach to treatment in psychiatry. Once the medications began to be developed in the 1950s, it was only a matter of time before the psychopharmacology revolution would lead to a neo-Kraepelinian restoration. Jaspers saw this link.

It is also notable that Jaspers does not reject psychopharmacology; his problem is not Kraepelin's biological attitude, but its absolutism. Jaspers would accept psychopharmacology 'as a matter of preference', meaning within some limits, as with all science; but not 'in an absolute sense'. Importantly, Jaspers is not simply rejecting psychopharmacology, in an absolute sense.

Ideal types

Much of Jaspers' nosology hinges on the concept of the ideal type, which is meant as a standard, or simplified version, of reality (Pepper 1963; Weber 1949). Let us take the example of the historian, because this is where the concept was developed (Makkreel 1992), but everything that is said here can apply to the psychologist or the psychiatrist when faced with clinical aspects of treating patients. The historian observes certain aspects of an historical event. He then takes those aspects that seem to be the most striking, those that are the most unique or interesting to him, and he abstracts them from the rest of the details of the event. Connected in the abstract, limited to the most salient aspects of the historical reality, the historian thus creates the ideal type for that event (Pepper 1963; Weber 1949).

The point of the ideal type is not to directly correspond to reality, but to highlight certain aspects of reality that might otherwise get lost in the varying details of concrete reality. The ideal type is not seen as a general theory either, which changes as more and more information on the empirical details of concrete reality is gathered. The ideal type is itself the standard to which concrete reality is compared (Pepper 1963; Weber 1949). By using the word 'ideal', Weber did not mean that the ideal type is the best type, or better than concrete reality; he meant to emphasize the fact that it is an abstraction, a conceptualization made away from concrete reality (Weber 1949).

A conceptual analogy to the ideal type is a ruler, by which objects are measured. The ruler is not made based on empirical comparisons to reality. It simply is created by us, by humans, stipulated to be a certain length, and then used to measure real objects. External validity is irrelevant; we create the ruler, and give it certain parameters, end of story. Similarly, ideal types are concepts created by historians, and the 'facts' of history are measured against them. The point of ideal types is to help us understand the meaning of those facts of history.

Some have suggested (Wiggins and Schwartz 1994) that the DSM system of nosology in psychiatry can be seen as utilizing the same method. The diagnoses in DSM are not 'real' entities; they are abstractions. No single patient exactly meets the specific criteria of any diagnosis; every patient is uniquely different in some way. This reflects the concrete uniqueness of human existence, that aspect of human cultural reality which Weber and his predecessors so emphasized. Thus, the DSM diagnoses are not meant to correspond directly and perfectly to clinical reality. Nor are they meant to represent general theories of diagnoses, which are to be changed as more and more empirical evidence is gathered.

The only question is whether there is any biological reality behind the ideal types. Many critics of psychiatry say no. Biological dogmatists would say yes. The DSM-IV leadership, following postmodernist 'pragmatism', doesn't care. Jaspers would say: Sometimes yes, and sometimes no—and it's up to science to tell us which is which.

Anti-Jaspersian DSM-III: the decline of neurotic depression

Four decades ago, a major controversy raged in the United Kingdom (Shorter 2007). Was depression one thing or many? The unifiers were led by Sir Aubrey Lewis, powerful head of the Maudsley Hospital. The dividers were led by Sir Martin Roth, the most prominent British exponent of Jaspers' ideas in modern times. Following his teacher Adolf Meyer, Lewis took a pragmatic approach to diagnosis; if clinical differences did not make a difference in practice, then there was no difference. Roth emphasized psychopathology: if clinical syndromes could be shown to be different phenomenologically, then they are different. The terms of the debate were endogenous versus exogenous depression: the first biologically and the second environmentally caused. Exogenous depression was synonymous with neurotic or reactive depression—associated with anxiety and mood reactivity, and highly sensitive to psychosocial stressors. Endogenous depression was melancholic, unreactive in mood, and non-anxious. Epidemiological studies in the 1960s and 1970s found that such divisions did not imply differences in outcomes; Lewis won, and his ideas were crowned posthumously (for him) in 1980 with DSM-III: all kinds of depression were lumped in one label—the almighty MDD.

Four decades later, we can pass a new judgement on the British debate. The large STAR*D study of antidepressant effectiveness found quite low long-term remission rates, despite reasonably good acute treatment response rates. If MDD is one entity, then it is not very responsive to antidepressant treatments. It is very possible that the low long-term response rates reflect a wide variation in treatment response given the various subgroups of depression, including neurotic depression (Ghaemi 2008).

Maybe Martin Roth had it right, but not in the exact terms of the old UK debate. The distinction is not between biological versus non-biological depressions (Lewis 1967). Most depressive conditions (non-bipolar) can be shown to be about equally genetic and environmental (Kendler and Prescott 2006). It is not their aetiology that distinguishes them; rather, in the tradition of Jaspers, it is their clinical presentation, and, in the tradition of Kraepelin, it is their outcomes. Neurotic depression has a completely different clinical picture than melancholia; it may also differ markedly in treatment response, melancholia being more, and neurotic depression less responsive to at least some antidepressants (like tricyclic agents or electroconvulsive therapy). And there may be a third subgroup, mixed depression—where manic and depression symptoms combine with marked irritability and psychomotor agitation (Koukopoulos and Ghaemi 2009)—which is also antidepressant non-responsive and neuroleptic responsive (see Figure 17.1).

Following Roth, I have proposed specific diagnostic criteria for neurotic depression (Ghaemi 2008) that can be used in practice and research (see Table 17.1), and Koukopoulos has proposed specific diagnostic criteria for mixed depression (Koukopoulos et al. 2007). Proposals for DSM-5 make initial steps in both directions, with new definitions for 'mixed anxious depression' and 'MDD with mixed features'.

The old debate is not over, but purist followers of DSM-III onwards pretend that it ended in 1980. The most important thing is to change the terms of the debate from 'pragmatism', following Meyer and Foucault and the postmodernists whose ideas ruled in DSM-IV, to phenomenology and science, in the tradition of Jaspers and Roth (and Kraepelin).

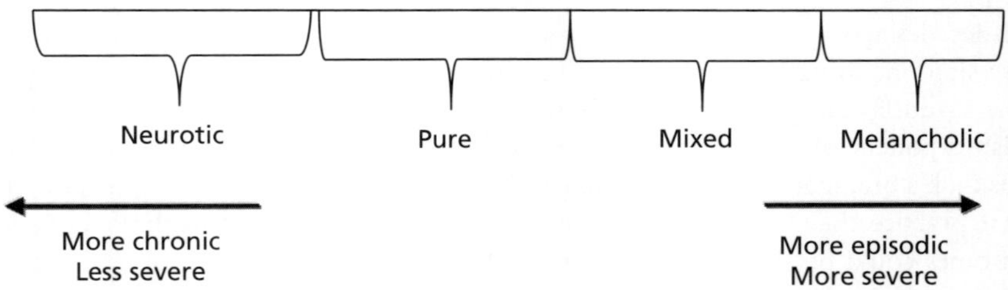

Figure 17.1 Subtypes of 'major depressive disorder'. Reprinted from *Psychiatric Clinics of North America*, 35(1), S. Nassir Ghaemi, Paul A. Vöhringer, and Derick E. Vergne, The Varieties of Depressive Experience: Diagnosing Mood Disorders, pp. 73–86, Copyright (2012), with permission from Elsevier.

Table 17.1 Proposed diagnostic criteria for neurotic depression

A. Depressed mood leading to severe subjective distress or marked functional impairment.
B. Meeting 2–4 of the following criteria: sleep decreased or increased, decreased interest in usual activities, decreased self-esteem, decreased energy, decreased concentration, decreased or increased appetite, suicidal ideation, but not meeting DSM-V criteria for a major depressive episode (i.e. subsyndromal major depressive episode symptoms)
C. Prolonged or frequent worries or anxiety nearly daily for most of each day, or sustained or frequently recurring multiple somatic symptoms (e.g. gastrointestinal distress, headaches, paraesthesias) with no secondary medical cause
D. Criteria A–C present over at least 6 months, during the majority of early every day
E. Mood or other symptoms apparently reactive to adverse or favourable changes in circumstances or everyday events
F. Absence of severe psychomotor retardation guilt, anger, agitation, or psychotic features
G. DSM-IV major depressive episode criteria are not met during more than half of the duration of features A–G

Adapted from *Bipolar Disorders* 10(8), S Nassir Ghaemi, Why antidepressants are not antidepressants: STEP-BD, STAR*D, and the return of neurotic depression, pp. 957–68 © 2008, John Wiley and Sons, with permission.

The diagnostic role of empathy

To most clinicians today, empathy is seen as therapeutic. One empathizes to help a patient. For Jaspers, empathy was diagnostic as well. The first step in his clinical work, and in his nosology, was to do the work of *Verstehen*—to extend empathy and meaningful understanding as far as one could go with a given patient; then, and only then, would diagnostic or therapeutic judgements be possible. He felt that the distinction between *Verstehen* and *Erklären* would provide one of the few organizing principles for nosology:

> The most profound distinction in psychic life seems to be that between what is meaningful and allows empathy and what in its particular way is un-understandable, 'mad' in the literal sense, schizophrenic psychic life (even though there may be no delusions). Pathological psychic life of the first kind we can comprehend vividly enough as an exaggeration or diminution of known phenomena and as an appearance of such phenomena without the usual causes or motives. Pathological psychic life of the second kind we cannot adequately comprehend in this way. Instead we find changes of the most general kind for which we have no empathy but which in some way we try to make comprehensible from an external point of view.... The affective illnesses appear to us to be open to empathy and natural but the various types of "madness" do not seem open to empathy and appear unnatural. (Jaspers 1959/1997: 577–578)

The psychiatrist Leston Havens, one of my teachers, introduced Jaspers to American psychiatry (Havens 1967), and in his own work, Havens extended the application of Jaspers' emphasis on empathy as both diagnostically and therapeutically important in clinical practice (Havens 1973/2004). By establishing a therapeutic alliance through careful empathic work (Havens et al. 2001), the psychiatrist can begin to understand what is, or is not, wrong with the patient. Only after that work can a proper diagnosis be made, which can include the simple application of Kraepelinian or even DSM-like criteria. But without the prior empathic work (Havens 1986), such diagnostic attempts will often be wrong simply because accurate information will not have been obtained. Such diagnosis is not simple question-and-answer interrogation; it is the difficult labour of getting to know someone; it is 'participant observation' where what is observed depends on how one assesses it (Havens

1983). After such diagnosis, biological treatments, even the least popular ones, can be given. None of this work precludes biological disease concepts or the use of medications. This is all biological existentialism, applied to psychiatry.

Sometimes this empathic beginning process is the ending process; sometimes the empathic work leads to the conclusion that there is no diagnosis to be made, and hence no biological treatment. There is instead the difficult work of being human (Havens 1994), and then, the empathic method becomes the existential treatment itself.

Existential despair and the therapeutic alliance

The experience of depression often involves the experience of despair. Sometimes this despair happens in the midst of the experience of a disease, like manic-depression; sometimes it happens without disease, as in neurotic depression. Hence despair, though clinically salient, is diagnostically non-specific. Its salience has to do with appreciating what it means to a person suffering from depression. A patient with bipolar depression still wants to be understood in terms of the existential impact of the depressive experience: he is in despair and needs to be understood that way. So too someone might experience great despair and yet not have bipolar illness or mixed depression or melancholia. In neurotic depression too, there can be times of great despair.

When the phenomenological sensitivity is lost, and the diagnostic complexity is ignored, then all these expressions of despair simply get labelled with the generic term 'depression', typically diagnosed with the generic MDD diagnosis, and treated with the generic antidepressant.

Jaspers' influence can help us learn to pay attention to existential despair as part of the varieties of depressive experience (Havens and Ghaemi 2005). The method used is empathy once more, beginning with the person, and then seeing if there is a disease that underlies the experience of the person or not.

Four decades ago, a psychiatrist was considered skilled if he could complete these tasks: first, he would elicit thoughts and feelings from patients using the free association method; then, he would organize these thoughts and feelings into a clinical formulation that demonstrated the unconscious motivations behind them. He would then present interpretations based on that formulation back to the patient in the course of treatment.

Today, a psychiatrist is considered competent if she has a different set of skills: she has to collect disease indicators so that she can define an entity that she can then either medicate or treat psychologically.

The problem now, as then, is that while both of these approaches have benefits, often clinicians do nothing else. It was not enough then to psychoanalyse; it is not enough now to diagnose and prescribe. What has been put aside is the relationship. Without it, all other diagnostic and treatment efforts are at the very least impaired, and, at worst, simply wrong.

Making the relationship primary to the diagnostic interview and the therapeutic process results in an approach to the interview that Havens has called 'soundings' (Havens et al. 2001).This idea emphasizes the fact that empathizing with mania or depression is not only a means of acknowledging the patient's strengths and hopes, and not only a means of strengthening the therapeutic alliance, but, in addition, it is also a means of accurately assessing the extent of a person's depression or mania. It entails making statements as diagnostic probes and then judging the patient's response to the statements. This contrasts with the standard question-and-answer approach of diagnostic interviewing, an objective-descriptive approach that tends to produce highly distorted results when used with manic or depressed patients. Using the soundings method, we like to respond to a depressing situation by responding with an experience of our own that is even more depressed. The patient is puzzled and surprised 'to find someone with him'.

Empathizing with mania

Too often, the history of mood disorders has involved an almost complete focus on depression. Mania, when studied, was seen as somehow uninteresting psychologically, or odd phenomenologically, or, in psychoanalytic thinking, a kind of false reaction to depression. In fact, mania may be the secret to all mood disorders; to turn around the psychoanalytic view, it might even be the secret to depression (Koukopoulos and Ghaemi 2009).

When one considers Jaspers' emphasis on empathy, it is important to realize that such empathy is not limited to depression. There is a great deal of empathy that can happen with mania, even though traditionally our field has assumed otherwise (Havens and Ghaemi 2005). Havens has suggested how this can be done, using the idea of counter-assumptive statements, derived from the work of Harry Stack Sullivan (Sullivan 1954). The basic idea of this counter-assumptive position is that 'sharing feelings reduces them' (Havens 1989). So the work of empathy is actually a way of diminishing even extreme psychiatric symptoms, like psychosis or mania.

So, when a manic patient makes a grandiose statement, it is more often than not best to agree with it, at least initially. Joining with elation, and not just depression, is an essential part of forming a human connection with the manic patient. In the old days, Havens used to teach, especially in the Boston area, young manic patients would aspire to be like that other Boston Irishman who made it big: patients used to say, and truly believe, that they were John F. Kennedy. Whether it is Kennedy or Christ (who never seems to fall out of favour), manic patients deserve at least some acknowledgement of their worthiness as human beings. If someone says, 'I'm Jesus Christ', Havens might respond: 'Well, I was hoping to meet him some day'.

A person's aspirations should not be discouraged or pathologized. This usually produces the opposite reaction: the manic person realizes she cannot connect with the clinician, and treatment ends. Or perhaps the manic patient accepts treatment, but at the price of giving up all her hopes. That chronic depression, which seems to be the most common course of patients with bipolar disorder despite our current best treatment (Judd and Akiskal 2003), may reflect such loss of hope.

Max Weber and the genius of manic-depression

Jaspers likely had a professional, not just a personal, relationship with Max Weber, who clearly had manic-depression. He had severe bouts of depression where he did not function, was extremely sad, uninterested in almost all activities, and frequently suicidal. Weber was psychiatrically hospitalized in the late 1890s, along with a severely melancholic first cousin who later committed suicide. His family was full of severe depression and psychosis; his sister committed suicide. Weber became extremely depressed around 1900, leading to the need to go on what today would be called disability support from the University of

Heidelberg for most of the next two decades. He rarely lectured, and worked and wrote in isolation and freedom from any other external responsibilities. Previous to that time, Weber had periods of marked increased energy, increased activity (especially creative writing), increased libido (with sexual liaisons), and decreased need for sleep (Mitzman 1970; Weber 1975). Jaspers saw these moods in Weber: 'I could always reach agreement with him in conversation about specifics, but the abyss of his despair was of a kind that made me sense he was charged with something I was not charged with. There was an explosive force in him that I lack' (Arendt and Jaspers 1992: 549). Though prior biographers describe these symptoms, they ascribe them to psychological explanations (Mitzman 1970), rather than the simplest and most scientifically supportable conclusion, admitted by his wife in her biography (Marianne Weber 1975): Weber had severe depressive episodes. I would add he had clear manic episodes, along with a family history of severe psychiatric illness consistent with manic-depression.

In his final years, the octagenerian Jaspers often mused about Weber in his correspondence with Hannah Arendt. Three years before his death, Jaspers went into great detail, comparing Weber repeatedly to Nietzsche and Kierkegaard:

> They were all three sick men, but Max Weber was different. He did not suffer from paralysis [meaning syphilis] or schizophrenia but from something as yet undiagnosed. He experienced in his life those elemental phases that are somehow grounded in biology: peaks of energy and productivity and then total collapse in which he couldn't even read anymore. In the last year of his life—we saw him during a last visit in Heidelberg, two months before his death—he was in a 'manic' but completely disciplined state. He said that he never had the sentences and concepts flow from his pen with such clarity, ceaseless continuity, and force ... He was incredibly prolific; he gave lectures that no student could forget. He was constantly making political trips and giving speeches; he glowed and suffered at the same time; that suffering seemed without limits. If he had remained alive, he probably would have had another collapse. (Arendt and Jaspers 1992: 637)

Jaspers saw the mania and the depression, but he put the pathology in quotes because he also saw the positive side. And so it is with manic-depression: mania enhancing creativity and resilience, and depression increasing realism and empathy. Sick and good, biological and existential, at the same time. The 80-year-old Jaspers, in the same letter, kept thinking about the meaning of the man who had died almost 50 years earlier:

> I have in recent years come to understand Max Weber better and more profoundly, or so I think ... He was truly serious about unlimited honesty. That is what made him the archetypal modern man who opens himself completely to absolute inner chaos, to the battle between warring powers, and who doesn't allow himself any secret cheating but lives passionately, struggles with himself, and has no goal. He felt that all of science and learning taken together was totally incapable of providing fulfillment in life ... Whoever thinks, as Max Weber did, not just theoretically, but who also lives out this human existence may well reach amazing heights but only momentarily; everything is called into question. And so his lifelong penchant for death, his inclination to thoughts of suicide. (Arendt and Jaspers 1992: 636)

Here, in a private letter, near the end of his life, Jaspers gives us a profound and personal description of manic-depression, of its strengths and its weaknesses, of its pathological nature and its existential power. Here we see mood illnesses diagnosed, understood, and—most importantly—appreciated.

References

Arendt, H., Jaspers, K. (1992). *Correspondence 1926–1969*. San Diego, CA: Harcourt, Brace and Company.

Baldessarini, R.J. (2002, 6 June). 'Historical Evolution of Kraepelin's Manic-Depressive Illness Concept', Presented at the Boston chapter of the Association for the Advancement of Philosophy and Psychiatry.

Berrios, G.E., Porter, R. (1999). *A History of Clinical Psychiatry*. London: Athlone Press.

Bracken, P., Thomas, P. (2001). 'Postpsychiatry: A New Direction for Mental Health', *British Medical Journal*, **322**(7288): 724–727.

Dennett, D.D. (1999/2000). 'Why Getting It Right Matters', *Free Inquiry*, 20(1): 40–43.

Foucault, M. (1988). *Madness and Civilization*. New York, NY: Vintage.

Frances, A. (2010). 'DSM in Philosophyland: Curioser and Curioser', available at: <http://alien.dowling.edu/~cperring/aapp/bulletin.htm> (accessed 8 November 2012).

Ghaemi, S.N. (2003). *The Concepts of Psychiatry*. Baltimore, MD: Johns Hopkins University Press.

Ghaemi, S.N. (2008). 'Why Antidepressants are Not Antidepressants: STEP-BD, STAR*D, and the Return of Neurotic Depression', *Bipolar Disorder*, **10**(8): 957–968.

Ghaemi, S.N. (2009). *The Rise and Fall of the Biopsychosocial Model: Reconciling Art and Science in Psychiatry*. Baltimore, MD: Johns Hopkins University Press.

Ghaemi, S.N. (2011). *A First-Rate Madness: Uncovering the Links Between Mental Illness and Leadership*. New York, NY: Penguin Press.

Ghaemi, S.N., Vohringer, P.A., Vergne, D.E. (2012). 'The Varieties of Depressive Experience: Diagnosing Mood Disorders', *Psychiatric Clinics of North America*, **35**(1): 73–86.

Goodwin, F.K., Jamison, K.R. (2007). *Manic Depressive Illness*. New York, NY: Oxford University Press.

Havens, L., Vaillant, G.E., Price, B.H., Goldstein, M., Kim, D. (2001). 'Soundings: A Psychological Equivalent of Medical Percussion', *Harvard Review of Psychiatry*, **9**(4): 147–157.

Havens, L.L. (1967). 'Karl Jaspers and American Psychiatry', *American Journal Psychiatry*, **124**(1): 66–70.

Havens, L.L. (1983). *Participant Observation*. Northvale, NJ: Jason Aronson.

Havens, L.L. (1986). *Making Contact: Uses of Language in Psychotherapy*. Cambridge, MA: Harvard University Press.

Havens, L.L. (1989). *A Safe Place*. Cambridge, MA: Harvard University Press.

Havens, L.L. (1994). *Learning to be Human*. Reading, MA: Addison-Wesley.

Havens, L.L. (2004). *Psychiatric Movements: From Sects Toward Science*. New Brunswick, NJ: Transaction Publishers. (Original work published 1973.)

Havens, L.L., Ghaemi, S. N. (2005). 'Existential Despair and Bipolar Disorder: The Therapeutic Alliance as a Mood Stabilizer', *American Journal Psychiatry*, 59 (2): 137–147.

James, W. (2011). *The Meaning of Truth*. Charleston, SC, CreateSpace Independent Publishing. (Original work published 1909.)

Jaspers, K. (1951). *Way to Wisdom*. New Haven, CT: Yale University Press.

Jaspers, K. (1986). 'An Autobiographical Account', in L.H. Ehrlich, E. Ehrlich, G.B. Pepper (eds), *Karl Jaspers: Basic Philosophical Writings*. Atlantic Highlands, NJ: Humanities Press, 5. (Original work published in 1957.)

Jaspers, K. (1997). *General Psychopathology*, Vol. 2. (7th edn) (J. Hoenig, M.W. Hamilton, trans.). Baltimore, MD: Johns Hopkins University Press. (Original work published in German in 1959.)

Judd, L.L., Akiskal, H.S. (2003). 'Depressive Episodes and Symptoms Dominate the Longitudinal Course of Bipolar Disorder', *Current Psychiatry Report*, **5**(6): 417–418.

Kaplan, E.A. (1993). *Postmodernism and its Discontents: Theories, Practices*. London: Verso.

Kendler, K.S., Prescott, C.A. (2006). *Genes, Environment, and Psychopathology: Understanding the Causes of Psychiatric and Substance Use Disorders*. New York, NY: Guilford Press.

Kirkbright, S. (2004). *Karl Jaspers: A Biography. Navigations in Truth*. New Haven, CT: Yale University Press.

Klerman, G.L. (1986). *Historical Perspectives on Contemporary Schools of Psychopathology, Contemporary directions in psychopathology: Toward the DSM-IV*. New York, NY: Guilford Press, 3–28.

Klerman, G.L., Vaillant, G.E., Spitzer, R.L., Michels, R. (1984). 'A Debate on DSM-III', *American Journal Psychiatry*, **141**: 539–553.

Koukopoulos, A., Ghaemi, S. N. (2009). 'The Primacy of Mania: a Reconsideration of Mood Disorders', *European Psychiatry*, **24**(2): 125–134.

Koukopoulos, A., Sani, G., Koukopoulos, A.E., Manfredi, G., Pacchiarotti, I., Girardi, P. (2007). 'Melancholia Agitata and Mixed Depression', *Acta Psychiatrica Scandinavica Supplementum*, 433: 50–57.

Leonhard, K. (1968). 'On Monopolar and Bipolar Endogenous Psychoses', *Nervenarzt*, 39(3): 104–106.

Leonhard, K. (1979). *Classification of Endogenous Psychoses and their Differential Etiology*. Berlin: Springer Verlag.

Lewis, A. (1967). *The State of Psychiatry: Essays and Addresses*. New York, NY: Science House.

Makkreel, R. (1992). *Dilthey: Philosopher of the Human Studies*. Princeton, NJ: Princeton University Press.

Menninger, K. (1963). *The Vital Balance*. New York, NY: Viking.

Mitzman, A. (1970). *The Iron Cage: An Historical Interpretation of Max Weber*. Piscataway, NJ: Transaction Publishers.

Olson, A.M. (1994). *Heidegger and Jaspers*. Philadelphia, PA: Temple University Press.

Pepper, G.B. (1963). 'A Re-Examination of the Ideal Type Concept', *American Catholic Sociological Review*, **24**: 185–201.

Phillips, J., Frances, A., Cerullo, M.A., Chardavoyne, J., Decker, H.S., First, M.B., *et al.* (2012). 'The Six Most Essential Questions in Psychiatric Diagnosis: A Pluralogue. Part 1: Conceptual and Definitional Issues in Psychiatric Diagnosis', *Philosophy, Ethics and Humanities in Medicine*, **7**(1): 3.

Rayner, T. (2007). *Foucault's Heidegger*. New York, NY: Continuum.

Rorty, R. (1991) *Objectivity, Relativism, and Truth: Philosophical Papers I*. Cambridge, UK, Cambridge University Press.

Sadler, J.Z. (2002). *Descriptions and Prescriptions: Values, Mental Disorders, and the DSM*. Baltimore, MD: Johns Hopkins University Press.

Schwartz, M.A., Wiggins, O.P. (1987). 'Diagnosis and Ideal Types: A Contribution to Psychiatric Classification', *Comprehensive Psychiatry*, **28**(4): 277–291.

Shorter, E. (1997). *A History of Psychiatry*. New York, NY: Wiley.

Shorter, E. (2007). 'The Doctrine of the Two Depressions in Historical Perspective', *Acta Psychiatrica Scandinavica Supplementum*, 433: 5–13.

Smith, D. J., Ghaemi, N.S. (2010). 'Is Underdiagnosis the Main Pitfall when Diagnosing Bipolar Disorder? Yes', *British Medical Journal*, **340**: 854.

Sullivan, H.S. (1954). *The Psychiatric Interview*. New York, NY: Norton.

Ungvari, G.S. (1993). 'The Wernicke-Kleist-Leonhard School of Psychiatry', *Biological Psychiatry*, **34**(11): 749–752.

Videla, P. (1994). 'On the Narratives of Science: The Critique of Modernity in Husserl and Heidegger', *Human Studies*, **17**: 189–202.

Weber, M. (1949). *The Methodology of the Social Sciences* (E.A. Shils, H.A. Finch, trans.). Glencoe. IL: Free Press.

Weber, M. (1975). *Max Weber: A Biography*. Piscataway, NJ: Transaction Publishers.

Wiggins, O.P., Schwartz, M.A. (1991). 'Is There a Science of Meaning?', *Integrative Psychiatry*, **7**: 48–53.

Wiggins, O.P., Schwartz, M.A. (1994). 'The Limits of Psychiatric Knowledge and the Problem of Classification', in J.Z. Sadler, O.P. Wiggins, M.A. Schwartz (eds), *Philosophical Perspectives on Psychiatric Diagnostic Classification*. Baltimore, MD: Johns Hopkins University Press, 89–103.

Chapter 18

Reaction and development of manic and melancholic-depressive patients

Alfred Kraus

In his *General Psychopathology* (1965, 1997), Karl Jaspers brought manic and melancholic-depressive disturbances together with notions that are still highly important for diagnostics, as well as for classification in the methodology of investigation. The notions handled here of reaction and development, along with those of process, situation, and personality, are partly new and more precisely determined by Jaspers.

Jaspers' concept of manic and melancholic-depressive disturbances

Generally, Jaspers contrasts 'emotional disturbance' (as 'a kind of natural psychic life') with 'mental illness, i.e. schizophrenic mental life. Simultaniously, in his diagnostic scheme he contrasts manic-depressive illness with 'schizophrenia', but calls both together the 'big psychoses' (Jaspers 1965: 508).[1] He describes thoroughly the symptomatology of 'pure mania' and of 'pure depression', as well as what he calls particularly characteristic 'melancholia', which is in his understanding an ideal type (Jaspers 1965: 499–501). For Jaspers, the old types of mania and depression are opposite syndromes. Pure mania is characterized by original, overflowing cheerfulness and a motiveless euphoria connected with a flight of ideas, a feeling of pleasure, heightened domination by one's physical desires, unwavering optimism, abundance of associations, and bodily feelings of well-being. For the manic person his own capabilities seem outstanding. In contrast, Jaspers understands pure depression as essentially determined by a motiveless, deep sadness accompanied by an inhibition of all mental processes. The patient feels this deep sadness as sensations in his 'breast and body as if [he] could grasp the sadness by these sensations' (Jaspers 1965: 500). Apart from these symptoms, patients describe self-reproaches, ideas of sin and of insufficiency, as well as ideas of destitution. According to Jaspers, symptoms of pure mania and of pure depression

[1] All page numbers marked that relate to our own translation of *Allgemeine Psychopathologie* are referred to by the publication date 1965 with original page numbers. English translations of Jaspers' *General Psychopathology* by Hoenig and Hamilton are referred to by the publication date 1997. In the German version of DSM, 'major depression' is translated as 'typical depression'. But this does not have the meaning of an ideal type (in Jaspers' sense) but rather means to be only relatively characteristic.

seem 'very natural because of an understandable continuous connection of the single traits' (Jaspers 1965: 500). If depression deteriorates, for example, when overvalued ideas or obsessional ideas become delusion-like, it can change into melancholia; many bodily sensations along with the highest degrees of depersonalization and disturbances of perception may follow. Since for Jaspers melancholia is a subcategory of emotional disturbances, everything he says about such disturbances is also applicable to melancholia. So in his view it is possible to intuitively understand melancholia, whereas he states that schizophrenic psychic life is, in a certain way, not understandable. The pathological psychic life in emotional disturbances is 'vividly conceivable as an increase or decrease of phenomena already known to us and as an occurrence of such phenomena without normal reasons and motives' (Jaspers 1965: 483). Thus, according to Jaspers the manic ideas as well as the melancholic delusions of sin, of destitution and of nihilism, are not delusions proper like schizophrenic delusion, but are merely delusion-like ideas (*wahnhafte Ideen*), which in contrast to schizophrenic delusion originate from different psychic phenomena, such as 'affects, drives, desires and fears' (Jaspers 1965: 89). So in delusion-like[2] ideas there is no alteration of the personality but merely a transient change of the whole psychic life. Jaspers posits conclusively that in delusion proper the delusional ideas cannot be sufficiently understood in terms of the personality or the situation; they are much more just 'symptoms of a disease process that can be identified by the presence of other symptoms as well' (Jaspers 1997: 107). In the categories of schizophrenic and affective disorders, the diagnostic manuals ICD-10-V/F (International Classification of Diseases, tenth revision, chapter V(F) (Dilling et al. 2005)) and DSM-IV-TR (*Diagnostic and Statistical Manual of Mental Disorders, Fourth Edition, Text Revision* (American Psychiatric Association 2004)) simply define delusion without Jaspers' differentiation between delusion-like ideas and delusion proper.

Regarding the course and outcome of the illness, traditionally the terms of attack (exacerbation), process, and defect are connected with schizophrenia, while those of phase[3] and restitution are connected with cyclothymia,[4] and those of reaction and development with neuroses and variations of character (cf. Häfner 1963: 394). Therefore, we have to explain why we question the significance of the terms of reaction and development in our contribution to manic and melancholic-depressive patients.

With regard to the term of reaction, not only Jaspers spoke of the possibility of reactive psychosis. Particularly around the time after the publication of *General Psychopathology*, the question regarding reaction to certain outer situations (respectively, of precipitation) was often the subject of scientific investigations, as well as in the context of endogenous depression, which was earlier seen as being non-reactive. This has led to clinical terms like 'reactive depression', 'endoreactive dysthymia', 'vitalized depressive reaction', etc. Among these terms in ICD-10, 'depressive reaction' is used in the category 'depressive episode' as well as in the category of 'adjustment disorder', whereas the notions of 'psychogenic' and

[2] Regarding depressive and manic episodes with psychotic symptoms in modern psychiatry, one speaks of delusion as on an equal footing with schizophrenia. The term delusion-like is no longer used. Delusional became the adjective of delusion.

[3] In German psychiatry, phase (Anglo Saxon psychiatry: 'episode') is contrasted to thrust.

[4] 'Zyklothymie', used by K. Schneider (1967) and his school, is synonymous with 'manisch-depressive Krankheit' and 'manisch-depressive Psychose'.

'reactive depression' are now considered as belonging only to the notion of a 'depressive episode'. This manual also explains a 'reactive depressive psychosis' and a 'psychogenic depressive psychosis' as belonging to a 'severe depressive episode with psychotic symptoms'. If the severe episode is without psychotic symptoms, then one solely requires the term 'melancholia', rather than the term 'reactive depression' to be inclusive. By means of inclusions, aetiological aspects came into the diagnostic manual of ICD-10. Because Jaspers' *General Psychopathology* has not only influenced the classification of schizophrenic disorders in diagnostic manuals considerably, but has also influenced classifications of affective disorders, the question arises: what does Jaspers understand by reaction?

Reaction as a normal as well as an abnormal mechanism

Jaspers begins his chapter on 'meaningful connections and their specific mechanisms' (1997: 364) with the statement that without these extra-conscious mechanisms as a substructure of our psychic life and without their intact functioning, no meaningful connections could ever be realized. The notion of reaction denotes normal as well as abnormal mechanisms. In any case, according to Jaspers, there is also always a reaction of the bodily organism implied, be it a reaction to the influences of the external world, a reaction of an organ, a reaction of the patient to a psychotic process of illness, or a reaction to an experience. Reactions become abnormal, when in 'their amount, degree and duration these go beyond what is usual […] Excitement becomes overexcitement, inhibition becomes paralysis […] Associations that have become mechanical habits turn into despotic and binding ties, into fixations […] If the whole psychic life is a continuous synthesis of something that has been separated, so the final and complete dissociation is something abnormal' (Jaspers 1997: 381). Such dissociation is found in psychogenic reactions, in hysterical phenomena, and in psychotic states no matter how different these reactions may be in their significance and implication. In addition to this mechanism of dissociation, Jaspers finds in abnormal states the mechanism of a switchover by which, through a certain jolt, an entirely different psychic state occurs as the condition for the appearance of new abnormal phenomena. Even if in these mechanisms the psychic excitement plays a contributory role, one must always search for their organic causes.

According to Jaspers (1997: 384), there are two kinds of pathological reactions: (1) a merely precipitated psychosis, the content of which has no meaningful connections with the experience.[5] An example would be the precipitation of a catatonia or of a circular depression in the case of bereavement. In this case, the psychic shake-up is exclusively the last and possibly dispensable provocation of the illness, be it a transient phase or the beginning of a process that could have finally emerged without this provocation and developed completely and independently following its own laws. From this kind of reaction we can differentiate that which Jaspers calls (2) a 'reaction proper', because here the content is meaningfully connected with the experience. This 'x' would never have occurred without that experience 'y;' the course of the reaction and whatever is connected with it remain dependent on

[5] The English language does not, in contrast to the German language, discriminate between *Erlebnis* and *Erfahrung*, and speaks of 'experience' in both cases. *Erfahrung* means that one or more *Erlebnis(-se)* have resulted in an *Erfahrung*, i.e. somebody has learned something through *Erlebnis(-se)*. In passages referred to earlier, Jaspers means *Erlebnis*.

the experience. A paradigm for this is the psychogenic reaction. If we were dealing with a reactive psychosis here, this would be related to a central experience (Jaspers 1997: 384). In contrast to this, in the case of a merely precipitated and spontaneous psychosis, we would observe a primary development of the illness without any relationship to the personal fate or experience of the patient. The content here occurs merely by chance, which means the experiences of earlier life would have no effects. A reactive psychosis may be an immediate reaction to an experience or occur only after some time of ripening. It is paramount for an understanding of Jaspers' term of a psychic reaction that, as we have already shown, reaction has an aspect of meaningfulness (experience and content), a causal aspect (change in what is extra-conscious), and a prognostic aspect (i.e. the change is transient). On one hand, we are dealing with psychoses bearing convincing, meaningful connections between the psychotic content and the experience (the reactive psychosis proper). On the other hand, we encounter merely precipitated psychoses, the content of which 'has no meaningful connections with the life-history' of the patient, even if, of course, the content must have been drawn from his former life. Regardless, the content's value as part of the patient's life is not the decisive reason for why 'it has merged into the psychotic content' (Jaspers 1997: 385) (i.e. pure phases or thrusts).

For Jaspers (1997: 385), this means that reactions in general are meaningful in three different ways: (1) they are meaningful as the 'extent of a psychic trauma as the adequate cause' (Jaspers 1997: 385) of any breakdown; (2) they have a meaning or purpose 'which the reactive psychosis sub-serves' (Jaspers 1997: 113) by which we understand the contents of the reactive psychosis in particular, i.e. the single traits of the illness are adequate for this meaning (this meaning can be, e.g. the fulfilment of wishes); and (3) they are meaningful in helping us understand the slide into a psychosis, or into a physical illness together with the contents (e.g. if anxieties, needs, hopes, and wishes appear as realized in a delusional or hallucinatory way).

Jaspers summarizes the meaningfulness of psychosis as follows: 'It serves as a defence, as a refuge, an escape, as a wish-fulfilment. It springs from a conflict with reality which has become intolerable' (Jaspers 1997: 389). However, Jaspers restricts this kind of understanding by saying that the mechanisms of transformation themselves and the extent of the causal significance of a shocking event are difficult to assess. In these psychoses, he posits that there are always more abnormal phenomena than those which can be included in an understandable context. In this context he mentions reactive depressive states, but also reactive manias (even if in his view these are rare).

In an overview of reactive states, Jaspers classifies these: (1) 'according to what precipitates the reaction' (Jaspers 1997: 389) (e.g. prison-psychosis, compensation-neurosis, after accidents, earthquakes, catastrophes, etc.); and (2) 'according to the type of psychic structure of the reactive state' (Jaspers 1997: 389) (such as the states of reactive depression and reactive mania; here sadness tends to grow naturally, cheerfulness may exceed all bounds and become unmanageable). If we knew the respective extra-conscious mechanisms, it might be possible to recognize the specific hysterical or paranoid reactions. However, as long as we do not, they remain hypothetical. Finally, we are able to classify reactive states (3) according 'to the type of psychic constitution which determines the reaction' (Jaspers 1997: 391).

Jaspers understands constitution as that which develops out of the original dispositions in the process of life. One might say, for example, as new dispositions of reacting in a certain way. In patients showing phases, he sees a swaying constitutional disposition when it comes to reacting. This 'swaying' total mental state fluctuates in phases quite spontaneously. It is further a result of experiences and physical events. The importance of this constitutional disposition for reacting with a circular depression is apparently the reason that Jaspers considers phases as being different from reaction proper. Thus, here he only speaks of a mere reaction in the way of precipitation, the content of which has no understandable connection with the experience, as for instance in the case of death (his own example). A psychic shake-up as the cause for a circular depression may be missing. The kind of psychosis may even be contradictory to the content of the experience. In fact, a case of death can precipitate a mania. Apart from this, in the case of depression we cannot presume that with the disappearance of the cause that the reason for the experience would also gradually disappear. Jaspers concedes, however, that because of the permanently given flowing interplay of connections (both causal and understandable connections) in a single case, it is not always possible to separate clearly the reaction proper from a phase (e.g. of a circular depression, *zirkuläre Gemütserkrankung*) or from a thrust (e.g. in schizophrenia).

Development and process as different categories

The notion of process, particularly as a characteristic of the course of schizophrenic psychosis, is closely connected with that of the incomprehensibility of primary delusion in the context of the question of development or process in Jaspers' thinking. It is also intricately connected with other psychotic phenomena. The theorem of a psychotic occurrence of process as well as that of incomprehensibility certainly belong to the most important, but at the same time most disputed, concepts of Jaspers' thought. Both concepts, that of process as well as that of incomprehensibility, are in sharp conflict with the fundamental historicity of human life—respectively, with Jaspers' concept of development and its far reaching comprehensibility. The lawfulness of motivation (*Motivationsgesetzlichkeit*) as well as the ripening of the personality in the course of life are the most comprehensible aspects of all. In this article, we cannot deal with all the different notions of process taken into consideration by Jaspers, for example, physical-organic processes in diseases of the brain, psychological processes characterized only by psychological features, and psychotic processes. Jaspers draws a sharp distinction between the psychotic occurrence of process and the development of an emotional reaction, along with the development of personality. Psychotic processes in schizophrenic patients are characterized by irreversibility as well as by the psychological criterion in its real sense, i.e. the occurrence of 'something new', of 'something alien which invaded the comprehensible development of the personality' (Häfner 1963: 396). In his attempt to replace this psychological criterion, which is dependent on the empathy of the diagnostician, with an objective criterion, Schneider (1967) spoke of an interruption of the 'lawfulness of meaning' (*Sinngesetzlichkeit*), of the 'continuity of meaning' (*Sinnkontinuität*) in the development of life, which should differentiate the psychotic process from both kinds of development mentioned earlier. What seems particularly important for our purposes is Jaspers' assumption that the development of life itself is a kind of process, a process in which man is submitted biologically to an ascending and a descending direction of ripening, thereby 'enforcing' a psychological-existential ripening that can be missed or not realized. This normal occurrence of a psychological process seems important to us, especially if we compare it with clinically relevant psychological and psychotic processes. This could, for Jaspers, have been the chance to conceive a concept of a psychopathology of development, which shows itself in some outlines of his work, but which remained undeveloped. Later, we will show how, for this purpose, modern empirically-based research could profit from his concept of antinomia and boundary situation (*Grenzsituationen*).

Before continuing, it is important to consider the following elements of Jaspers' differentiation of the development of a person as a whole. The development consists in: (1) the biological process of life; (2) the factual psychic history of life, which at this stage is not yet connected with insight about oneself; (3) 'the self-reflected awareness', with which the history of life enlightens itself; and (4) the 'existential basis of decision and acceptance of the given for a more thorough appropriation of it' (Jaspers 1997: 694). It can be questioned as to how far Jaspers was influenced by Binswanger's article (1961) about 'function of life and history of life', which had already been published in 1910 (the first edition of *General Psychopathology* was published in 1913), in the development of this concept. In any case, he differentiated and completed Binswanger's concept. One example of a single additional category is, among others, the acquisition of new automatisms (e.g. learning to walk, constructing a world, adapting to a certain stable surrounding first life-event).

Development and understanding of personality according to Jaspers and modern concepts of the manic-depressive spectrum of personality

Jaspers considers the notion of development to be the development of personality. The personality or character of man encompasses that which he is from birth, as well as the becoming and the having become of oneself (i.e. the development of oneself by oneself). These aspects are visible in one's biography, which comprises of one's life history with all its possibilities and decisions (Jaspers 1997: 358). Although Jaspers starts from a fundamental differentiation between personality (or character) and psychosis, different to Kretschmer (1961), an important topic for him is the relationship of personality to psychosis (i.e. personality to phase as well as to process), instead of just the relationship of the original personality to its pathological development (in psychopaths). Simultaneously, he only thematizes the relationship of personality to phase, for example, that of mania or depression, with respect to the disposition of temperament and mood of the patient. He quotes investigations by Reiss (1910: 536), who, for example, found a cheerful disposition in manic states of mood disorders and a depressive disposition in sad mood disorders. The conspicuous disposition of mood alteration before the onset of or between manic and depressive phases was also observed by Kraepelin and Kretschmer, a fact which is now under thorough investigation by Akiskal (1996) and his group of researchers. To what extent these are minor expressions of a depressive or manic-depressive illness cannot yet be decided.

Concerning the personality of patients on the manic-depressive spectrum, we will focus on the typus melancholicus and typus manicus and their further development. We consider these to be salient because they seem to correspond with what Jaspers described by the opposing (antinomic) structure of mental life in general and the significance of this concept for comprehensive psychology. They also seem to correspond to his notion of characterology for the understanding of psychopathological phenomena (Jaspers 1965: 283–289).

Jaspers was well aware that particularly among psychoanalytic authors, going back to Abraham (1911) and Freud (1967) but also classical authors like Shimoda in Japan (see Kraus 1971a), an anankastic personality was often ascribed to melancholic patients, which showed a strong similarity to the so-called 'typus melancholicus' of Tellenbach (1983a). For instance, Freud stated (1967) that 'a formerly well behaved, efficient woman is more prone to get ill from melancholia than the "good-for-nothing"' (Freud 1967, vol. X: 432). Typus melancholicus, when compared with a disposition to alterations of temperaments and moods, is often exhibited in a premorbid personality, which is (without a doubt) responsible for the precipitation of melancholic episodes in many cases. In monopolar manics, a somewhat opposite personality type, the typus manicus, seems to be prominent, whereas in bipolars a combination of both types appears in a different form (see Dörr 1986; von Zerssen 1982, 1996b, 2001). Unfortunately, we cannot go into detail here about this research; it is instead our hope to point out the definition of the typus melancholicus by Tellenbach (1983), who was the first to describe this type extensively. According to him, the typus melancholicus is extremely industrious in terms of social behaviour, hardworking, oriented to order in a meticulous way, and inclined to a symbiotic and dependent relationship with others. Many research groups have since confirmed these personality traits with different empirical instruments and with a prevalence of around 50%, plus 25% (with reservation) in patients with endogenous depression (Mundt et al. 1997). Other empirical studies were carried out by von Zerssen (1982, 1996a, 1996b, 2001), Sato (1992), Ueki et al. (2006), and Kronmüller (2002; Kronmüller et al. 2002). We, along with Schwartz and Wiggins (2000) and Kraus (1977, 1995, 1996, 2007a, 2007b, 2011), showed that, regarding the aspect of their motivation melancholic persons differ in regards to the 'idionomic' behaviour of anankastic persons. Typus melancholicus patients are strongly oriented to the social norms of society and the surroundings in which they live. They are over-identified with these norms. Due to this over-identification with the respective norms, we spoke of hypernomic behaviour (nomos in Greece means norm, law, rule) as the essential characteristic of the typus melancholicus. This particular relationship of their behaviour to external social norms has also been confirmed by empirical studies (see Hecht et al. 1998; Heerlein et al. 2002; Mundt et al. 1997; Stanghellini and Mundt 1997; von Zerssen 1996a, 1996b, 2001). The hypernomic and, according to psychoanalytic authors, conformist behaviour (see Arieti 1962 Cohen et al. 1954; Matussek and Feil 1983) is in our view the consequence of an insufficient ego-identity.

The other side of the typus melancholicus concept—a symbiotic relationship with others—consists mainly in a being-for-others in the form of an achievement for others according to Tellenbach. As with other precipitating situations, the main endangering factor to become depressed is any kind of disorder or violation of this order of being-with-others. Because of the high sensibility for order (e.g. in Tellenbach's view), divorce is for these patients primarily a loss of order.

However, there are also other personality features of manics and melancholics to be considered. In several articles, we described a cognitive and emotional intolerance of ambiguity in these patients (Kraus 1977, 1988, 2011). Cognitive and emotional tolerance of ambiguity was conceived by the sociologist Frenkel-Brunswik (1949/1950) to be a general variable of personality. Applied to the personality type of melancholic and manic patients we already find an intolerance of ambiguity prior to the onset and between the phases, as well as particularly within the phases. For instance patients with a typus melancholicus personality have a tendency to attribute mainly negative qualities to themselves, whereas they may simultaneously idealize family members or other persons with whom they have important or intimate relationships. For the manic type of personality an inverse tendency can be observed. Connected with this one-sided tendency towards cognitive intolerance of ambiguity, we find an emotional intolerance of ambiguity—a person's incapacity to develop an ambiguity of emotions for himself or for others. Thus, over-goodness, overfriendliness, helpfulness, being overcritical to oneself, low aggressivity, peace at any prize, avoiding the perception of disappointing traits of others (melancholic type) can all be opposed to reckless, demanding, violating behaviour, and critical or pejorative evaluation of others (manic type). These characteristics have also been confirmed by empirical studies (see Baer 1975; Hell 1982; Heerlein and Richter 1991; Heerlein et al. 1996; Matussek and Feil 1983; Matussek et al. 1965; Mundt et al 1997).

The consequence of the intolerance of ambiguity is not only a loss of reality in one's relationships with others but also with oneself. The melancholic person typifies himself with this reduction of the complexity, which is a reduced complexity not only of the representation of others but also of himself in combination with the hypernomic behaviour in its extreme orientation to outer norms, thereby negating his own wishes and aims (Kraus 1977: 77). This behaviour leads to a loss of individuality. Thus, the patient with melancholia appears as a 'real type' when met in person as opposed to an individual. With respect to the awareness of the melancholic person towards himself, Stanghellini (2004: 107) spoke of an *idioagnosia*, which in our understanding is particularly prominent in melancholic delusions (e.g. the particular delusion of insufficiency). It is in our view a loss of empathy not only for others but also a loss of empathy for oneself as a precondition of realistic self-reflection. If we compare the hypernomic behaviour of the typus melancholicus with the antinomic, rebellious behaviour of the typus manicus we recognize a mutual exclusion of reality. For this reason, we have also referred thus far of an intolerance of ambiguity in the behaviour of both types.

When Jaspers speaks about the comprehensibility of personality (Jaspers 1965: 283–289) particularly in his *Psychology of World Views* (Jaspers 1925), he comes very close to counting tolerance of ambiguity as a concept to be counted as a general personality variable, which we have applied as intolerance to the personality of melancholic, manic, and bipolar patients. Unfortunately, Jaspers did not relate his concept to manic and melancholic patients but merely to schizophrenic and neurotic ones (see Fuchs 2008). For Jaspers, there exists a fundamental tension as a consequence of opposite feelings, moods, thoughts, etc., which are normally standardized (*vereinheitlicht*) by choice or synthesis. Accordingly, abnormality results if this synthesis or standardization fails, for example, in the case of the ambivalence of positive and negative emotions regarding the same object at the same time. Even if the notion of ambiguity has some relationship to that of ambivalence, these notions are not the same because tolerance of ambiguity according to Frenkel-Brunswik is not a failure of synthesis but of the capability to tolerate ambiguous feelings and to perceive positive as well as negative qualities of the same object or person. Jaspers maintains that opposite tendencies, in principle, belong together but can also separate from each other. If these opposite tendencies, as basic, dialectical possibilities, are synthesized, they can result in productive tensions and in establishing harmonic unities. For example, we showed the significance of the concept of tolerance of ambiguity for the creativity of bipolar persons and their relatives (Kraus 2007b).

The recognition of the precipitation of melancholic and manic episodes as well as of schizophrenia in general depends very much on knowledge of the vulnerability of the respective personality. By now recognizing that typus melancholicus and typus manicus extend to hyernomic and antinomic behaviour, we think that we are in a much better position to recognize precipitating situations.

Precipitation of psychosis according to Jaspers

We have already mentioned how Jaspers differentiated precipitated psychosis from reactive psychosis proper. Because he dealt with both psychoses under the heading of reaction, this can easily lead to confusing the reader. The difference for Jaspers consists in a different connection of psychosis with experience. In the case of a precipitated psychosis there is: (1) no comprehensive connection to be found between the psychosis and the experience, and (2) if there is a precipitating experience, the psychosis is not dependent in its development on the experience of the event insofar as the psychosis is not relieved when the external situation is removed. The development of the illness can only be explained by reference to a bodily process. Thus, the precipitated phase lacks any understandable connection with the life-history and the content of the respective experiences. This does not exclude that the psychic destabilization was caused by a shake-up in experience, which then became the final cause for the outbreak of the illness. Very similarly, Schneider (1967: 128) concedes that sometimes a cyclothymic psychosis is started by an experience. However, what matters in these cases is not the content of the experience but the effect of an emotion on the body (Schneider 1967: 128). The precipitating event here is not effective as a meaningful experience but as a 'vital power', as a 'vital blow'. The effect of the emotion is blind concerning its meaning (*sinnblind*; Schneider 1967: 128). Schneider warns against being persuaded by the contents to assume a psychogenic relationship. Even today, this view is widespread, determining life event research in the context of affective disorders above all. This research does not primarily start from the experience of an event but from the event as such, to which a general affective reaction of stress is supposed. Here I can only point to the fact that the stimulus-reaction as such, taken from organic medicine, suggests immediate drastic causal effects by violent irritations.

Apart from its concrete application to endogenous psychosis, Jaspers developed a differentiated concept of the term for a situation in general. Apart from being part of society through particular social roles, every person finds himself in his own world and he himself produces a world, grasping or missing chances in various situations.

In *Psychology of World Views* (1925), Jaspers developed his profound concept of 'boundary situation' (*Grenzsituationen*). He begins with the anthropological concept that man is fundamentally exposed to certain boundary situations, which are 'unavoidable' and 'intolerable' (Jaspers 1925: 229) because they are 'insolvable' as such (Jaspers 1925: 232). At the border of everything that man can achieve there is the experience of 'chance (*Zufall*), death and guilt' (Jaspers 1925: 230). There are no absolute values; everything is relative and divided into opposites. Everywhere antinomies are felt, experienced, and thought at the borders of our being. In a certain sense, they influence every real situation in life. Jaspers differentiates between antinomies on the side of the object and antinomies on the side of subjectivity (Jaspers 1925: 238). The former are antinomies of thinking and recognition, the latter are those of opposite drives, feelings, and opposite characterological qualities.

There are different kinds of possible reactions to these antinomies about which one is more or less conscious. First, he might be destroyed by them, for example, if he wants to fulfil all antinomies to the point of paralysis from ever acting (Jaspers 1925: 240). Second, he might dodge the antimonies, for example, by always neutralizing the other contradictory aspect of something. Or finally, he might gain power. This last kind of reaction is possible in two ways: one may ignore one aspect of the antinomies and gain power in spite of existing antinomies by awaiting them; or, one may gain power by the existing antinomies. According to Jaspers, this is the case only in great personalities who are able (in a certain sense) to solve real antinomies by a process that entails much suffering. In the first possible reaction, there is a connection between the ruin of man (by trying to fulfil all expectations) and the delusion of negation (e.g. Cotard syndrome) in severe melancholic psychosis. Jaspers describes this severe type of melancholic psychosis as follows: nothing really exists; all people feel that they and others are dead; the world itself even ceases to exist in such absolute nihilism. There is also a connection with the third possible reaction to manic states, when the patient gains power by ignoring the opposite aspect of that in which he is presently engaged.

During Jaspers' lifetime, other important and new concepts of the notion of situation were developed in psychiatry by the phenomenological-anthropological approach, often in confrontation with the stimulus-reaction model. These concepts (summarized by Kraus 1971b, 1996) remained unknown for a long time in Anglo-Saxon psychiatry. We only mention the concept of the representative meaning of dramatic events by Straus (1978), the notion of situated genesis (*Situagenie*) by von Baeyer (1966), and the concept of lived situation, which in its genetic meaning is not known by the patient but gets its individual meaning 'unconsciously' by the personality structure of the respective patient (i.e. from his structure of personality) (*gelebte Struktur*) by Janzarik (1988). It is common in all three of these concepts that they refer explicitly not only to the experience but also to the lived situation. The lived situation gets its specific (traumatic) meaning from the respective personality engaged in it. That means the individual may be aware of the traumatic meaning of the situation on a pre-reflexive level without reflecting consciously about it. Taking the lived situation into consideration within the context of the precipitation of depressive and manic phases is of particular importance because the withdrawal of the real traumatic meaning of an event (leaving the consciousness void) seems to be an integral part of melancholic and manic phases. Even Freud (1967, Vol. X: 431) viewed melancholia as different from bereavement due to its relation to the loss of an object, which is inaccessible to consciousness: for example, in the case of someone's death, the melancholic person 'knows whom but not what he has lost' (Freud 1967, Vol. X: 431). Thus, the melancholic person is not conscious of what is really depressing him and so is unable to communicate it to other people. This withdrawal of the real traumatic meaning of an event does not seem to be caused by a repression, such as in neuroses, but is a result of the particular kind of missing meaning (e.g. the loss of identity). In this way, the concept of a lived situation has fundamentally changed the understanding of the connection between event and melancholic or manic phases.

Identity-theoretical aspects of 'antinomic structure' and '*Gehäuse*'

A significant deficit in empirical research on typus melancholicus, as well as in empirical research on personality in general, is that investigations focus primarily on psychological qualities, behavioural assessments, and statistical correlative connections between them. The problem is that this method makes it impossible to show the inner connections of the structure or essence of a type. Assessments of the constitutive, fundamental structure of the typus melancholicus as 'being fixed to orderliness' (*Festgelegtsein auf Ordentlichkeit*) (Tellenbach 1983), or, in the psychoanalytic view, fixed to 'anankastic behaviour', or as we would say fixed to 'over-identification with the social role', do not immediately follow from single typological characteristics themselves. At most, they can be suggested by these constitutive structures. However, in order to substantiate these genetic terms, further methods and empirical assessments need to be pursued. These terms of structure and essence are of great significance. Monti and Stanghellini (1996: 203) call these 'psychopathological organizers' or, respectively, 'meaning organizers'. They are important for the diagnostics and therapy of psychopathological disturbances in general. These synthesized schemes 'of comprehension […] are aimed at collecting different psychopathological experiences into a unitary core of meaningfulness' (Monti and Stanghellini 1996: 203). With this in mind, we now return to what we have already said about the typology of manic and depressive patients. Taking the melancholic and the manic type of personality from the perspective of their identity formation, we find many parallels to Jaspers' term, the 'antinomic structure of being' (1925: 232) and to what he calls 'dwellings of being' (*Gehäuse des Seins*) (1925: 305) when speaking about his famous concept of boundary situations (*Grenzsituationen*). Our goal here is to enrich our concept, along with Jaspers' own, of manic-depressive illness. In the last few years, many articles on boundary situations have been published. Here we mention only those relating to concepts of psychiatric topics. These are those of Kick (2009), of Fuchs (2008), and of Schlimme (2011).

Hypernomic and conformistic behaviour, as well as cognitive and emotional intolerance of ambiguity, serve an identical purpose for melancholic persons in maintaining their role-identity(ies), i.e. the identity found in their respective social roles. Role identities are particularly important in compensating for a lack of ego-identity and ego-achievements. A strong dependency on one's role-identity(ies) is, firstly, shown in the rigidity or being fixed in the kind of behaviour just mentioned and, secondly, in the precipitating situation of melancholic and manic phases. These are often situations of changes and losses in general, but also changes and losses of social roles in particular.

First, we mention situations called situations of 'social ambivalence' by sociologists (Merton and Barber 1963). These are very common situations of daily life. They can be situations in which normatively legitimated expectations of different social roles are fixed in the same person at the same time, for example, the person's professional role and her role as a housewife, mother, and partner (inter-role conflicts). Also, conflicts may arise within one role, for example, if somebody is simultaneously the superior of one or many role partners and the subordinate of other role partners (intra-role conflicts). Such situations of conflicting demands of role expectations can only be solved by a certain role-distance to these expectations, by flexibility and perspectivity, or in short, by the application of ego-achievements. The term sociological ambivalence does not mean subjective ambivalence, rather an objective ambivalence of the outer situation, even if it can lead to subjective ambivalence. However, it is very common that melancholic patients in these situations do not come to such ambivalence. Instead, they may tend to fulfil all normative and value-oriented expectations as thoroughly as possible, i.e. in an exaggerated way to the point of exhaustion. It is evident that hypernomic behaviour, which in our view substitutes for a lack of ego-achievements, is particularly unfit to solve such situations of conflicting norms and values. This overtaxing of role expectations can endanger or even lead to a breakdown of one's role identity and also to a breakdown of identity as a whole, with the consequence of a melancholic or manic phase. This breakdown can happen in particular when bodily strength is weakened by age or bodily illness. Many so-called somatic depressions, for example, a depression in the wake of a cerebral stroke, a *contusio cerebri*, a heart attack, influenza, and so on, show this dynamic in patients with a typus melancholicus structure. In most of these cases, depression is not a symptom of the respective somatic illness, but is precipitated by it in the context of the typus melancholicus behaviour. In these cases we do not think speaking of somatic depression as justified. It is important to recognize that hypernomic behaviour, as a substitute of lacking ego-achievements, is not so much the expression of particularly strong strivings for high achievements as such or *Selbstanspruch des Leistens*, according to Tellenbach (1983), or of narcissistic needs, as some authors believe, but a consequence of the needs of a typus melancholicus to maintain his role-identity in particularly demanding objective situations. It has, in our view, nothing to do primarily with narcissisms, as long as we understand it as autoeroticism in the way of self-love or other kinds of hypercathexis of the self (i.e. to be loved by the super-ego, etc.).

The personality trait of cognitive and emotional intolerance might have a similar consequence as hypernomic behaviour for the precipitation of manic or depressive episodes. Let us assume that for a long time, a patient has been exploited or deceived by somebody with whom he had an intimate relationship and has idealized this person on the basis of this trait of intolerance of ambiguity. Finally, he could no longer avoid recognizing the negative aspects of this person and as a consequence experienced a severe crisis of his identity found in the relationship with this person. In this case, an identity crisis is particularly severe because of the strong dependency needs of melancholic patients according to Nietzel and Harris (1990).

Losses and changes of social roles, the acquisition of new roles (Finlay and Brown 1981; Glassner et al. 1979) are other typical situations for the precipitation of melancholic and manic episodes. Many of these situations have a strong relationship with a certain developmental stage of the personality and, thus, with the age of the patient. This is expressed in various denominations of depression: for example, the gestational and postpartum depression, depression in consequence of manic behaviour or marital divorce, depression following promotion or success, empty nest depression (when children leave home), retirement depression, depression after bereavement or loss of somebody with whom an intimate relationship existed, etc. Most of these situations to which a depressive episode refers are so-called 'exit events' (Paykel 1982), which imply a new stage or break of development connected with a loss of (role-)identity. Even if the precipitating situation is an entrance event, or a desirable one like a promotion or a success, it can imply a loss of identity before the new one has been acquired. Even if the strong impact of these situations on one's identity is not conscious, it is the individual meaning of the situation that determines the depressive episode in many ways. Thus, Jaspers' sharp division of precipitating reaction and reaction proper cannot be maintained without restriction.

It is well known that melancholic and manic episodes mostly occur at a later age than the first episode of a schizophrenic disorder. According to Huber (1999), affective psychoses mostly become manifest in the third, fourth, and fifth decades, whereas schizophrenic disorders in more than half of the cases (55%) start before the third decade. This late manifestation responds to the fact that in affective disorders we are dealing more with exit events than entrance events precipitating these disorders. In schizophrenic disorders with an earlier incidence of psychosis, entrance events are more prominent.

Patients with affective disorders in general do not have greater difficulties in building up social role-identities (professional role, marital role, etc.). In contrast, schizophrenic persons are mostly so-called non-starters (Goldberg and Morris 1963), having severe problems with the so-called secondary socialization. Often their first episode starts when they try to get rooted in society by entering into a social role (for example, engagement catatonia). After the remission of their episodes, most melancholic and manic patients are able to return to their former roles or build up new ones, whereas with schizophrenic patients these social roles for the most part do not exist. This could have a strong impact on the different course of both disorders (phases against thrusts).

Recent research on the early relationship between mother and child has pointed to the possibility of particular sensitivity for depression in persons who experienced failures to develop primary attachments to their mother or losses in childhood. It can also be supposed, however, that the different mechanisms of intolerance of ambiguity, particularly hypernomic behaviour as vulnerability factors for depression, are the consequence of particular styles of education and relationships in the family (see Stierlin et al. 1986).

If we now return to Jaspers' (1925) antinomic structure of being, we are dealing with an 'objective' structure of our lifeworld, as well as of ourselves. As long as we are confronted by it, the antinomic structure always makes our individual statements about it a particular challenge. According to Jaspers, the boundary situation (*Grenzsituation*), characterized by opposites like life and death, coincidence and necessity, fight and mutual help, are principally intolerable and unsolvable. Thus, it remains a secret not answered by Jaspers as to how, in concrete individual life, it is nevertheless possible to produce a certain synthesis and unity between these antinomies. Their synthesis leads to the construction of certain houses or dwellings (*Gehäuse*), which offer foundation and stability, but always have to be given up anew on account of certain life circumstances and, thereby, must perennially be rebuilt. But there is also a danger that these *Gehäuse* are castles of escape, which are built to avoid exposure to the antinomies or, in the extreme case, to deny them completely. Thus, the *Gehäuse* have a positive as well as a negative aspect.

According to Jaspers, the antinomies have a strong impact on the development of the personality. Jaspers says: 'What man in his true nature is and can become has its origin in the experience, acquisition and overcoming of boundary situations […] A basic structure of mental development is the movement between opposites, to proceed from opposites to synthesis or to decision, in short it is a dialectic unfolding' (Jaspers 1965: 271). In order to develop at all, a 'man must enter into the opposites' (Jaspers 1965: 589). Here Jaspers' biographical model of an interconnection of biologically determined factual processes of life, life history, and existential decisions appear again.

We already spoke about our patients' dependency on role-identities because of a lack of ego-identity. We also detailed the consequences that arise if they are confronted with situations of contradicting expectancies or changing roles. But these were only some examples of their insufficiency to react in an adequate way to ambiguous situations. Every loss implies a kind of 'bereavement reaction' (*Trauerreaktion*), which is characterized by contradicting tendencies of a bonding with the lost object and at the same time a readiness to break away from somebody or free oneself from something. It is precisely the achievement of this vacillating attitude, however, which proves impossible for these patients. The primary reason for this has to do with different mechanisms of intolerance of ambiguity or over-identification with the respective, representative object of one's identity, which we furthermore see as a general feature of the identity-structure of melancholic patients. Thus, this over-identification can be understood as a general tendency to include oneself in the respective *Gehäuse* of one's identity. This means that the mechanisms of intolerance towards ambiguity can be understood as avoidance of the antinomies with which the patients are confronted in the respective situation, which precipitates their episodes. By comparison, schizophrenic patients have a problem of building up protective and stabilizing *Gehäuse* at all. Consequently, the result is either an independence of one tendency from the antinomic opposite tendency, or the simultaneous occurrence of opposite tendencies, for example, simultaneous feelings of love and hate for one person in the sense of Bleuler's ambivalence (which Jaspers also demonstrated). Such a differing relationship to the '*Gehäuse*' could also be shown in particular by attention to close connections between melancholic, depressed persons and 'common sense'. Common sense, here, shows itself already in the hypernomic behaviour opposed to the loss of natural self-evidence, which is not rooted in the common sense of persons with schizophrenia (Blankenburg 1969). Thus, in cases with melancholic and manic persons, as well as schizophrenic persons, one can assess a different deficiency of development of the individual. We assume that this deficiency makes up an essential part of the illness, particularly concerning the different courses of the illness in schizophrenic patients and affective episodes.

So far we have treated the intolerance of ambiguity of melancholic and manic persons on the level of their typical behaviour as personalities. We have connected it with the antinomic structure (according to Jaspers' sense) by showing that, because of their intolerance, the patients avoid grappling with the antinomies presented by Jaspers, or are incapable to cope with them. This manifests itself particularly in the situations precipitating their episodes and leading to a crisis of identity. Now, we want to compare the manic and the melancholic phenomena as such under the aspect of intolerance of ambiguity. What we have recognized is that the melancholic and the manic phase (in mutual relationship) exclude the experiences and behaviours of the opposite phase in an intolerant way. The following oppositions can be highlighted: in melancholic mood disturbances, seen as a whole, a predominant experience of being thrown (*Geworfenheit*) can be contrasted to that of being constantly designed by oneself in a new way in mania (*Entwurfscharakter des Seins*). The experience of severity of the living conditions and burdens of being stand in sharp contrast to the easiness of life in mania (*Leichtigkeit des Seins*). Brooding about everything is contrasted by a flight of ideas in which no idea can be deepened, and everything is equated as representing the same great importance. The ego wanders from one thing to the next. Melancholic patients feel themselves as separated and excluded from others, alienated from their surrounding and from daily life; by contrast, manic patients, so long as they are not in a state of a secondary irritated mania, feel themselves as being in an almost magical communion and agreement with others and the world. Dependency and a feeling of being determined by external rules and norms in melancholia become self-determination and autonomy in mania. An absolute nihilism in the melancholic state mentioned by Jaspers (1925: 300) stands in contrast to an absolute 'positiveness' and optimism in a manic episode. A globalization of relationships between oneself and the world in a certain direction of intolerance with which the patient is almost totally identified in the respective episode seems to be particularly characteristic of this. While intolerance of ambiguity was only a behavioural tendency in the premorbid state, it is now completed in the respective psychotic episode and out of the patient's control. This over-identification with the respective kind of being, which is expressed in melancholic and manic episodes by contrasting states of mood, cognitions, and strivings, is the real pathological mechanism depriving the patient of every possibility of taking an opposite antinomic reflexive stance to the respective state in which he is presently involved (according to identity theory). Jaspers characterizes abnormal mechanisms generally as those that, firstly, overstep the usual mark, degree, and length of the respective period; that, secondly, exaggerate the usual associations and inhibit one via paralysis; and that, thirdly, change the normal psychic life, which consists in a continual keeping-together of what tends to separate, into a complete and insurmountable split. Jaspers does not clarify exactly what the split methodologically and systematically constitutes; regardless, a switch of the state of consciousness is taking place not only in hysterical but also in psychotic states by which, like in a jolt, a completely different psychic state is present.

It is impossible to show here the extent of the phenomena in the clinical episodes that can be understood as a kind of depersonalization in melancholia and of hyperpersonalization in mania. If possible, this would underline the coherence of characteristics of identity formation in the premorbid personality and in both clinical states with the same mechanisms to lock oneself in a *Gehäuse*. Even if the *Gehäuse* of melancholia and mania are different, due to the fact that the antinomies that are normally related to each other are split into opposites in both states, the patient is cut off from the experiencing of and coping with boundary situations, for example, in the case of the death of a loved one. Whereas in normal mourning a dialectical movement binds one to the lost person and simultaneously allows one to let him go, in similar cases with melancholic persons this dialectical movement is missing in the depersonalized quality of their mood alterations. According to DSM-IV, this is 'distinctly different from the kind of feeling experienced in mourning'. In order to break new ground for the practice of psychotherapy for melancholic and manic disturbances, the exact and actual meaning of Jaspers' metaphor, *Gehäuse*, should be clarified. This attempt might do well by thinking, for example, in terms of identity theory.

References

Abraham, K. (1911). 'Ansätze zur psychoanalytischen Erforschung und Behandlung des manisch-depressiven Irreseins und verwandter Zustände', *Zentralblatt für Psychoanalyse*, **2**: 302–315.

Akiskal, H.S. (1996). 'The Temperamental Foundations of Affective Disorders', in C. Mundt, M.J. Goldstein, K. Hahlweg, P. Fiedler (eds), *Interpersonal Factors in the Origin and Course of Affective Disorders*. London: Gaskell, 3–30.

American Psychiatric Association (2000). *Diagnostic and Statistical Manual of Mental Disorders, Fourth Edition, Text Revision, DSM-IV-TR*. Washington, DC: American Psychiatric Association.

Arieti, S. (1962) 'The Psychotherapeutic Approach to Depression', *American Journal Psychotherapy*, **16**: 397–406.

Baer, R. (1975). *Die sozialpsychiatrische Prognose der zyklothymen Depression*. Stuttgart: Thieme.

Baeyer, von W. (1966). 'Situation, Jetztsein und Psychose. Bemerkungen zum Problem der komplementären Situagenie', in W.K. Baeyer (ed), *Conditio Humama*. Berlin: Springer, 14–34.

Binswanger, L. (1961). 'Lebensfunktion und innere Lebensgeschichte', in *Ausgewählte Vorträge und Aufsätze*, Bern: Bd. I. Francke, 50–73.

Blankenburg, W. (1969). 'Ansätze zu einer Psychopathologie des "Common Sense"', *Confinia Psychiatrica*, **12**: 144–163.

Cohen, M.B., Baker, G., Cohen, R.A., Fromm-Reichmann, F., Weigert, E.V. (1954). 'An Intensive Study of 12 Cases of Manic-Depressive Psychosis', *Psychiatry*, **17**: 103–137.

Dilling, H., Mombour, W., Schmidt, M.H. (eds) (2005). *ICD-10-V(F)* (5th edn). Göttingen: Huber.

Dörr, O. (1986). 'Perspectiva fenomenologica de los trastornos de personalidad', *Revista de Psiquiatría*, **3**: 117–127.

Finley, J.R., Brown, G.W. (1981). 'Types of Stressful Life Event and the Onset of Anxiety and Depressive Disorders', *Psychological Medicine*, **11**: 803–815.

Frenkel-Brunswik, E. (1949/1950). 'Intolerance of Ambiguity as an Emotional and Perceptual Personality Variable', *Journal of Personality*, **18**: 108–143.

Freud, S. (1967). *Trauer und Melancholie. Collected works, Vol. X* (4th edn). Frankfurt: Fischer, 427–446.

Fuchs, T. (2008). 'Existenzielle Vulnerabilität. Ansätze zu einer Psychopathologie der Grenzsituationen', in S. Rinofner-Kreidl, H.A. Wiltsche (eds), *Karls Jaspers Allgemeine Psychopathologie zwischen Wissenschaft, Philosophie und Praxis*. Würzburg: Königshausen & Neumann, 95–107.

Glassner, B., Haldipur, C.V., Dessauersmith, J. (1979). 'Role Loss and Working-Class Manic Depression', *Journal of Nervous and Mental Disease*, **167**: 530–541.

Goldberg, E.M., Morrison, S.L. (1963). 'Schizophrenia and Social Class', *British Journal Psychiatry*, **109**: 758–802.

Häfner, H. (1963). 'Prozeß und Entwicklung als Grundbegriffe der Psychopathologie', *Fortschritte der Neurologie, Psychiatrie und ihrer Grenzgebiete*, **31**: 393–438

Hecht, H., van Calker, D., Berger, M., von Zerssen, D. (1998). 'Personality in Patients with Affective Disorder and their Relatives', *Journal Affective Disorder*, **51**: 33–43.

Heerlein, A., Richter, P. (1991). 'Ambiguitätsintoleranz bei affektiven und schizophrenen Störungen', *Nervenarzt*, **62**: 269–273.

Heerlein, A., Rentería, P., Santander, J., Richter, P. (2002). 'Persönlichkeitsaspekte bei Zwangskranken und endogen Depressiven', in T. Fuchs, C. Mundt (eds), *Affekt und affektive Störungen. Phänomenologische Konzepte und empirische Befunde im Dialog*. Paderborn: Ferdinand Schönigh, 215–230.

Heerlein, A., Santander, J., Richter, P. (1996) 'Ambiguitätsintoleranz bei endogenen Psychosen aus transkultureller Sicht', *Fortschritte der Neurologie, Psychiatrie*, **64**: 358–361

Hell, D. (1982). *Ehen depressiver und schizophrener Menschen*. Berlin: Springer.

Huber, G. (1999). *Psychiatrie* (6th edn). Stuttgart: Schattauer.

Janzarik, W. (1988). *Strukturdynamische Grundlagen der Psychiatrie*. Stuttgart: Enke.

Jaspers, K. (1925). *Psychologie der Weltanschauungen* (3rd edn). Berlin: Julius Springer.

Jaspers, K. (1965). *Allgemeine Psychopathologie* (7th edn). Berlin: Springer.

Jaspers, K. (1997). *General Psychology* (7th edn) (J. Hoenig, M.W. Hamilton, trans.). Baltimore, MD: Johns Hopkins University Press.

Kick, H. (2009). 'Grenzsituation und Wertebildung—eine prozessdynamische Interpretation nach Karl Jaspers', in D. von Engelhardt, H.J. Gerigk (eds), *Karl Jaspers im Schnittpunkt von Zeitgeschichte. Psychopathologie, Literatur und Film*. Heidelberg: Mattes, 73–88.

Kraus, A. (1971a). 'Der Typus melancholicus in östlicher und westlicher Forschung (der japanische Beitrag M. Shimodas zur prämorbiden Persönlichkeit Manisch-Depressiver)', *Nervenarzt*, **42**: 481–483.

Kraus, A. (1971b). 'Situationstheoretische Aspekte der Auslösung manisch-depressiver Phasen', in W. Walcher (eds), *Probleme der Provokation depressiver Psychosen. International Symposium in Graz*. Wien: Brüder Hollinek, 117–123.

Kraus, A. (1977). *Sozialverhalten und Psychose Manisch-Depressiver*. Stuttgart: Enke.

Kraus, A. (1988). 'Ambiguitätsintoleranz als Persönlichkeitsmerkmal der Krankheitsphänomene Manisch-Depressiver', in W. Janzarik (ed), *Persönlichkeit und Psychose*. Stuttgart: Enke, 140–149.

Kraus, A. (1995). 'Psychotherapy based on identity problems of depressives', *American Journal of Psychotherapy*, **49**: 197–212.

Kraus, A. (1996). 'Role Performance, Identity Structure and Psychosis in Melancholic and Manic-Depressive Patients', in C. Mundt, M.J. Goldstein., K. Hahlweg, P. Fiedler (eds), *Interpersonal Factors in the Origin and Course of Affective Disorders*. London: Gaskell, 31–47.

Kraus, A. (2007a). 'Der Typus melancholicus als Nomopath', in H. Lang, H. Faller, M. Schowalter (eds), *Struktur, Persönlichkeit, Persönlichkeitsstörung*. Würzburg: Königshausen & Neumann, 193–209.

Kraus, A. (2007b). 'Manisch-depressives Spektrum und Kreativität', in D. Borchmeyer (ed), *Melancholie und Heiterkeit*. Heidelberg: Winter-Verlag, 189–220.

Kraus, A. (2011). 'Identitätsorientierte Psychotherapie Melancholischer', in H. Faller, H. Lang (eds), *Depression, Klinik, Ursachen, Therapie*. Würzburg: Königshausen & Neumann, 149–164.

Kretschmer, E. (1961). *Körperbau und Charakter* (23rd/24th edn). Berlin: Springer.

Kronmüller, K.T. (2002). 'Einfluss von Persönlichkeitsfaktoren und -struktur auf den Verlauf der Major-Depression', *Nervenarzt*, **73**: 255–261.

Kronmüller, K.T., Backenstrass, M., Kocherscheidt, K., Hunt, A., Unger, J., Fiedler, P., *et al.* (2002). 'Typus Melancholicus Personality Type and the Five-Factor-Model of Personality', *Psychopathology*, **35**: 327–334.

Matussek, P.A., Feil, W.B. (1983). 'Personality Attributes of Depressive Patients', *Archives of General Psychiatry*, **40**: 783–790.

Matussek, P.A., Halbach, A., Troeger, U. (1965). *Endogene Depression*. München: Urban & Schwarzenberg,

Merton, R.K., Barber, E. (1963). 'Sociological Ambivalence', in E.A. Tiryakian (ed), *Sociological Theory, Values and Sociocultural Change*. New York, NY: Free Press, 91–120.

Mundt, C., Backenstrass, M., Kronmiller, K.T., Fiedler, P., Kraus, A., Stanghellini, G. (1997). 'Personality and Endogenous/Major Depression: An Empirical Approach to Typus Melancholicus. 2. Validation of Typus Melancholicus Core-Properties by Personality Inventory Scales', *Psychopathology*, **30**: 130–139.

Nietzel, M.T., Harris, M.J. (1990). 'Relationship of Dependency and Achievement/Autonomy to Depression', *Clinical Psychology Review*, **10**: 279–297.

Paykel, E.S. (1982). 'Life Events and Early Environment', in E.S. Paykel (ed), *Handbook of Affective Disorders*. Edinburgh: Churchill Livingstone, 171–184.

Reiss, E. (1910). 'Konstitutionelle Verstimmung und manisch-depressives Irresein', *Zeitschr ges Neurol Psychiatrie,* **II**: 348–628.

Rossi Monti, M., Stanghellini, G. (1996). 'Psychopathology: An Edgeless Razor?', *Comprehensive Psychiatry*, **37**(3): 196–204.

Sato, T., Sakado, K., Sato, S. (1992). 'Differences Between Two Questionnaires for Assessment of Typus Melancholicus, Zerssen's F-List and Kasahar's Scale: The Validity and Relationship to DSM-III-R Personality Disorders', *Japanese Journal of Psychiatry and Neurology*, **46**(3): 603–608.

Schlimme, J.E. (2011). 'Karl Jaspers und Psychopathologie und Psychotherapie', in H.R. Yousefi, W. Schüßler, R. Schulz, U. Diehl (eds), *Karls Jaspers Grundbegriffe seines Denkens*. Reinbek: Lan-Verlag & Handel K.G., 229–250.

Schneider, K. (1967). *Klinische Psychopathologie* (8th edn). Stuttgart: Thieme.

Schwartz, M.A., Wiggins O.P. (2000). 'Pathological Selves', in D. Zahavi (ed), *Exploring the Self.* Amsterdam: John Benjamins Publishing Co, 257–277.

Stanghellini, G. (2004). *Disembodied Spirits and Deanimated Bodies: The Psychopathology of Common Sense.* Oxford: University Press.

Stanghellini, G., Mundt, Ch. (1997). 'Personality and Endogenous/Major Depression: An Empirical Approach to Typus Melancholicus', *Psychopath*, **30**: 119–129.

Stierlin, H., Weber, G., Schmidt, G., Simon, F.B. (1986). 'Features of Families with Major Affective Disorders', *Family Process*, **25**: 325–336.

Straus, E. (1978). *Geschehnis und Erlebnis. Zugleich eine historiologische Deutung des psychischen Traumas und der Renten-Neurose.* Berlin: Springer-Verlag.

Tellenbach, H. (1983). *Melancholie. Problemgeschichte, Endogenität, Typologie, Pathogenese, Klinik* (4th edn). Berlin: Springer.

Ueki, H., Holzapfel, C., Sakado, K., Washino, K., Inoue, M., Ogawa, N., *et al.* (2006). 'Prevalence of Typus Melancholicus in Healthy Germans', *Psychopathology*, **39**: 113–119.

World Health Organization (1992). *The ICD-10 Classification of Mental and Behavioural Disorders: Clinical Descriptions and Diagnostic Guidelines.* Geneva: World Health Organization.

Zerssen, D. von (1982). 'Personality and Affective Disorders', in G.S. Paykel (ed), *Handbook of Affective Disorders.* Edinburgh: Churchill Livingstone, 212–228.

Zerssen, D. von (1996a). 'Forschungen zur prämorbiden Persönlichkeit in der Psychiatrie der deutschsprachigen Länder: Die letzten drei Jahrzehnte', *Fortschritte der Neurologie, Psychiatrie*, **64**: 168–183.

Zerssen, D. von (1996b). 'Melancholic and Manic Types of Personality as Premorbid Structures in Affective Orders', in C. Mundt, M.J. Goldstein, K. Hahlweg, P. Fiedler (eds), *Interpersonal Factors in the Origin and Course of Affective Disorders.* London: Gaskell, 65–88.

Zerssen, D. von (2001). 'Personality and Affective Disorder', in N. Sartorius, F. Henn, H. Helmchen, H. Lauter (eds), *Specific Psychiatric Disorders.* Berlin: Springer, 279–296.

Author index

Index entries appear in letter-by-letter alphabetical order.

J

K

L

M

N

P

Q

R

S

T

V

W

Subject index

Index entries appear in letter-by-letter alphabetical order.

F

G